Outline Guide to

Chinese Herbal Patent Medicines in Pill Form -

with Sample Pictures of the Boxes

An Introduction to Chinese Herbal Medicines

Margaret A. Naeser, Ph.D. (Linguistics), Dipl.Ac. (NCCA)
Licensed Acupuncturist, Massachusetts

Department of Neurology
Boston University School of Medicine

Boston Chinese Medicine

Library of Congress Catalog Card Number: 90 - 80264
International Standard Book Number: 0 - 9625651 - 1 - 3
Printed in the United States of America

Second Edition, Third Printing
Paperback
April, 1991

Cover design by Marcel Leblanc
(The herb on the cover is Jin Qian Cao, used in the treatment of urinary tract infection, kidney stones or gallstones, hepatitis with jaundice, or cirrhosis of the liver. See Chapter 10, #10.1)

Formatting by Margaret Naeser
(MacWrite software on an Apple Macintosh computer and a LaserWriter Plus printer)

Printed by Edwards Brothers, Inc.
Ann Arbor, Michigan

Published and distributed by
Boston Chinese Medicine
P. O. Box 5747
Boston, MA 02114

Pre-paid orders may be sent to the above address.
Cost, $24.95 (Massachusetts Residents add $1.25 for Sales Tax)
Shipping (Book Rate) and Handling Fee per Book is $3.00. Checks payable to
Boston Chinese Medicine

This book is dedicated to my teacher

Chun-Han Zhu, O.M.D.

Oriental Medical Doctor, Brighton, Massachusetts

Acknowledgments

The author would like to thank Li-Zhao Wang, Ph.D., for providing the calligraphy. I also thank Jie-Lan Zou, from Beijing, China, for providing additional information on the Patent Medicines including their history, manufacture and laws regulating their production and use. I am also grateful to Ted Kaptchuk, O.M.D., Andrew Gamble, O.M.D., and Dan Bensky, O.M.D., for their help and encouragement throughout the process. I have special thanks for Marlene Meyer, M.D., Esq., for helping to make this manuscript a reality. I also thank Dorothy Donovan, R.N, Sylvia and Lionel Goddu, Winter and Michael Robinson, Mona Lisa Schulz, Beth Leimkuhler, Ph.D., and my family in Virginia and Colorado, for extra help. I am grateful to Kenneth Lubowich, Dipl.Ac. and Bob Flaws, DOM, CMT, Dipl.Ac. for help with translation. I also thank Barry Levine, Dipl.Ac., Maxine Shapiro, Lic. Ac., Joyce Singer, Lic. Ac., Roger Ray, Carole Palumbo, Jessica Lydon and Neva Frumkin, Ph.D., for support and assistance in preparation of the manuscript. I am grateful to Marcel Leblanc for designing the cover; and Reena Patel (Copies Now, Brookline, Mass.), and Joe Thomson and Tommie Kennepohl (Edwards Brothers, Framingham, Mass. and Lillington, N.C.) for help with the printing.

M.N.
Boston, MA
June, 1990

The author and publisher make no warranties as to the efficacy or appropriateness of any product or treatment described in this book. The author and publisher have made every effort to list accurately and completely the contents of the products contained herein, but the reader is urged to refer directly to the product for final authority regarding the contents. The book is based on historical information and is not intended as advertising, in any way, for any product listed herein. This book is not meant to replace medical advice and consultation.

Most of these products are best used following consultation with an Acupuncturist or Herbalist. A list of Certified Acupuncturists in the U.S. may be obtained from the American Association of Acupuncture and Oriental Medicine, 1424 16th Street, N.W., Suite 501, Washington, D.C. 20036. (202) 265-2287

How to Use This Book

This book is organized so that the reader can easily take it to the herb store, point to the appropriate picture, and readily locate the appropriate Patent Medicine. Chinese characters are written clearly at the top of each page for each Patent Medicine; a general English translation is provided for each character.

Over 175 Patent Medicines are explained in this book; the following information is provided for most:

1. **Historical Source** for the Patent Medicine

   Where and when the formula was first used.

2. **Function** of the Patent Medicine

   Function within Traditional Chinese Medicine, i.e., Tonify Kidney Yin; Clear Heat, etc.

3. **Application** of the Patent Medicine

   Which conditions the formula is used for.

4. **Ingredients** of the Patent Medicine

   Each constituent ingredient is listed with the following format: Chinese Name (e.g. Dang Gui); Pharmaceutical Name (e.g., Radix Angelicae Sinensis); percent in the formula; and Traditional Chinese Medicine Function (e.g., Tonify Blood).

   The spelling of the Chinese name (written in Pinyin) and the Pharmaceutical name are taken from the book by D. Bensky and A. Gamble: Chinese Herbal Medicine, MATERIA MEDICA, Seattle, Eastland Press, 1986. Readers are referred to this text for more information regarding major known biochemical properties of the herbs; and pharmacological and clinical research with the herbs.

   All terms used in this book regarding Traditional Chinese Medicine diagnosis and treatment are taken from the book by T. Kaptchuk: The Web that has No Weaver: Understanding Chinese Medicine, New York, Congden and Weed, 1983. Readers are referred to this text for further explanation of Traditional Chinese Medicine diagnosis and treatment terminology.

5. **A Sample Picture** of the Box for the Patent Medicine

   These pictures (black & white) are presented to show the general front-design of the box, for each Patent Medicine. Wherever possible, they show both the English side and the Chinese side of the box. (Formulas listed on the box may vary somewhat from the formulas listed in this book; formulas often vary with different manufacturers.) The unique lettering and design on each box distinguish the various Patent Medicines from each other.

Patent Medicines which are listed in this book have a chapter and item number preceding or following the Patent Medicine name, such as Yin Qiao Jie Du Pian, #1.4 (Chapter 1, Item 4). Some Patent Medicines which are not listed in this book are mentioned in discussions regarding comparisons of Patent Medicines throughout the book.

There are 14 chapters in this book; some chapters contain only one Patent Medicine. This is because other Patent Medicines which would be included in these chapters are not currently available in the U.S. When additional Patent Medicines become available, they will be added to future editions of the book.

Table of Contents

Chapter 6. Treat Tremors and Spasms due to Wind 135

(Includes Patent Medicines used with stroke cases; also some used to reduce itching)

Chapter 7. Clear Heat 151

(Includes Patent Medicines used to reduce infections, sore throat; treat wounds, etc.)

Chapter 11. Regulate Qi 213

(Includes Patent Medicines used with some Digestive Disorders; Liver/Gall Bladder dysfunction, etc.)

Chapter 12. Regulate Blood 229

Section A. **Promote Blood Circulation and Remove Blood Stasis**

Section B. **Stop Bleeding**

Section C. **Regulate Menstruation**

Chapter 13. Tonics 257

(Includes Kidney and Lung Tonics; Tonics used to Strengthen Qi, Blood, Yin and Yang)

Part I: Introduction

Section I: History, Manufacture, and Chinese Drug Control Regulations Act

Explanation of Patent Medicines

Patent Medicines are one form of Traditional Chinese Medicine (TCM). They are made with standard herbal formulas and a standard method of production. The first medical book in Chinese History, the Huang Di Nei Jing, Han Dynasty 206 B.C - 220 A.D. listed 13 herbal formulas, and 9 of these were Patent Medicines including pills, powders, plasters and tinctures. Thus, the history of Patent Medicines spans more than 2000 years. Some of the Patent Medicines still in use today date from the text, Shang Han Lun, 219 A.D.

Patent Medicines are used by physicians in clinical practice using Traditional Chinese Medicine diagnosis. The patient obtains the Patent Medicines in one of two ways: 1) The patient is given the Patent Medicine in the clinic or the hospital, where the medicine is dispensed by prescription from the physician or 2) The patient obtains the Patent Medicine from the herbal pharmacy directly, unless the herbal formula in the Patent Medicine requires a prescription.

There is a tradition in the Chinese Herbal Pharmacy where the pharmacist answers questions from the patients, and the pharmacist may give the patients suggestions regarding which kind of Patent Medicines to use. In some of the larger herbal pharmacies, a special area of the store may be devoted to patient questions where a diagnosis is made and a suggested prescription is given. Usually a senior physician or a senior pharmacist is available for consultation, and the prescription is given to the patient at no cost. The patient pays only for the herbal medicines.

Another tradition in the Chinese Herbal Pharmacy is to provide services 24 hours a day. For example, someone will answer the door and provide services at any time during the night; someone is always on duty. There is no extra charge for this service, although the patient will pay for the herbal medicines.

The TCM term for Patent Medicines is Zhong Cheng Yao. The meaning of Zhong Cheng Yao is the following: Zhong means "Chinese;" Cheng means "ready to be taken" (i.e. "prepared"), Yao means "medicine." Cheng Yao means "prepared medicine." Cheng Yao is the term used most commonly for Patent Medicines; Yin Pian is the term used for "loose herb formulas." The Yin Pian requires cooking or boiling of the herbs before they can be taken; the Cheng Yao requires no special preparation and can be taken in the prepared form.

Another term for Patent Medicines is Wan Yao. The English translation of Wan is "round, spherical pill." The term Wan Yao is commonly used because most Patent Medicines are available in round pill form.

Another term for Patent Medicines is Wan San Gao Dan. The translation of these four words is as follows: Wan means "round pill;" San means "powder;" Gao means "plaster;" and Dan means "a form of Patent Medicine containing minerals." This term is also commonly used for the Patent Medicines because these four words refer to the four forms in which the Patent Medicines are available - e.g. pills, powders, plasters and medicine containing minerals. This term for Patent Medicines is often used on a sign in front of a Chinese Herbal Pharmacy, thus indicating that these four forms of the Patent Medicines are sold there.

In China, the Herbal Pharmacy will also prepare into "ready to take form" a special herbal formula different from the standard Patent Medicines, which an Oriental medical doctor has prescribed. This "prepared form" is used when the physician feels that the pill or powder form is more appropriate than the herbal tea form. The "prepared form" will be made by the Herbal Pharmacy into pill form (sugar-coated, for example), or powder form, etc. according to the directions from the physician. It takes about a week to make the prescribed pills.

Since the late 1950's, there has been a great deal of research in China regarding herbal medicines. This research has yielded information regarding the use of herbal medicines in relation to Western medicine disease diagnoses. Therefore, some Chinese herbal medicine pharmaceutical manufactories have cited this research in their publications and have suggested the use of some of the Patent Medicines with Western medicine diseases. Therefore, the suggested use for some of the Patent Medicines does not have any relationship to the TCM diagnoses. One example of this is Patent Medicines made with the herb Shan Zha (Fructus Crataegi), an herb used to treat cardiac angina and decrease cholesterol levels in the blood. Another example is Patent Medicines made with Wu Wei Zi (Fructus Schisandrae Chinensis), an herb used to treat hepatitis because it will lower SGPT levels. Another example is Patent Medicines made with Ge Gen (Radix Puerariae), an herb used to treat coronary heart disease with angina as well as to treat symptoms such as headache, dizziness, stiff neck and numbness in the limbs associated with chronic hypertension.

History of Patent Medicines

In the 1970's in China, archeologists discovered an ancient tomb built during the Han Dynasty (206 B.C - 220 A.D.) in the area called Ma Wang Dui, Hunan Province. Inside this tomb, a medical book was discovered which is believed to have been written during the Warring States period (403 B.C. - 221 B.C.). The name of this medical book is Wu Shi Er Bing Fang (Formulas for the Treatment of Fifty-two Diseases). Some Patent Medicines were in this book. This is the earliest record thus far discovered containing information on Patent Medicines.

The first classical medical text in Chinese History, the Huang Di Nei Jing (Canon of Medicine written by Huang Di), Han Dynasty (206 B.C. - 220 A.D.), contains several formulas for making Patent Medicines. Most of the contents are concerned with TCM theory and methodology; 13 herbal medicine formulas are mentioned and 9 are in the Patent Medicine form. These 9 Patent Medicines are not in use today, but the same forms (pills, powders, plasters, etc.) have been in continuous use for over 2000 years.

The earliest Patent Medicines which are still in use today date from the Shang Han Za Bing Lun (Treatise on Fevers and Miscellaneous Diseases), 219 A.D. This text is considered to be the primary source for Chinese herbal medicine formulas. This book contains 113 herbal formulas; more than 60 of them are Patent Medicines. Some of these Patent Medicines are still in common use today, such as Wu Ling San (powder form), and Jin Gui Shen Qi Wan, a Kidney Tonic, #13.22, p. 299 in this Outline Guide. In addition, some formulas used in the Shang Han Lun as herbal tea, are currently produced by Chinese herbal medicine manufactories as Patent Medicines. For example, an herbal tea formula in the Shang Han Lun used to treat cough, Ma Xin Shi Gan Tang, is now used in the Patent Medicine form as Zhi Sou Ding Chuan Wan, #3.17, p. 96.

During the Han Dynasty (206 B.C. - 220 A.D.), a well-known physician Hua Tuo developed an herbal powder (Ma Fei San) which was used successfully as an anesthetic for surgery. The powder was dissolved in a small amount of wine, the patient drank it and fell into a sleep that was deep enough to permit removal of an abdominal tumor, for example. Although the exact ingredients are not known today, it is believed it was either Da Ma (Cannabis Sativae) or Wu Tou (Radix Aconti) or Yang Jin Hua (Datura metel L.).

The first book in Chinese medical history which is devoted to Patent Medicines is the Tai Ping Hui Min He Ji Jiu Fang (Formulas of the People's Welfare Pharmacy), Song Dynasty (960 - 1279 A.D.). There are 788 Patent Medicines in this book; it also introduces the procedures used to produce the Patent Medicines. Many Patent Medicines still in use today, were first introduced in this book. Thus, many Patent Medicines listed in this Outline Guide were first described in the Tai Ping Hui Min He Ji Jiu Fang, almost 1000 years ago.

During the Ming Dynasty (1368 - 1644 A.D.) and the Qing Dynasty (1644 - 1911 A.D.) Capitalism was introduced into China from European countries. Thus, many herbal pharmacies were opened as investments. Different herbal pharmacies produced different Patent Medicines. Some Patent Medicines were secret and they were produced only by one particular herbal pharmacy. One of the oldest and most famous herbal pharmacies in China today, is the Tung Jen Tang Pharmacy, in Beijing. This pharmacy was formally founded in 1669. The Tung Jen Tang Pharmacy is famous for several Patent Medicines, including Hu Gu Jiou (Tiger Bone Liquor for Rheumatism).

During the Ming and Qing Dynasties another school of thought was developed, the Wen Bing School (Seasonal Febrile Diseases School). This Wen Bing School produced many Patent Medicines. Several of these Patent Medicines from the Wen Bing School are still in common use, including two of the "Three Treasures Medicines," 1) An Gong Niu Huang Wan, #5.2 (pill form), and 2) Zi Xue Dan, #5.1 (powder form). These Patent Medicines are referred to as "Treasure Medicines" because they are used to reduce high fevers and coma, and produce results no other formulas can. Some other Patent Medicines used today which are made with formulas from the Wen Bing School include Sang Ju Gan Mao Pian, #1.3, and Yin Qiao Jie Du Pian, #1.4.

During the past 30 years the government of the People's Republic of China has focused on the standardization of Patent Medicine formulas, including standardization of the production methods. In 1957, 2,782 Patent Medicines were included in the text, Wan San Gao Dan Ji Cheng (The Collection of Patent Medicines). In 1963, the Yao Dian (Chinese Pharmacopoeia), published by the Chinese Government, contained 197 Patent Medicines. This is the first time in China that the Patent Medicines appeared in the Chinese Pharmacopoeia. In 1977, the Chinese Pharmacopoeia included 270 Patent Medicines. When a Patent Medicine is listed in the Chinese Pharmacopoeia, a pharmaceutical manufacturer producing that Patent Medicine must follow that formula and use that standard method of preparation.

Why Patent Medicines were Produced

There are three reasons why Patent Medicines were produced. In Chinese, these three reasons are summarized with the words, Yan Bian Lian. Yan means "effective;" Bian means "convenient;" Lian means "economical."

1. Yan, effective

The Patent Medicines are considered to be effective because in some cases it is more appropriate to use a plaster locally, for example, than to drink an herbal tea which would have a more general effect on the whole body. In addition, it is important that some of the medicines be dissolved slowly so that the effect will last longer. Also, it is important that some of the medicines dissolve slowly to prevent too much of the medicine from suddenly being released into the system. If too much of the medicine is suddenly released into the system, negative side-effects could develop. Some Patent Medicines are particularly appropriate to use following chronic disease or recovery following a long illness because the herbal concentrations are small and therefore they can be used over a long period of time.

Some Chinese Herbal Medicines cannot be used in the loose herbal teas because the herbs cannot be cooked or boiled at high temperatures without losing their effectiveness. For example, Bing Pian (Borneol), and She Xiang (Secretio Moschus moschiferi) are two herbal ingredients that would lose their potency if cooked or boiled.

2. Bian, convenient

The Patent Medicines can be obtained easily throughout China, even in the more remote areas where loose herbs or Western drugs are not always available.

Some Patent Medicines are useful for emergency conditions, and therefore they are ready to use and can be used in much less time than that which would be required to prepare an herbal tea formula. Some of these Patent Medicines have been used by the military throughout recorded Chinese history. This includes the use of some of these medicines to control epidemic diseases. A large number of Patent Medicines are mentioned in two books which discuss Chinese medical history, Wai Tai Mi Yao, (The Medical Secrets of a Military Official), 752, A.D.; and Zhou Hou Bei Ji Fang, (The Formulas for Emergency Conditions should be Kept Nearby (behind the elbow), Jin Dynasty, 1115 - 1234, A.D. Thus, the Patent Medicines were widely used by the military and considered especially important for use in emergency conditions. Even today, the Patent Medicines are commonly used by persons practicing Martial Arts, to treat injuries including, bruises, sprains, strains, and broken bones as well as to stop bleeding in emergency situations.

It is easy to use Patent Medicines to treat common diseases frequently encountered in a large population such as the common cold, flu, cough, stomach ache, gastric disorders and diarrhea. In such instances, large numbers of people have the same symptoms. When the Patent Medicines are used correctly, the effect is obvious.

Patent Medicines are especially convenient to use to treat children's diseases because most children are reluctant to take the herbal teas which are sometimes bitter.

3. Lian, economical

When expensive ingredients are required as part of an herbal tea formula, the same effect can be obtained if only a small portion is used in the Patent Medicine. Some of the expensive ingredients including Xi Jiao (Cornu Rhinoceri), Ling Yang Jiao (Cornu Antelopis) , Ge Jie (Gecko), and Niu Huang (Calculus Bovis) are usually made in the Patent Medicines only.

In addition, the Patent Medicines are more economical because the pharmaceutical manufactories can mass produce the formulas at a reduced cost, as opposed to individually purchasing the ingredients necessary for each patient for each formula. In addition, for common diseases and disorders, patients can easily purchase the Patent Medicines without the additional cost of consulting the physician.

How Patent Medicines differ from Traditional Herbal Tea Formulas

In China, when a patient visits a Traditional Chinese Medicine clinic for treatment, 80% of the time, the patient will be given an herbal tea formula; the patient expects this when he or she visits the clinic. For the most part, the herbal tea form is stronger than the Patent Medicine and the herbal tea form is absorbed more rapidly than the Patent Medicine. The remainder of the the time, the patient will be given a Patent Medicine. The Patent Medicines are very common in China, however, and for the most part, the patient is able to find out which Patent Medicine to use from the herbalist at the Chinese Herbal Pharmacy. For more serious disorders, of course, the patient visits the clinic and is seen by the physician.

Many Patent Medicines are made with the same formulas which are used in the herbal tea formulas. The herbal tea formulas chosen for use in the Patent Medicines include primarily those which are most effective. This attribute plus the three-word phrase, Yan Bian Lian (effective, convenient, economical) summarize the assets of Patent Medicines.

In some cases, when an original herbal tea formula is used in the Patent Medicine, a few changes are included by the pharmaceutical manufactory. For example, in the herbal tea formula for common cold, flu, Yin Qiao San, there are nine ingredients and it is required that the Lu Gen (Rhizoma Phragmitis Communis) be fresh. In the Patent Medicine, Yin Qiao Jie Du Pian, produced by the Tientsin Drug Manufactory, Tientsin, China, there are ten ingredients and the Lu Gen is not fresh, because it is already prepared into pill form. The extra ingredient in the Patent Medicine is Ling Yang Jiao (Cornu Antelopis), which has been added to increase the effectiveness. The Patent Medicine Yin Qiao Jie Du Pian produced in Beijing has the original nine ingredients; the Prepared FormulaYin Qiao Jie Du Pian produced in Xi An also has the original nine ingredients.

Another example is Zhi Sou Ding Chuan Wan, a Patent Medicine which has the same ingredients as Ma Xing Shi Gan Tang, an herbal tea formula. However, when using the herbal tea formula Ma Xing Shi Gan Tang, the Chinese herbalist can change the relative doseage of the two major ingredients, Ma Huang (Herba Ephedrae) and Shi Gao (Gypsum), depending upon whether the patient has asthma with or without sweating.

Use of Patent Medicines Today versus in the Past

The earliest history regarding the use of Chinese Patent Medicines is found in the book, Wu Shi Er Bing Fang, (Formulas for the Treatment of Fifty-two Diseases), Warring States Period (403 B.C. - 221 B.C.). In this book, there are a total of 189 formulas. At that time, when people took Patent Medicines in pill form, usually they first broke-up the pills, then mixed this in wine, then drank the wine containing the medicine. This differs from the manner in which most people take the Patent Medicines today, e.g. with water.

During the Warring States Period (403 B.C. - 221 B.C.), the people also began to make powders for internal use. There were 13 formulas in this text for making powders for internal use. Two of these powders were to be taken with water; eleven of them were to be taken with wine. Today, most powders are taken with water.

In addition, during that time, the people began to use powders externally to treat skin diseases or open wounds. This book contained 8 formulas for making these types of powders. When the powder was processed, the herbal medicine was first carbonized (turned to black powder). The powder was then used on the affected area, directly. This method of processing differs from that used today.

Since the 1950's, the Patent Medicines have become more developed than at any other time in Chinese history and overall, they are used much more widely, than ever before. This is due to the following four reasons.

1) The production of Patent Medicines has become more regulated and standardized by the Chinese Government. Before this, the manufacturers of the Patent Medicines kept them a secret. Some of the formulas were kept in families as secret formulas; in addition, some of the methods of preparation were kept a secret. Even within one family, only certain family members were allowed to know the secret

Societies

formula or preparation. This would sometimes mean that the information was only passsed down to the next son when the father was near death, or when he felt it was an appropriate time. Also, the father would rather pass the information on to a daughter-in-law, rather than his own daughter. This is because the daughter-in-law is considered to be a part of the family, whereas the daughter marries into another family.

In the 1950's, the Chinese Government started to re-organize the production of Patent Medicines. Several meetings were held in different regions where the same medicines were produced by different manufactories with different methods of preparation. The best method of production was agreed upon, and eventually the method of preparation has become standardized.

The 270 Patent Medicines included in the Pharmacopoeia of the People's Republic of China, 1977, have a standard method of preparation established by the Chinese Government. Thus, any Patent Medicine which is produced using a formula from this book, must conform to the standards fo the Chinese Government. In addition, several large cities and provinces have their own standards which are unique to their geographical region. For example, separate standards have been established in Beijing, Shanghai and Tianjin.

2) Some of the traditional Patent Medicines have been modified for use in the treatment of some specific Western medicine diseases. For example, Guan Xin Su He Wan, #5.4, is used for the treatment of coronary heart disease. It has been observed in China to improve the blood circulation in the coronary arteries. This formula is a modification of the traditional Chinese Patent Medicine, Su He Xiong Wan (Song Dynasty, 960 - 1279 A.D.), which is still used widely to treat unconsciousness, coma and stroke. The traditional formula in Su He Xiong Wan contains 15 ingredients; the modified formula in Guan Xin Su He Wan, #5.4, contains only 6 ingredients. The modified formula is not commonly used to treat unconsciousness, coma and stroke.

3) During the past few years, a great deal of research has been done on each separate herb in the formulas. This research has shown that some separate herbs are effective in treating some Western medicine diseases. Thus, originally, a laboratory produced some pills or powders made with only one herb. This was then studied in laboratory research and in clinical trials before the manufactories were allowed to produce the Patent Medicine containing only primarily one herb. An example is Yu Feng Ning Xin Pian, made with Ge Gen (Radix Pueraria) which has been shown through research to improve blood circulation to the brain. Another example is Dan Shen Pian, #12.1, made with Dan Shen (Radix Salviae Miltiorrhizae) which has been shown through research to be helpful in the treatment of coronary heart disease by improving circulation through the coronary arteries. Another example is Jie Du Xiao Yan Pian made with Chuan Xin Lian, #7.27 (Herba Andrographis Paniculatae), used to treat infections. None of these are traditional herbal formulas.

Over the past 20 or 30 years, some new Patent Medicines have been developed with more complex formulas written by prominent physicians. Some of these new formulas were also developed through laboratory and clinical research. None of these formulas had previously been used. Because the formulas are effective, they are now being produced by various manufactories. The formulas used in the Patent Medicines Shen Jing Suai Ruo Wan, #13.9, and Jiang Ya Wan, #7.15, were written by a prominent contemporary physician Shi Jin-mo. Bi Yan Pian, #1.10, a Patent Medicine used to treat rhinitis and sinusitis was developed through clinical research.

4) The form of the Patent Medicines has improved over the past thirty years. Prior to this time, the term Wan San Gao Dan (pills, powders, plasters) referred to the forms in which Patent Medicines were available. Even though Patent Medicines have the assets of Yan Bian Lian (effective, convenient, economical), usually the patient still had to take large amounts of the Patent Medicine pills or powders. In the 1950's, through the development of science and technology, it has become possible to extract the formulas in greater concentration into the pill or liquid form. In the 1950's, the Tung Jen Tang Pharmacy in Beijing, was the first herbal pharmacy which started to use this method to produce pills or tablets with higher concentration, such as Niu Huang Jie Du Pian, #7.8. Thus, since that time, it has become possible to obtain the same effect, for example, with only two small tablets vs. one large pill.

In the 1960's, modern techniques were used to produce the injection form of some Chinese herbal medicines. Thus, it became possible to use Chinese herbal medicines in injection form to treat emergency cases where it is absorbed by the body much faster. For example, an injection form has been made with Chai Hu (Radix Bupleuri) where it is used to lower high-grade fevers. Each time, only 2cc is injected. The temperature drops down smoothly without any side effects including no excess sweating or agitation. Another injection form is made with Chan Su (Secretio Bufonis) used intravenously to treat shock by increasing blood pressure in a critical condition. Chan Su is also used to treat respiratory failure. Dan Shen (Radix Salviae Miltiorrhizae) is used intramuscularly or intravenously to treat coronary heart disease.

Production of Patent Medicines Today versus in the Past

The history of the production of Patent Medicines spans over 2,000 years, as mentioned above. It dates back to the time of the first herbal formula which appeared in the Huang Di Nei Jing (Han Dynasty, 206 B.C. - 220 A.D.). At that time, however, the Patent Medicines were only made for patients on a case by case basis. The first factory to mass-produce the Patent Medicines dates back to the Song Dynasty (960 A.D. - 1279 A.D.). During the late 11th century, the centralized Chinese feudal empire set up a special Imperial hospital for use by the royal family. A Chinese herbal pharmacy was established in this hospital. The herbal pharmacy was called, Shu Yao Suo (Shu means "processing of medicine;" Yao means medicine;" Suo means "place"). Later, the name was changed from Shu Yao Suo to He Ji Ju (He Ji means "to compound a prescription;" Ju means "bureau"). In the He Ji Ju herbal pharmacy, many Patent Medicines were produced. The formulas were collected by a famous physician at that time, Chen Shi-wen and 788 of these formulas were published in the text, Tai Ping Hui Min He Ji Ju Fang (Formulas of the People's Welfare Pharmacy), 1151 A.D. During this time, all pharmacies were run by the Chinese Government; there were no private pharmacies.

Later, during the Ming Dynasty (1368-1644) and shortly thereafter, private pharmacies began to develop. One of the first of these private pharmacies was Tung Jen Tang in Beijing, founded in 1669. Because there was competition among the various private herbal pharmacies, each pharmacy produced its own special formulas in an attempt to produce more business. Some of these special formulas are still in use today.

Until recently, throughout Chinese history, the Patent Medicines were always made by hand, or with simple tools. Therefore, it was not possible to produce the Patent Medicines in large quantities. During the past 30 years, the Chinese Government has emphasized the development of Chinese herbal medicines. In addition, progress in science and technology has contributed to developments in producing the machinery necessary to mass-produce the Patent Medicines. Mass-production of Patent Medicines today is also, of course, related to the large population in China, approximately one billion people, who need to be served by these over-the-counter herbal medicines. The mass-production of Patent Medicines is considered to be a successful industry in China.

The Major Manufacturers of Patent Medicines in China

Today, the largest manufacturers of Patent Medicines in China are the following: Tung Jen Tang in Beijing; Hangzhou Second Traditional Chinese Pharmaceutical Works in Hangzhou; Shanghai First, Second and Third Traditional Chinese Pharmaceutical Works in Shanghai; Da Ren Tang in Tianjin; and Zhong Lian Traditional Chinese Pharmaceutical Works in Wuhan, Hubei Province.

The Beijing Tung Jen Tang Pharmacy, one of the largest pharmacies in China, was formally established in 1669 and has been managed by members of the same family for over 317 years. It is located in a busy business section of Beijing on a narrow street (Da Zha Lan) where there is not even enough space for cars. Tung Jen Tang has been located at this address since 1702.

Since the time when this herbal pharmacy was first established over 300 years ago, every owner has concentrated on the production of Patent Medicines, "Wan San Gao Dan" (pills, powders, plasters) and "Yao Jiou" (medicinal liquors). The original owner had a position in the Imperial hospital in Beijing. Therefore, this provided an opportunity for him to collect many secret Imperial herbal medicine formulas for use as Patent Medicines. It has always been believed that Patent Medicines produced by Tung Jen Tang are special formulas and they have higher quality herbal contents. During the 19th century, the Tung Jen Tang pharmacy had a "Royal Contract" with the Imperial Palace and members used only Patent Medicines produced by the Tung Jen Tang pharmacy.

The manager of Tung Jen Tang today, Zhao Cong-ru, states the following reasons why the Patent Medicines from Tung Jen Tang are special: 1) Most formulas were originally from the Imperial Palace or they are formulas which have been observed to be effective over many years. 2) The herbs used in these formulas are always very high quality and must be grown in special geographic areas. For example, Huang Lian (Rhizoma Coptidis) must be grown in Szechuan Province; Chen Pi (Pericarpium Citri Reticulatae) must be from Xin Hui county, Guangdong (Canton) Province; Dang Gui must be from Min county, Gan Su Province; Sheng Di (Radix Rehmanniae Glutinosae), He Nan Province. 3) The production methodology must be followed precisely according to the specific process as specified in the prescription including special processing for expensive ingredients. Over the 300 years, the pharmacy has had many different managers, but the preceding stipulations have always been followed by all of them.

An example of the high standards that have been maintained in the Tung Jen Tang pharmacy for over 100 years is presented in the following report. When the pharmacy was originally established in 1669, it was in a different location from where it is today. The original location has continued to be used as a warehouse, however, for the Patent Medicines, including those produced today. In the Februray 14, 1985 issue of the Jian Kang Bao (Health News Newspaper), it was reported that upon doing an inventory of the Patent Medicines in this warehouse, some workers found some Patent Medicines which had been prepared over 130 years ago, including Da Huo Luo Dan, #6.3; Su He Xiang Wan; and Ren Shen Zai Zao Wan, #6.4. The herbal ingredients were examined and determined to be fresh and still usable. They had been prepared in the Honey Pill form and were sealed inside a wax ball. They had been kept over 130 years at room temperature.

The number of employees in the Tung Jen Tang factory in 1949 was only 40. Today, there are 2000 employees who work in three Tung Jen Tang factories and one store. One factory specializes in producing Patent Medicines; one factory, medicinal liquors; and another factory, extracts for Patent Medicines. In 1984, the output was 417 times the output in 1948. Some specific pills have been increased in production number by as much a 1000 fold since 1949. For example, 10 million Niu Huang Qing Xin Wan (#6.6), pills were produced in 1986, which is a 1000 fold increase from 1949.

At this time, the Tung Jen Tang pharmacy produces 495 Patent Medicines and they specialize in making Patent Medicines to treat specifice disorders and diseases (as opposed to specializing in Tonics). Some of the Patent Medicines with an especially high reputation which traditionally have been produced by Tung Jen Tang, include An Gong Niu Huang Wan, #5.2; Wu Qi Bai Feng Wan, #12.12; Niu Huang Qing Xin Wan, #6.6; and Hu Gu Jiou. The ten most famous Patent Medicines produced by Tung Jen Tang are the following: Niu Huang Qing Xin Wan#6.6; An Gong Niu Huang Wan, #5.2; Zai Zao Wan, #6.4; Shen Rong Wei Sheng Wan; Su He Xiang Wan; Zi Xue Dan, #5.1; Da Huo Luo Dan, #6.3; Ju Fang Zhi Bau Dan; Niu Jin Dan; and Hu Gu Jiou.

Also, in Tung Jen Tang, there are strict regulations regarding quality control of the Patent Medicines. For example, when choosing the loose herbs, the herbal pharmacy will inspect the quality two times, before deciding if it is high enough to use in the Patent Medicines. Also, when making a complex formula, each step is always checked over twice. Before the Patent Medicine is placed on the shelf for sale, the box and contents are again checked for quality and freshness. This is always done by a senior herbal pharmacist with at least 40 or 50 years of experience. This herbal pharmacist can often tell by looking, smelling and tasting the medicine, where it has come from and whether it is of high quality. This is especially true for the rare and expensive medicines.

After Tung Jen Tang, the second most famous Traditional Chinese Medicine Manufacturer is the Hangzhou Second Traditional Chinese Pharmaceutical Works in Zhejiang Province. This is an outgrowth of the Huqing Yutang Pharmacy which was first established in Hangzhou in 1874. This manufactory is primarily known for producing Patent Medicine Tonics for general health. Their two most famous Tonic Patent Medicines are Ching Chun Bao and Shuang Bao Su., #13.12 Ching Chun Bao is used to maintain health and promote longevity. Shuang Bao Su is a general Tonic Patent Medicine similar to Ren Shen Feng Wang Jiang (Ren Shen Royal Jelly). (See #13.1 and #13.12.)

The Hangzhou Second Traditional Chinese Pharmaceutical Works was recently commended by the Chinese Government for its speed of growth in comparison to the other 500 Traditional Chinese pharmaceutical manufactories. In 1972, its first year, it paid over 450,000 Yuan tax on its profits to the State, ranking 300th among the Pharmaceutical Works. In 1985, it paid 10.7 million Yuan tax, occupying first place. This factory produces over 90 kinds of Patent Medicines with modern equipment and there are over 1000 employees. It is becoming a center for tourists to visit who are interested in learning more about the production of Patent Medicines. (Source: China Daily, November 20, 1986, Jielan Zou.)

Chinese Drug Control Regulations Act, July 1, 1985

In China, as of 1986, there were 6,499 different Patent Medicines which were produced. Of these, 1,000 are considered to be commonly used. This large number of Patent Medicines produced by many different manufactories without uniform standards had caused confusion. Several formulas were produced with the same name, but contained different formulas; or the same formula was produced with different names. For example, the formula used in Chuan Xin Lian Pian varied according to the various regions in which it was produced or by the various manufactories. This Patent Medicine had nine different names. In another example, the name Ren Shen Zai Zao Wan (used to treat stroke patients with paralysis) was used for twenty different formulas from different manufactories. The most popular formula used to expel Summer Heat, Ren Dan, is also used as a popular drink in the summertime. The name, Ren Dan, had eight different formulas, throughout the country. This confusion was brought to the attention of the Chinese Government and was the primary reason that a Drug Control Regulations Act was issued by the Chinese National Administrative Bureau of Drugs on September 20, 1984 and became effective July 1, 1985. Qi Mou-jia, director of the National Administrative Bureau of Drugs stated that the purpose of the Drug Control Regulations Act is to guarantee the quality of drugs (China Daily, July 3, 1985).

This federal law is named the Administrative Law of Medicine of the People's Republic of China. This law states in Chapter 1, Article 3, that the People's Republic of China encourages the development of both Modern Medicine and Traditional Chinese Medicine. Also, the Chinese Government will protect the geographical source of the herbs and encourage the cultivating of Chinese herbal medicines. In Chapter 2, Article 4, the law states that the Chinese Government will license a manufactory to produce medicines. This license to produce medicines has an expiration date and before that time, the manufactory must be inspected again, in order to renew the license to continue to manufacture. The law states in Chapter 2, Article 5, that any factory which produces medicines must have specific personnel such as pharmacists, engineers, technicians, etc., who must have proper space, buildings and equipment, etc. which are suitable to produce specific medicines for which the manufactory is licensed. In addition, the manufactory must have the necessary equipment and professional personnel to inspect the quality of the medicines which have been produced. Chapter 2, Article 6, states that the process of producing Chinese Herbal Medicines must follow the requirements of the Pharmacopoeia of the P.R.C. or the requirements issued by the local government. Chapter 2, Article 7, states that the materials and supplementary materials used to produce the medicine, as well as the container holding the medicine, must conform to certain regulations. Chapter 2, Article 8, states that the medicine must be inspected for quality control before it leaves the factory. If the medicine fails the inspection, it cannot be released.

Chapter 5, Article 33, states that it is illegal to state that a Patent Medicine with a specific name contains ingredients which are not on the list approved by the local or federal government for that specific Patent Medicine. It is also illegal to use additional ingredients which are not medicinal ingredients; or medicinal ingredients which are substituted for other specific medicinal ingredients in the formula. Some medicines are considered to be illegal, such as those medicines which have been banned by the Chinese Government. It is also not legal to use medicines which have been produced by factories which did not have the proper license. Chapter 5, Article 34 states that certain standards must be met in terms of herbal quality. This means, for example, that if an herbal formula requires 10% Ginseng, it is illegal to make the formula with 7% Ginseng. In addition, it is illegal to use herbal medicines which have exceeded an expiration date. Chapter 5, Article 35, states that the clinical personnel who come into contact with the herbal medicines must have annual health exams to insure protection of the herbal contents from any contamination.

Chapter 10 includes the legal responsibilites of the manufactory. The manufactory has the legal responsibility to comply with the law.

One year after the Drug Control Regulations Act went into effect, the June 19, 1986 edition of the China Daily reported that in the latest round of inspections (March, 1986), 1,763 of China's 1,950 pharmaceutical factories were certified as complying with the law's standards, as were 19,095 out of 24,944 sales and distribution companies. Under the law, uncertified factories must bring all products up to standared to continue production and uncertified sales and distribution centers are denied access to products from factories. During this first year after the law became effective, the Chinese Government destroyed poor quality or expired medicines (both Modern Medicines and Traditional Chinese Medicines) which were worth over 180,000,000 R.M.B. Yuan which did not meet the Chinese Government standards. In September, 1986, as a result of this law, several people who were involved in the production and sales of fake medicines in Jinjiang Province were given prison sentences up to 11 years (Beijing People's Daily, September 12, 1986). Liu Yong-gang, Deputy Director of the State Pharmaceutical Administration stated in the June 19, 1986 China Daily that the law guarantees the safety and effectiveness of medicine in China. "Control of the quality of medicine will be our top priority for the rest of the decade," he said.

Drug Advertisement Regulations Act, September 17, 1985

These regulations were issued by the Chinese National Industrial and Commercial Administration and the Health Ministry in 1985. In China, medicines are advertised in medical journals, general and medical newspapers, television, radio and even billboards along the sidewalks and streets. This law pertains to all advertisements of medicines, regardless of the type of medium used.

This law states that if the person making the advertisement is also the drug manufacturer, he must have a permit to produce the medicine. If the person making the advertisement is only in sales and distribution, and not involved in the manufacturing, he must have the proper license to sell the medicines. In addition, he must have a business license. Also, anyone advertising the sale of medicines must have approval from the local Public Health Administration. Anyone advertising the sale of a specific medicine must present to the local Provincial Public Health Administration and the local Provincial Industrial and Commercial Administration the permit number of the manufactory which is producing that particular medicine. In addition, they must show the leaflet explaining the medicine and the trademark of the medicine. If this medicine has received any awards or prizes for its effectiveness, this information must also be included. The content of the advertisement cannot be changed after the advertisement has been approved. If changes are necessary, the process must be initiated again.

Article 9 states that the Provincial Public Health Administration has the right to stop any advertisement which has been published in the media with changes which were not approved. Additional conditions which may result in withdrawal of an advertisement by the local authorities are listed below: 1) If clinical treatment trials have found this medicine to have serious side effects or unexpected side effects. 2) If the quality of the medicine is poor and cannot reach the level required by the Chinese Pharmacopoeia. 3) If the manufactory has ceased to produce this medicine or if the permit for the manufactory to produce this medicine has been cancelled. Today, the advertisement of Chinese medicines is taken as a serious matter in China.

The factual information in Section I was obtained from the following sources:

Liu De-yi: Zhong Yao Cheng Yao Xue, (Traditional Chinese Patent Medicines Textbook), Tianjing, China: Science and Technology Press, 1984. Nankai University, Tianjing, China.

Zhong Yao Zhi Ji Shou Ce, (The Handbook of Traditional Chinese Medicine Preparation), Written by The Institute of Traditional Chinese Herbal Medicine within The Academy of Traditional Chinese Medicine, Beijing, China: The People's Medical Publishing House, Second Edition, 1975.

Ma Ji-xing: The Success of Traditional Chinese Herbal Medicine Pharmacology in the Medical Book found in the Ma Wang Dui Tomb, Han Dynasty. Zhong Yi Za Zhi (Journal of Traditional Chinese Medicine), Vol. 27, No. 8, August, 1986; 57-58.

Li Jing-wei: Brief Introduction to Anesthesia and Surgery in Chinese History. Zhong Yi Za Zhi (Journal of Traditional Chinese Medicine), Vol. 26, No 5, May, 1985; 63-65.

Section II. **The Forms of The Patent Medicines**

Traditional Forms of Patent Medicines

A. Pills

The pill form has a round, spherical shape. It takes some time for the pills to be dissolved after they have been taken. Therefore, the effect from the pills may be somewhat slow to begin, but the effect will be longer lasting. The pills are made with a powder of herbs in a medium. There are a variety of mediums and the pills may be of a different type depending on the medium which is used. For example, if the medium is water, it is called a "water pill." If the medium is honey, it is called a "honey pill." If the medium is a paste (rice flour), it is called a "paste pill." If the medium is wax, it is called a "wax pill." These latter two forms, paste and wax, are not commonly used today. The rate of absorption of these pills is as follows: the water pill is the fastest; the honey pill is next, followed by the paste pill and then the wax pill.

The pills are in a solid form. It is easier to take these and store them than to use the herbal teas. Also, there is no unpleasant taste or odor associated with the pill form, whereas the herbal teas can sometimes have an unpleasant taste or odor. The pills are difficult for small children to swallow, however, and several formulas are available for them in syrup form.

1. Water Pills

The water pills are made with boiled water which has cooled to room temperature as the medium. The size of these water pills is usually somewhat smaller. The water pills dissolve faster than pills made with other mediums. Thus, the pills used to disperse food mass; improve appetite; Clear Heat or Disperse Fire, are usually made with the water pill form. The water pill contains only a small amount of water, 5 to 7%; there are no additional ingredients. Thus, the percentage of the medicine is higher in the water pills and the effect is faster. Because the percentage of the water medium is so low, only 5 to 7%, the cost is also lower with more active ingredients per pill.

2. Honey Pills

The honey pills are made with cooked honey. Usually each honey pill weighs 6 to 9 grams. When the weight is below 3 grams, it is called a small honey pill. The honey itself is considered to be a tonic medicine. For example, it will moisten the lungs and stop coughing; it will also moisten the intestines and treat constipation. Therefore, when honey is used as the medium in a Tonic Patent Medicine, it will strengthen the Tonic effect. It will also sweeten the taste, which is useful when herbs are used with a poor taste. It will also be absorbed somewhat slower than the water pill, for example. Therefore, the honey pill is usually used as a medium in Tonic Patent Medicines. When children's medicines are made into honey pill form, it is easy to cut the pills into any size as needed.

Some formulas which contain rare medicines or very expensive medicines or aromatic medicines usually are made with honey as the medium. This is because the honey will help to maintain the effect of the medicinal properties. In the honey pills, the medium is usually 50%. Therefore, the actual medicinal content of a honey pill is only about 50%. If a honey pill is stored over a long period of time, the pill may harden because the moisture from the honey has been lost. Some honey pills are therefore sealed inside a wax shell or packed in a box that is sealed with wax.

3. Water-Honey Pills

These pills have a mixture of water and honey as the medium. They are harder than the honey pills, because after they are made, they are dried in an oven with low heat or dried by ventilation. Therefore, the pills are solid and hard. These pills have a variety of sizes ranging from small to large. The water-honey pills are the most common pills sold in glass containers; they are usually about the size of small black beans. The effect of the water-honey pills lasts longer than either the water or the honey pills, alone, because these pills are dissolved more slowly than the honey pill. It is easier to store and keep this pill because there is less moisture.

4. Pills made with Flour-base Paste

These pills are very hard and dissolve more slowly than either the honey pills or the water pills. The flour is usually a rice flour or a wheat flour and it is 1/10 to 1/3 the weight of the whole pill. This form is able to decrease the stimulation of the stomach in dissolving the pills. This form is sometimes used when the herbal medicine used contains some toxic substances; it will help to reduce the toxic side-effect. Because this paste medium will decrease the rate of absorbtion of the herbal medicine, it will prolong the effect of the herbal medicine.

5. Pills made with Wax

Pills made with a wax medium take the longest to be absorbed. They are made with beeswax. The beeswax is a solid form at room temperature, but it softens after being taken internally. These pills dissolve very slowly, thus producing a long-lasting effect. This form is also sometimes used when the herbal medicine used contains some toxic substances; it will help to reduce the toxic side-effect. Pills made with beeswax as the medium are usually those used to detoxify poisons or stop pain by dispersing Blood Stagnation. There are two sizes of pills made with beeswax, one is larger and one is smaller. The larger pill weighs 3 grams and should be dissolved in hot water or hot wine and then cooled down to a warm temperature before taking. The smaller pill may be taken directly, with warm water.

B. Powders

The powder form consists of herbal medicines which have been mixed very well. There are two kinds, one is for internal use and one, for external use. The powder form for internal use can either be taken directly, or mixed with water to form a tea and then taken. The powder form for external use can be applied into an orifice such as eyes, mouth, ears, or throat directly. Or, the powder may be mixed with a medium such as alcohol, vinegar, sesame oil or water, to make a paste. This paste is then applied locally on the affected area. Some powders may be used both internally and externally.

The absorbtion of the herbal medicines in the powder form is rapid. It is faster than the pill form but slower than the herbal tea form. More recently it has become common to take the powders internally by first putting the powder into gelatin capsules.

C. Plasters

The Chinese word for "plaster" is "gao." The word gao also means "ointment" and it also means "syrup." Hence, there is are two forms of gao used externally, a plaster form and an ointment form; and there a gao used internally, a syrup form. The types of gao for external use are discussed below:

1. Ointment

There are two methods of preparation of ointments. The first is to use vegetable oil; the second is to use pork fat or beeswax. The herbal medicine is then fried in the oil, fat or wax, allowing the substances from the herbal medicines to get into the medium. The ointment is then used as an external medicine. Another method is to mix the herbal medicine powder into the ointment base, which was usually pork fat or beeswax. The ointments are usually used to treat skin infections, skin diseases or bruises and sprains.

2. Plasters

The plaster form of herbal medicine is a paste which is held in a piece of cloth or some animal skin. At room temperature, this paste is in a solid or hard form, but when exposed to higher temperature, the paste softens. Many herbal plasters are made by placing the herbal medicines on one half of a piece of material and then folding the other half on top. Before use, this sort of plaster must be warmed up with heat, to soften the herbal medicines. As soon as the plaster becomes sticky inside, it is opened up and placed face down onto the skin. The plaster form is often able to retain the heat in the affected area and prevent the area from cooling down. This form of plaster will improve the circulation of Blood and Qi to the affected area. Usually, the medicine in the plaster is designed to stop muscular pain on the back or limbs; or to stop pain in the abdomen due to Cold; or to treat pain related to gynecological disorders. Some plasters are also used to treat carbuncles on the skin.

D. Dan Form

The word dan means "red color" in Chinese. Originally, the Dan Form was invented by the Taoists. They believed this form of medicine would help them to live forever. The Taoists always used Zhu Sha (Cinnabaris), which has a red color, in preparing their herbal medicine powders. The Taoists always cooked their formulas for more than a day. These formulas often contained many minerals including the red colored mineral, Zhu Sha (Cinnabaris). Sometimes, when the cooked formulas would turn to a white colored powder, they were still labelled "Dan," a red color. In Chinese Patent Medicines, some pills may be coated with the cinnabar. Thus, these pills are always red in color, and are often called "Dan." Some Patent Medicines do not contain any cinnabar, but do contain some other minerals and are also labelled "Dan." Today, these are labelled Dan, largely for commercial purposes, because medicines labelled Dan are considered to be especially effective and valuable.

During the "cultural revolution" many pills which used to be labelled "Dan" (with or without cinnabar) were re-labelled "Wan," meaning pills. This was done because during that time, any reference to religious practices (the Taoists) was forbidden. Today, some medicines which contain cinnabar still use the term Wan, which was changed from Dan during the "cultural revolution." In addition, some formulas which originally contained cinnabar and were formerly called "Dan," have been changed to "Wan," because the cinnabar is now omitted. It is necessary to read the contents on the label, to know if cinnabar is in the formula of a given Patent Medicine.

E. Gelatin Form

This form is made with animal parts, especially the skin, bone, horn or shell (turtle shell). Usually the gelatin form is a Tonic medicine. This is good for elderly people or those with a long illness or patients with general weakness. The gelatin can be taken alone, or made into pill form with other herbs or made into an herbal tea. The gelatin is simmered in wine or water until it is melted, and then the liquid is taken, alone, or mixed into an herbal tea.

F. Liquor Form

The liquor form is made with a white wine. The percent alcohol is 60 to 65%. The liquor is used as a solvent to absorb the herbal medicines. Also, the alcohol is able to improve the Blood circulation and to Expel Cold, thus the alcohol will reinforce the effect of the herbal medicines. This form of herbal medicine is used primarily to treat the disorders known as Bi Syndrome (joint pain; muscle pain; rheumatism pain). Also, some Tonic medicines are used in the liquor form as a Tonic beverage.

G. Water-base Form

Some Patent Medicines are made into a water-base form and most of them contain some percentage of alcohol. It is called water-base form because it has been traditionally labelled that. This form is not called "liquor form" because it is not made with yellow wine. The percentage of alcohol varies according to the different medicines made with the water-base. This form also cannot be called "tincture form" because tinctures contain a specific percentage of alcohol; the water-base form again has various percentages of alcohol. Alcohol is included with the water-base form because the herbal contents are dissolved into the alcohol more rapidly than water alone and in addition, the alcohol is absorbed more quickly in the body.

For example, Shi Di Shui (meaning "ten drops of water"), Liu Shen Shui, #2.4 (meaning "six spirit water") and Yuen Xiang Jing are water-base Patent Medicines. This kind of medicine is usually used to treat acute gastric disorders such as vomiting or diarrhea.

In addition to these, there are some water-base water medicines for external use only, which are used to treat certain skin diseases. These water-base medicines which are prepared for external use only may contain some poisons which are included, for example, to kill a fungus, etc.

H. Distilled Form

This form is made from the conversion of a liquid into vapors which are reconverted to liquid form as a means of eliminating contaminants from the original solution. This form is not commonly used because most medicines cannot be prepared in this form. It is only used when the medicine contains a high percentage of volatile oil.

I. Tea Form

The tea form of Patent Medicines is made with herbal medicine and regular green tea leaves. Some of them may be made without the regular tea. The ingredients are mixed into a rough powder form; or a medium is used to form a cube shape. When this form of herbal medicine is used, a certain amount is broken off and placed into boiling water and cooked briefly; then the liquid is swallowed as a regular tea. Examples of this form are Wu Shi Cha, #1.2, and Shen Chu Cha, #2.3

J. Liniment Form

This is an oil-base medicine in liquid form. Most of these are for external use. For example, Wan Hua You, #12.7, and Chu Feng You are both herbal medicines in liniment form for external use.

K. Ding Form

These are herbal medicines in pill form which are prepared using the medicine as a powder which is mixed with a medium such as honey or some starch paste. These pills may have various shapes including round, oblong, etc. Most of these are for internal plus external use, although some are for internal use only and some are for external use only. Examples of the Ding form are Zi Jin Ding, #7.30, and Wan Ying Ding.

Newer Forms of Patent Medicines

During the past three decades, the Patent Medicines have been produced in many new forms. The newer forms were developed, for example, so that larger doses could be contained within the pills. In addition, the newer forms have a better taste and can be more rapidly absorbed by the body. Western medicine techniques were applied to develop the new tablet and injection forms. The new forms of Patent Medicines are as effective as the traditional forms of Patent Medicines and there are none of the previous shortcomings.

A. Tablets

Tablets are made with herbal medicine powder, and an herbal extract in liquid form which is used as a medium. In addition, starch may be used in some cases as the medium. The relative proportion of the herbal medicine powder and the extract result in three forms of tablets: 1) Raw material medicine tablets which are made with herbal medicine powder only. These tablets are very large. 2) Extract material medicine tablets which are made with the concentrated herbal extract only, plus some starch. These tablets have a smaller size, but there are some shortcomings. For example, when the weather is very humid, the tablets may soften because they easily absorb moisture from the air. An example of the extract material medicine tablet is Ji Xue Teng Jin Gao Pian, #4.2. 3) Semi-extract material medicine tablets which are made with herbal extract and herbal medicine powder under specific proportions. Most tablets are this type. Usually, these are small or medium in size. An example of this form is Yin Qiao Jie Du Pian, #1.4.

Tablets may be either uncoated or coated. An example of the uncoated form is Niu Huang Jie Du Pian, #7.8, in the packages where 8 tablets are in each vial. The sugar- coated form may improve the taste and make the tablets easier to swallow. In addition, the sugar-coated form may have a specific color which makes the Patent Medicine easier to identify. An example of the coated form is Niu Huang Jie Du Pian, #7.8, in the packages where 20 tablets are in each bottle. Additional examples include Li Fei, #3.13, and Chuan Bei Jing Pian, #3.1.

The sugar-coated tablets are especially easy to swallow and more rapidly absorbed than the honey pills, starch pills or concentrated pills. They are not as rapidly absorbed, however, as the water pills. Usually, a dose of four tablets are equal to one honey pill.

B. Concentrated Pills

The concentrated pills are an improved form of the traditional water pills. When these pills are made, the herbal medicine powder and herbal extract are mixed. This mixture is then made into a small pill form with a round shape; they are very hard on the outside. This kind of pill usually has a coating made from one of the ingredients in the formula, such as an herbal powder or cinnabar. These concentrated pills will have different colors depending on the color of the coating. For example, if talc is used as the coating, the color will be white; if cinnabar is used, the color will be red. The concentrated pills may easily absorb moisture and become damp; therefore, it is important to keep the bottle containing these concentrated pills away from moisture. Because the herbal medicine dose in the pills is in concentrated form, one usually has to take only a few pills at a time. An example of concentrated pills is Jian Nao Wan, #14.2.

C. Dissolvable Granules

This form is made with a fine herbal powder or herbal extract in dried granular form. This form maintains some of the special attributes of herbal tea. When the granules are dissolved in hot water, some honey or sweetner may be added, to improve the taste. An example of this is Gan Mao Twe Re Chun Ji, #1.5.

D. Syrup Form

A syrup is made from a high concentration of herbal tea mixed with honey or sugar syrup. The syrup form always has a sweet taste and the medicinal effect is milder. Thus, it is easily taken and easily absorbed. Some of the syrup forms contain 10 to 20% alcohol. Usually, Blood Tonification medicine or Nourish Yin medicine or cough medicine is made in this form. An example of this is Chuan Bei Bi Ba Gao, #3.14. The syrup form for children contains either no alcohol or much less alcohol; an example is Qi Xing Cha, #9.2.

E. Injection Form

The traditional Patent Medicine injection form was made with herbal medicine extract using the standard procedure required by the Chinese Pharmacopoeia. This procedure required sterile water and the production of a clear or semi-clear solution. The newer Patent Medicine injection form is still prepared according to the Chinese Pharmacopoeia. The injection form has a rapid and obvious effect. For example, Chai Hu injection form is used to decrease high-grade fever due to bacterial or viral infection.

The Chinese herbal injection form requires quality control and sterile procedure. Some of the injection forms require a skin test where only a small amount of the solution is first injected to test for a possible allergic reaction before the standard amount is injected.

F. Adhesive Plasters

The Chinese herbal medicines are mixed into the adhesive formula to form the medicinal plasters. These plasters are applied externally to reduce pain and decrease inflammation. Specific plasters may be applied onto specific acupuncture points to treat specific internal medicine diseases such as asthma. Although the effect of the plaster may be obvious soon after the plaster has been applied, in many cases the plaster must be re-applied, as specified for each type of medicinal plaster. The adhesive plaster may cause an allergic reaction for a few patients. The plasters should not be applied to an open wound or to a inflammed area of skin where exudate is present.

G. Capsule Form

The herbal medicine powder is sometimes placed into clear capsules. This form is used when the herbal medicines cannot be made into tablet or pill form. The capsules are easily taken and the herbal medicine is easily absorbed by the body. Examples of this are Guan Xin Su He Wan, #5.4, and Ge Jie Da Bu Wan, #13.4. Sometimes herbal medicines in liquid form are inserted into the capsules; only a few Patent Medicines are available in this form.

Section III. **Explanantion of the Leaflet which is Included with Each Patent Medicine**

The Patent Medicines should be selected for use according to the Oriental medical diagnosis which has been made by an herbalist or acupuncturist who is trained in Oriental medicine. However, for some mild conditions, or for some chronic conditions which are stable, or during recovery from a chronic illness, some patients may purchase the Patent Medicines directly from the herbal pharmacy. This is not the best way to use Patent Medicines, however, since patients who are untrained in Chinese medicine are not able to choose the best Patent Medicine, or the best combination of Patent Medicines for their particular condition. Thus, it is preferable to purchase the Patent Medicines after consulting with an herbalist.

A flier is inserted with most Patent Medicines, explaining that particular Patent Medicine. It is important to carefully read the instructions and to properly understand the meaning of the instructions. For example, there are many Patent Medicines which may be used to treat cough. Many of these cough medicines state that they are effective to treat cough, stop asthma, eliminate phlegm in the chest and nourish the lungs. However, when the ingredients are compared across several cough medicines, it is observed that they contain many different ingredients. The different herbs used in these different cough medicines will have different clinical effects. For example, some will Warm the Lungs and stop cough; some will Clear Lung Heat and stop cough; some will Nourish Lung Yin and stop cough. Different typse of cough medicine are used to treat cough with Wind Cold syndrome (symptoms including in part, clear or white, thin sputum) or cough with Wind Heat Syndrome (symptoms including in part, yellow, thick sputum) or cough with Def. Yin syndrome (Excess Dryness). Different types will present with different symptoms which belong to different syndromes. Thus, the correct diagnosis must first be made to determine to which type of syndrome the cough belongs.

After the correct diagnosis is made, then the correct Patent Medicine is chosen to obtain the best clinical effect. If the incorrect Patent Medicine is chosen, it may make the cough worse. For example, if the cough is due to Def. Yin and Excess Dryness, but a cough medicine was chosen which is used to treat a cough caused by Wind Cold, this type of cough medicine will contain Warm Property herbs, and these herbs may even Damage the Yin and develop more Dryness.

The leaflet that comes with the Patent Medicine usually discusses the Function and Indication/Application of that Patent Medicine. These two items are important, and they are inter-related. The information contained in the Function is related to the prinicple medical effect of the medicine. The information contained in the Indication is related to the treatment of major symptoms or diseases. A Patent Medicine can only be used to obtain maximum effect when both the Function and the Indication of a particular Patent Medicine are well understood. Understanding of both the Function and the Indication enables the clinician to have a complete understanding of the Patent Medicine.

In addition, it is suggested that the clinician carefully study the Ingredients listed on the leaflet in order to be familiar with the different ingredients of each different Patent Medicine. Some persons may refer only to the Indications; however, these are usually only very brief and simple in the leaflet. If one only refers to the Indications, this may lead to confusion. For example, one may ask the question, "Does the patient have to have all of the listed symptoms, or only one of these symptoms, to be able to use a particular Patent Medicine?" The patient does not have to have all of the listed symptoms, but he must have the most important symptoms.

For example, Yin Qiao Jie Du Pian, #1.4, is used to treat the flu, fever, chills, body aches, headache, cough, swollen and painful sore throat, parotitis. It is not necessary for the patient to have all of these symptoms to be able to use Yin Qiao Jie Du Pian, however, there are some symptoms which the patient must have to be able to use it. In order to know which symptoms the patient must have, it is important to study both the Function and Ingredients portions of the leaflet, as well as those included in this text. The ingredients used in this Patent Medicine are from herbal medicines in the "Clear Heat category" and "mild diaphoretic category." Therefore, the Function of this medicine is to Clear Heat and Expel Wind; i.e. it is for the treatment of Wind Heat syndrome.

In Chinese Medicine theory, the Wind Heat syndrome indicates that the patient has the following basic symptoms: The patient has a fever (sometimes even only a low-grade fever); there are no obvious chills; the patient is thirsty; sore throat is present. These above-mentioned symptoms are the most important symptoms to be considered when using Yin Qiao Jie Du Pian. This Patent Medicine can always be used to treat a patient who has these symptoms (Wind Heat symptoms); it is not necessary, for example, for the patient to have parotitis. On the other hand, if the patient has obvious chills, no thirst, no swollen, sore throat; and may or may not have fever or body aches or headache, it is not appropriate to use Yin Qiao Jie Du Pian. These symptoms belong to Wind Cold, or another syndrome, and they should not be treated with Yin Qiao Jie Du Pian. To obtain the best results, herbal medicine must be studied seriously.

Names of the Patent Medicines

Several Patent Medicines have similar names, but not the same name, and not the same function. For example, Yin Qiao Jie Du Pian, #1.4, and Ling Chiao Jie Du Pian, and Xi Ling Jie Du Pian, #1.7, all have similar names, but the function is not exactly the same for all three. Some Clear more Heat; some Clear more Lung Heat, some Clear more Lung Heat plus Heart Heat. Another example is Niu Huang Qing Xin Wan, #6.6, and Wan Shi Niu Huang Qing Xin Wan, #5.3. The former is used to Clear Heat in the Heart, Eliminate Wind Phlegm and stop spasm (this includes using it with stroke patients who have paralysis and speech problems). The latter is used to Clear Heat and Detoxify Fire Poison and revive a patient from unconsciousness due to Heat in the Heart. Another example is Ren Shen Gui Pi Wan, #13.8, and Ren Shen Jian Pi Wan, #9.1. The former is used to Tonify Blood and Calm the Spirit. The latter is used to Remove Food Mass. Another example is Liu Shen Wan, #7.9, and Liu Shen Shui, #2.4. The former is used to treat more serious cases of throat infection. The latter is used to treat digestive disorders. Another example is Da Huo Luo Dan, #6.3, and Xiao Huo Luo Dan, #4.7. The former is used to stop Wind syndrome (treat stroke patients with paralysis). The latter is used to treat Cold Bi syndrome and sports injuries and stop pain. For all of these examples, the names are similar, but the functions are different. Thus, when using these Patent Medicines, it is important to double-check the complete name.

Some medicines with the same formula may have several different names. The names will vary according to the manufacturer and the region where it is produced. Chuan Xin Lian Pian, #7.27, has nine names, but they all contain the same formula.

Some names are used several times with several different formulas. For example, the name Ren Shen Zai Zao Wan, #6.4, has twenty different formulas. The names vary according to the different geographical regions where the Patent Medicines are produced. The function is about the same, however, for these different formulas which have the same name. This situation is due to the fact that these Patent Medicines have been produced for over a thousand years, thus there are many examples of "historic precedence" for the use of a particular name. The Chinese Government is trying to re-organize the situation and it may take several years to resolve the issue of exactly which formula produced in which geographic location should be allowed to use which particular name. (Jian Kang Bao, Health News, April 13, 1986)

Thus, when using Patent Medicines, it is important to not only read the name, but also read where the medicine is produced - i.e. which factory. Also, it is important to know the size and form of the medicine. Some pills are 0.6 grams, some are 0.3, etc. It is important to read the flier which is included with each medicine. In addition to the Function, Indications and Ingredients, the flier will state the proper dose for that specific Patent Medicine.

Special Procedures to Follow When Taking Certain Patent Medicines

Some Patent Medicines require they be taken at a certain time of the day. For example, when taking an herb for intestinal parasites (Roundworm), Shi Jun Zi, it is important to take the seeds early in the morning, when the stomach is empty.

Dose

Most Patent Medicines require that the medicine be taken twice a day; some require three times a day. Only a few require once a day. The dose listed on the leaflet should be followed; or the dose recommended by the clinician. The patient should not increase the dose by himself, nor should the patient increase the frequency with which the medicine is taken, in an attempt to obtain faster results. It is especially important to follow the correct dosage with children and older people.

monastory

Section IV. **How to Take the Patent Medicines**

This section explains how to take the Patent Medicines internally and how to use them externally. Taking Patent Medicines correctly is an important aspect of their proper use. There are several methods for taking Patent Medicines which are listed below:

1) Taking Patent Medicines internally.

A. Taking Patent Medicines with liquid.

This method refers to taking the Patent Medicine with water or a Yao Yin. The type of Patent Medicine or the special requirement of the medicine may require a special liquid.

a. Boiled water which has cooled to a lukewarm or room temperature.

Most Patent Medicines for internal use should be taken in this way. This includes tablets, pills, powder and Dan forms as well as some Patent Medicines in liquid form. In China, it is necessary to boil the water before drinking it; in the U.S., most tap water is potable, therefore, it is not necessary to boil the water. Ordinary drinking water or spring water can be used; ice water is not recommended.

b. Yao Yin (an herbal "guide" medicine)

The term Yao Yin refers to a kind of medicine which is easy to find, easy to use and can be prepared at home by the patient himself. Many of the Yao Yin are ordinary foods found in the kitchen. In ancient times, all Patent Medicines were taken with Yao Yin. Many of the Patent Medicine leaflets contain directions for which Yao Yin to use, for best results. Today, the use of the Yao Yin is not as common as before. However, studies in China have shown that better results are obtained when Patent Medicines are taken with the Yao Yin. Directions for the preparation of eight Yao Yin are given below:

1. Sheng Jiang (Ginger)

Sheng Jiang has the function to Expel Wind Cold, Warm the Middle Warmer, and stop vomiting. Thus, when the Patent Medicine is used to treat Wind Cold Syndrome, or to stop vomiting or nausea due to Cold Evil in the Stomach, or to stop abdominal pain and diarrhea due to Cold Evil, Sheng Jiang is commonly used as a Yao Yin. To prepare the ginger tea, cut 3 to 5 thin slices of the ginger (10 to 15 grams) and cook it in boiling water for 10 minutes to make one cup of tea. Use this tea to swallow the Patent Medicine.

2. Lu Gen (Rhizoma Phragmitis Communis)

For best results, use fresh Lu Gen; however dried Lu Gen from the herbal pharmacy is also effective. Lu Gen has the effect to Clear Heat, increase body fluid and stop thirst and stop vomiting. When the Patent Medicine is used to treat Wind Heat Syndrome or to treat skin rash (including beginning measles skin rash), Lu Gen is used as the Yao Yin. If Lu Gen tea is used to swallow Yin Qiao Jie Du Pian, #1.4, the effect will be better. The usual dose is 10 to 15 grams for one cup of herbal tea. The Lu Gen should be boiled for 15 to 20 minutes; strain the liquid off and take the pills with the remaining tea.

3. Wine

Use yellow wine or white wine. The wine has a pungent taste and hot property. It will promote meridian circulation and expel Wind Cold. It is commonly used with Patent Medicines such as Da Huo Luo Dan. #6.3, or Qi Li San, #12.3, to treat Bi syndrome (muscular pain or joint pain caused by Wind Cold Dampness); or with Patent Medicines used to treat amenorrhea due to Blood Stagnation due to Cold; or with Patent Medicines used to treat sports injuries (bruises). The wine should be taken at room temperature or preferably heated a little. The dose should vary according to the size and sex of the person, as well as according to the sensitivity of the patient to the alcohol. The common dose for the Chinese yellow wine is 25 to 50 cc's. The common dose for the white wine is less than that for the yellow wine because the white wine is stronger. The patient should be careful not to take too much wine.

4. Salt

According to the Five Element Theory, salt has the effect of leading the Patent Medicine to the Kidney. Therefore, when using Patent Medicines to nourish Kidney Yin, for example, Liu Wei Di Huang Wan, #13.19, or Jian Bu Hu Chian Wan, #13.18, slightly salty water should be used as the Yao Yin. Use 2 grams of salt to one-half cup of warm water.

5. Rice Gruel

When rice is cooked where extra proportions of water are used, the water which remains after the cooking, is the rice gruel. The rice gruel has the function of protecting the Stomach Qi. Some medicines with a bitter taste (Cold Property) may damage the Stomach Qi. For example, some purgative medicines may damage the Stomach Qi. In these conditions, rice gruel is used as the Yao Yin. The patient should use the gruel to swallow the medicine. There is no limitation for the dose.

6. Dark Brown Sugar

Dark brown sugar has the function to Expel and Eliminate Cold; Promote Blood circulation and Nourish Blood. When using Patent Medicines to treat gynecological disorders due to Deficient Blood and Cold, such as dysmenorrhea or amenorrhea or hypomenorrhea, the dark brown sugar is often used as the Yao Yin. Each time, use 25 to 50 grams of the sugar to one cup of hot water.

7. Fresh Lotus Rhizoma Juice

This medicine has the effect of stopping bleeding due to Excess Heat. If the fresh lotus rhizoma juice is not available, fresh daikon juice may be used as a substitute. Clean the lotus rhizoma or daikon; chop into pieces; add a small amount of cold water; use a presser to squeeze out the juice. Use the juice to take the Patent Medicine He Ye Wan, a stop- bleeding medicine which contains lotus leaves.

8. Cong Bai (Herba Allii Fistulosi)

Cong Bai is the white part of a green scallion. Cong Bai has the effect of promoting Yang Qi and eliminating Cold Evil. When using a diaphoretic medicine to treat Wind Cold syndrome, Cong Bai may be used as the Yao Yin. This will help the Patent Medicine to induce sweating. Chop the white part of two or three scallions into pieces and simmer in water for 10 minutes; one cup of liquid should then remain to use as the Yao Yin.

Additional Yao Yin:

When using Patent Medicines as a laxative or when Nourishing Lung Yin and stopping Dry Cough, use one tablespoon of honey dissolved in one cup of warm water as the Yao Yin.

When using Patent Medicines which tranquilize, Suan Zao Ren (Semen Ziziphi Spinosae, dried form) may be used as the Yao Yin. Use 10 grams of Suan Zao Ren to make one cup of herbal tea; simmer for 10 to 15 minutes; strain off the liquid and drink it as the Yao Yin.

Da Zao (Fructus Zizyphi Jujubae) is commonly used as a Yao Yin for Patent Medicines which are able to strengthen the Spleen and Stomach. Use 5 to 10 pieces to make one cup of herbal tea; simmer for 30 to 45 minutes; strain off the liquid and drink it as the Yao Yin.

When using Patent Medicines to treat dysuria (painful or difficult urination due to Excess Heat), use Zhu Ye (Herba Lophatheri Gracilis), 6 grams; plus Deng Xin Cao (Medulla Junci Effusi), 6 grams; to make one cup of herbal tea; simmer for 15 minutes and strain off the liquid to use as the Yao Yin.

B. Patent Medicines taken without any liquid or only a small amount

These Patent Medicines are taken with only the small amount of water which is necessary to swallow the medicine, or they are chewed and/or then swallowed. The patient should not drink any liquid for one hour after taking the Patent Medicine. The liquid would dilute the Patent Medicine too much after it reached the stomach. Most Patent Medicines which require this method are those which Warm the Middle Warmer and stop stomach ache. An example of a Patent Medicine which is taken in this manner is Sai Mei An, #11.7.

emphasize

C. Patent Medicines taken with a Mixture

The Patent Medicine is mixed with milk or a syrup and then taken. This method is commonly used with children because the mixture will make the Patent Medicine taste better.

D. Patent Medicines dissolved slowly in the Mouth

With this method, the Patent Medicine is slowly dissolved in the mouth and then swallowed. This method is usually used to treat patients with a sore throat or tonsillitis. An example is Liu Shen Wan, #7.9, or Qing Yin Wan, #7.11.

E. Patent Medicines dissolved slowly with Heat

This method is used to prepare the gelatin form of a Patent Medicine, such as A Jiao (Gelatinum Asini). If the patient is taking the gelatin as a Patent Medicine and the gelatin is the only ingredient, the medicine should be placed in yellow wine in a double boiler. The gelatin should be melted into the wine from the heat in the double boiler. The patient then drinks the liquid (wine and gelatin mixture).

Note, Patent Medicine pills which have been made with wax as the medium should also be prepared using this method before taking.

F. Patent Medicines dissolved in Water

Some Patent Medicines are produced in a hard block form which is actually a fixed formula which is taken as an herbal tea. The herbs used in the formula have been pounded into a small hard block form. Shen Chu Cha, #2.3, is an example of a Patent Medicine in block form. The block is placed into a cup of cold water which is then brought to a boil and cooked down to 2/3 of a cup over a 10-minute period. The liquid can be taken cold or hot.

2) Using Patent Medicines externally

A. Topical Application of Ointment or Lotion

Before using the medicine, the local area should be cleaned. Examples include Jin Wan Long, #7.33, an ointment used for burns and Chu Feng You, an ointment used with arthritis.

B. Topical Application of Powders

The powder is placed on the affected area. Usually this kind of medicine is used to decrease inflammation, stop bleeding, cause astringent action, promote tissue regeneration and stop pain. An example is Yun Nan Bai Yao, #12.10, used to stop severe bleeding.

C. Mixtures for External Use

With this method, a powder is mixed with a liquid to form a paste. This paste is then applied to the affected area. The liquids for common use are the following: 1) Regular tea. This form is used with powders to make a paste to decrease inflammation, Detoxify Fire Poison and stop pain. 2) Liquor. The liquor used is a clear liquor (the percent alcohol should be 60 to 65%). This form is used to Remove Stuck Blood, Promote Blood circulation and stop pain. 3) The oil which has been used to fry a Szechuan pepper. The oil should be a cooking oil. The mixure made with this oil is used to treat itchy skin and Dry Dampness. 4) In addition to the above three, several other liquids may be used to prepare the mixture. For example, dark sesame oil may be used which can keep the skin moist and prevent dryness. Another example is vinegar, which will give the mixture a dry property so that it will decrease mucous and decrease fluid. Another example is milk, which has nourishing and tonic properties which will help prevent skin dryness.

D. Use of Blowing Technique to blow the Medicine onto a Specific Area.

When treating ear disorders, the powder form of a Patent Medicine can be gently blown into the ear, for example, to treat an infection, boil or eczema. Another application is to blow the Patent Medicine powder directly onto infected areas of the throat. Inflammation, hoarseness, or sore throat may be present. An example of this is Xi Gua Shuang, #7.10. Another application is to blow the Patent Medicine powder onto the gum area to treat a toothache. The method used for blowing the powder is as follows: Use a straw and cut one end of the straw at an angle. Use this end as a spoon to pick up the powder. Gently blow the powder onto the selected area from the other end.

E. Powders used for the Eyes.

Some Patent Medicines for eye disorders are made into powder form. This powder is a very fine grain of powder. When this medicine is applied, a small solid glass rod is used. The top of the glass rod should first be moistened with water. Then the rod is placed into the powder and the powder is applied to the inside of the lower eyelid.

F. Plasters for the Skin

The traditional plaster form requires that the outside of the folded plaster first be heated to soften the medicinal ingredients which are inside. After heating, the plaster is opened and applied to the skin. An example of the traditional form is Gou Pi Gao, #4.9. The modern plaster form has the medicinal ingredients attached to an adhesive patch which is applied directly to the skin without first heating. An example of the modern form is Shang Shi Bao Zhen Gao, #4.11.

G. Medicines which require Special Application

Some medicines require vinegar to be mixed with them which will release heat from the medicine. The vinegar paste can be applied to the affected area, where rheumatism or arthritis is present. An example of this form of medicine is Kan Li Sha.

Section V. How to Combine Patent Medicines with Herbal Tea Formulas and with Other Patent Medicines

Use of Patent Medicines with Herbal Tea Formulas

The combination of a Patent Medicine with a complete herbal medicine tea formula should be prescribed by a qualified Oriental Medical Doctor. The herbal tea is then used to swallow the Patent Medicine, instead of water. This combination method is commonly used with some specific or expensive Patent Medicines such as An Gong Niu Huang Wan, #5.2, Ju Fang Zhi Bao Dan, Zi Xue Dan, #5.1, Zai Zao Wan, #6.4, or Da Huo Luo Dan, #6.3, etc. This method is also used sometimes to treat cases who need a Patent Medicine to assist the function of an herbal medicine tea. Usually these patients take the Patent Medicine during the day, and herbal tea at night. In ancient Chinese medical texts, several physicians added the Patent Medicines into the herbal tea ingredients and cooked them all together. Because this method requires knowledge of both herbal tea formulas and the Patent Medicines, it will not be discussed here.

Use of Patent Medicines with Other Patent Medicines

It is common to use two or more kinds of Patent Medicines to treat a patient. This method has been used since ancient times. Generally, two different types of combinations are used which are explained below:

1) Combination of Patent Medicines which have a similar function and effect. Using this approach, the clinical outcome will be better than if either Patent Medicine alone, were used. For example, when treating toothache or sore throat with breath odor due to Stomach Heat, Niu Huang Jie Du Pian, #7.8, plus another Clear Stomach Heat Patent Medicine such as Qing Wei Huang Lian Wan may be used. When treating skin rash or erruption or itching caused by Wind Dampness, Fang Feng Tong Sheng Wan (Clear Heat and Expel Wind) plus Lian Qiao Bai Du Pian (treat skin disorders) are used. When treating hoarseness caused by Deficient Lung Yin, Yang Yin Qing Fei Wan or Yang Yin Qing Fei Tang Jiang, #3.12 (Nourish Lung Yin and increase body fluid) plus Qing Yin Wan, #7.11 (treat hoarseness caused by Dryness) are used. When treating amenorrhea with distension in the hypochrondiac region due to excess anger, Fu Ke Zhong Zi Wan, #12.15 (Nourish Blood, Regulate Menses, Remove Blood Stagnation) plus Shu Gan Wan, #11,1 (Move Stuck Liver Qi) are used.

2) Combination of Patent Medicines which have different indications and effects. Using this approach, the two Patent Medicines which are used complement each other and improve the overall effect. When treating Wind Heat syndrome with cough as a major symptom, use Yin Qiao Jie Du Wan Pian, #1.4 (Clear Wind Heat) plus a cough medicine such as Chuan Bei Jing Pian, #3.1 (stop cough) or a cough medicine such as Zhi Sou Ding Chuan Wan, #3.17 (stop cough, Open Lung Qi) are used. When treating menstrual disorders combined with poor digestion due to Deficient Qi and Deficient Blood, Fu Ke Ba Zhen Wan, #13.10 (Strengthen Qi and Blood; Regulate menses) plus Xiang Sha Liu Jun Zi Wan, #11.4 (Strengthen Middle Warmer Qi and improve digestion) are used. When treating abdominal pain due to Internal Cold plus diarrhea, Fu Zi Li Zhong Wan, #8.1 (Warm the Middle Warmer and stop abdominal pain) plus Huo Xiang Zheng Qi Wan, #2.1, (Regulate Stomach and Intestines; stop diarrhea, vomiting, nausea) are used.

In addition, various other combinations have been used by Chinese physicians and found to be effective through anecdotal experience. Three examples of these anedcotal combinations are given below: 1) To treat headache on the side of the head due to Wind Heat, Yin Qiao Jie Du Wan Pian, #1.4 plus Shu Gan Wan, #11.1 are used. 2) To treat leg or back pain due to Def. Kidney and Liver with debility of walking, Jian Bu Hu Chien Wan, #13.18 plus Shu Gan Wan, #11.1 are used. 3) To treat a serious Def. Qi case with OPI, Yin Qiao Jie Du Wan Pian, #1.4 plus Bu Zhong Yi Qi Wan #13.6 are used. (Zhong Yao Cheng Yao Xue, 1984).

Section VI. Contraindications with Patent Medicines

Patent Medicines which are not appropriate for use with certain cases

Patent Medicines which have the effect of Moving Qi, Moving Stuck Blood, or Promoting Blood circulation or those which are strong purgatives should not be used with pregnant women. A strong diaphoretic medicine should not be used with a patient who has serious Def. Yin or a patient who has serious loss of body fluid, including loss from vomiting, diarrhea, or bleeding. A patient should not take a Tonic medicine, only, when an OPI (Common Cold, flu; acute viral or bacterial condition) is present. In this case, if a Tonic medicine, only, is taken, the Tonic medicine may worsen the condition or cause the illness to last longer. In some instances it is possible to use both a Tonic medicine and an OPI medicine when treating a weaker patient who has contracted an OPI condition.

Special Dietary Cautions to Observe while Taking Certain Patent Medicines

A few Patent Medicines have dietary cautions referred to as Ji Kou; Ji means "forbidden" and Kou means "mouth." Thus while taking some Patent Medicines, it is important not to eat certain foods. For example, while taking Du Zheng Hu Gu Wan,#4.3, a medicine used to treat chronic Bi syndrome (pain in the joints due to Wind-Cold and Dampness), patients are advised not to eat beans (including soybeans) or seafood. Another example is while taking any Clear Heat medicine, it is important not to eat oily or spicy foods. Another example includes Shen Ling Bai Zhu Wan, #13.7 and other medicines used to treat poor digestion. These medicines require that the patient refrain from eating cold food, oily food or raw food while taking them. Another example is while taking medicines which Regulate Liver Qi, it is recommended that the patient try to avoid stressful situations. In addition, some Tonic medicines which are used to Strengthen the Kidney require that the patient refrain from sex for a certain period of time.

It is important to read the leaflet which is enclosed with each Patent Medicine to learn about the specific contraindications and cautions which are appropriate for a specific medicine. The contraindications are also mentioned for each Patent Medicine contained in this book, where appropriate. They are listed before the Dose section for each Patent Medicine.

Section VII. Use of Patent Medicines with Babies and Children

When the children's dose is discussed on the leaflet with most Patent Medicines, it is not always fully explained. However, the children's dose is very important because if it is too small, the expected results will not be obtained, and if it is too large, it may damage the Qi.

Children's Doses for Patent Medicines Designed Specifically for Children

When using a medicine that is designed specifically for children, the dose for the new-born infant to one month should be one-third that used for the one-year old child. When using a medicine that is designed specifically for children, the dose for the infant who is one month to six months should be two-thirds that used for the one-year old child; between six months to one year, use a dose that is between two-thirds and a full dose for a one-year old child. At one year of age, a full children's dose can be used.

Children's Doses for Patent Medicines Designed for Children and Adults

The dose on the label for medicine which is used both by children and adults is usually given for children and adults, but sometimes it is only given for adults. For example, if the dose for an adult is three pills, the dose for a child age seven is half the adult dose, i.e. one and one-half pills. A child who is age three to seven should be given one-third to one-half the adult dose. A child under age three should be given less than one-third.

Additional factors which are important in adjusting the dose for children include the following: overall strength of the child; the severity of the disease; the season; and the response of the child to a particular medicine during previous illnesses. For example, a child who is weaker or who has not developed properly, or who is underweight, should be given a smaller dose. If the disease is more severe, the dose should be larger. In the summertime, do not use too many Warm Property medicines; in the wintertime, do not use too many Cold Property medicines. If the child has shown a good response to a small dose in the past, continue to use as small a dose a possible which will effect a good clinical response.

There are a variety of methods which can be used to give the medicine to children. The most common problems encountered concerning taking the medicines are that the child refuses to take the medicine or the child vomits after taking the medicine. These problems are usually due to improper feeding of the medicine to the child. The parents should first be patient with the child and not force the child to take the medicine. Otherwise, the child will develop a fear of the medicine. When feeding the medicine to an infant, the medicine should be prepared into a liquid mixture, with a small amount of warm water or milk; some honey or sugar may be added. If the child has vomiting after taking the medicine, it is more appropriate to feed only a small amount each time, and use several administrations of a small amount of the medicine over a period of time. This will vary according to how small the dose needs to be or how often it needs to be given to insure that no vomiting occurs.

With children who are able to understand and talk, it is important to explain to them why it is necessary to take the medicine and help them to understand the situation. If the pill is large, especially the honey pill form, it may be cut into several small pieces and give the child only one or two of these small portions. If too many are given, vomiting may result. If children frequently have vomiting after swallowing the medicine, the parents may massage the acupuncture points NeiGuan (PC 6) and HeGu (LI 4) for the child.

Special Uses of Patent Medicines for Children's Disorders

Wu Ling San cooked together with an herbal tea made from Yin Chen as the Yao Yin is used for new-born hemolytic jaundice caused by Cold Dampness.

Fu Zi Li Zhong Wan, #8.1, cooked together with herbal tea made from Yin Chen as the Yao Yin is also used for newborn hemolytic jaundice.

Xi Gua Shuang, #7.10, is used in powder form applied topically to stop pain and reduce inflammation for stomatitis.

Hu Po Bao Long Wan, #6.5, is used to Clear Damp Heat and stop spasm and seizures due to high grade fever; treat pneumonia, meningitis.

legitimate

Sang Ju Gan Mao Pian, #1.3, is used to Expel Wind Heat; treat sore throat, fever, headache, cough associated with flu, or virus infection. Children's dose is 2 to 4 tablets, 3 times a day. For children less than three years, reduce the doseage.

Lian Qiao Bai Du Pian, #7.29, is used to treat eczema, boils or constipation.

An Gong Niu Huang Wan, #5.2, is used to treat high grade fever and spasms due to central nervous system infection including meningitis. The dose for children age 3 and over is half a pill, twice a day. Reduce the dosage for children under age 3.

Zi Xue Dan, #5.1, is used to treat high-grade fever and spasms due to central nervous system infection including meningitis. The dose for children age 3 and over is 0.5 to 1 gram, twice a day. Reduce the dosage for children under age 3.

Qing Qi Hua Tan Wan, #3.6, is used to treat cough due to Damp Heat with thicker, yellow phlegm. Nausea and full sensation in the chest may be present. The dosage is one-half to two-thirds the adult dose, twice a day. Reduce the dosage for children under age 3.

Qiou Li Gao, #3.16, is a syrup used to Tonify the Lungs and stop chronic cough. This is used to treat dry mouth, dry throat and hoarseness. Each time use 10 grams dissolved in hot water; drink it while it is warm. Use twice a day.

Jia Wei Xiang Lian Pian, #7.5, is used to treat dysentery and diarrhea with abdominal pain. Use half-dose. Reduce the dosage for children under age 3.

Qing Fei Yi Huo Pian, #3.4, is used to Clear Heat and treat cough with thick yellow sputum; sore throat, constipation or nasal bleeding. Use 2 to 4 tablets, twice a day, age 3 and over. Reduce the dosage under age 3.

Jin Gui Shen Qi Wan, #13.22, is used to treat edema due to Damp Cold, feeling of Cold in the limbs, and nephritis. Use half-dose, twice a day. Reduce the dosage for children under age 3.

Zhi Bao Ding is used to treat Wind Cold syndrome which has turned to Heat where fever, cough, asthma and phlegm (yellow) are present. The dosage is 1 honey pill, twice a day. For children under 1 year of age, decrease the dose.

Shen Ling Bai Zhu Wan, #13.7, is used to treat Def. Spleen with chronic diarrhea and poor appetite. The doseage is one-half to two-thirds for children age 3 and over. Reduce the dosage for children under age 3.

Fu Ke Ba Zhen Wan#13.10, is used to treat children with Def. Qi and Def. Blood due to Def. Spleen The child may have malnourishment and be underdeveloped. The dosage is one-half to two-thirds, twice a day. Reduce the dosage for children under 3.

Ren Shen Gui Pi Wan, #13.8, is used to treat children who have poor appetite, spontaneous sweating day or night, poor sleeping, and general deficiency. The dosage is one-half to two-thirds, twice a day. Reduce the dosage for children under age 3.

He Che Da Zao Wan, #13.17, is used to treat Def. Qi and Def. Blood in children who have abnormal mental or physical development. The dosage is one-half to full dose, twice a day. Reduce the dosage for children under age 3.

Bu Zhong Yi Qi Wan, #13.6, is used to treat Def. Qi and Def. Blood syndrome and diarrhea due to Def. Spleen with feeling of Cold. The dosage is one-half to full dose, twice a day. Reduce the dosage for children under age 3.

Long Dan Xie Gan Wan, #7.12, is used to Clear Liver Heat and treat stomatitis or mouth ulcer; acute tinnitus due to Liver Heat (Excess Yang). The dosage is one-half to full dose, twice a day. Reduce for children under age 3.

Chuan Xin Lian Pian, #7.27, is used to treat viral or bacterial infection such as flu; or gastric enteritis. The dosage is one-half to full dose, three times a day. Reduce for children under age 3.

Shi Di Xue is used to treat nausea, vomiting, due to Summer Heat. The dosage is 3 to 5 cc, as necessary. Reduce for children under age 3. This medicine has also been used successfully to treat heat rash. A solution is made with one part Shi Di Xue to ten parts warm water.

Liu Wei Di Huang Wan, #13.19, is used to treat children who have crying during the night. The dosage is one-half to full dose. Reduce the dosage for children under age 3. This formula is also used with children and babies who have developmental delay, see Notes under # 13.19.

Part II. The Patent Medicines

Chapter 1. Treat Exogenous Conditions
(Includes Patent Medicines used with Common Cold, Flu Conditions)

1.1 川 芎 茶 調 丸

Chuan	Xiong	Cha	Tiao	Wan
--------Ligusticum-------		tea	adjust	pills

Source: Tai Ping Hui Min He Ji Ju Fang, (Formulas of The People's Welfare Pharmacy), Song Dynasty, 960-1279.

Function: 1. Expel OPI Wind-Cold
2. Stop Headache due to Wind-Cold

Application: 1. Use to treat headache due to OPI Wind Factor.

2. Use to treat headache as well as Wind-Cold syndrome with symptoms such as chills, fever, stuffy nose.

3. Use to treat OPI headache in any of the following meridians - Xiao Yang (sides of head); Jue Yin (top of head); Tai Yang (back of head; neck, upper back); Yang Ming (forehead).

4. Use to treat headache due to nasal disorders such as rhinitis, sinusitis.

Contraindication: Do not use in a case where the headache is due to Deficiency. Do not use with a weak patient who has Def. Qi, Def. Blood or Def. Yin, where the Yang has ascended to cause the headache.

Dose: 8 pills, 2 or 3 times a day.

Chuan Xiong Cha Tiao Wan is manufactured as "Chuan Qiong Cha Tiao Wan" by the Lanzhou Chinese Medicine Works and the Shanghai Chinese Medicine Works in bottles of 200 small pills.

Pinyin Name	Pharmaceutical Name	Percent	TCM Function
Bo He	Herba Menthae	32	Expel Wind
Chuan Xiong	Rhizoma Ligustici	16	Promote Blood Circulation; Expel Wind; Stop pain, especially Xiao Yang, Jue Yin headache
Jing Jie	Herba seu Flos Schizonepetae Tenuifoliae	16	Expel Wind
Fang Feng	Herba Radix Ledebouriellae Sesloidis	8	Expel Wind
Qiang Huo	Rhizoma et Radix Notopterygii	8	Expel Wind-Cold; Stop pain, especially Tai Yang headache
Bai Zhi	Radix Angelicae	8	Expel Wind-Cold; Stop pain, especially Yang Ming headache
Gan Cao	Radix Glycyrrhizae Uralensis	8	Harmonize other herbs
Xi Xin	Radix Herba Asari cum Radice	4	Expel Wind-Cold, Stop pain

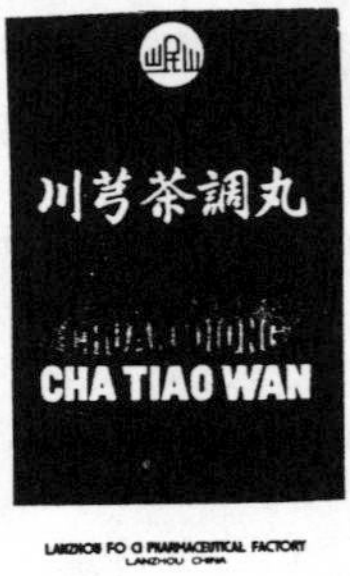

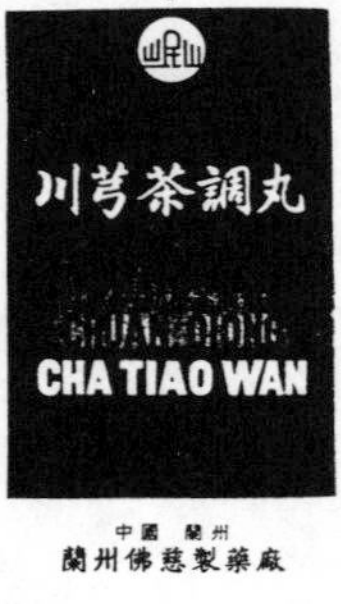

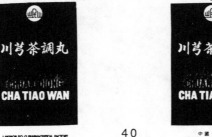

1.2 午 时 茶

午	时	茶
Wu	**Shi**	**Cha**
noon	time	tea

Source: Chen Xiu-Yuan Yi Shu Quan Ji, (Dr. Xiu-Yuan Chen's Complete Medical Book), Qing Dynasty, 1644-1911.

Function: 1. Expel Wind-Cold
2. Disperse Food Mass, Strengthen Stomach

Application: 1. Use to treat Wind-Cold syndrome such as the flu or common cold. Symptoms: chills, fever, headache, stuffy nose, full sensation in the chest, stomach distension due to food mass, diarrhea, vomiting.

Dose: Each block weighs 9 grams. Each time use two blocks, one or two times per day.
Either soak the blocks in 8 oz. boiled water, or place the blocks in 8 oz. water and boil for 2 minutes. Let the water cool to a warm temperature, and drink; discard the debris.

The contents are grouped below into 6 groups, according to their Traditional Chinese Medicine function.

Pinyin Name	Pharmaceutical Name	Percent	TCM Function
Group 1			
Huo Xiang	Herba Agastaches seu Pogostemi	2.13	Expel Wind-Cold;
Bai Zhi	Radix Angelicae	2.13	Induce sweat (diaphoretic);
Zi Su Ye	Folium Perillae Frutescentis	2.13	Stop headache
Fang Feng	Radix Ledebouriellae Sesloidis	2.13	
Qiang Huo	Rhizoma et Radix Notopterygii	2.13	
Chai Hu	Radix Bupleuri	2.84	
Group 2			
Zhi Shi	Fructus Citri seu Ponciri Immaturus	1.42	Regulate Qi;
Chen Pi	Pericarpium Citri Reticulatae	1.42	Remove Qi Stagnation;
Shan Zha	Fructus Crataegi	1.42	Strengthen Spleen;
Mai Ya	Fructus Hordei Vulgaris Germinantus	2.13	Remove Food Mass
Shen Qu	Massa Fermentata	21.98	
Group 3			
Hou Po	Cortex Magnoliae Officinalis	2.13	Eliminate Dampness;
Cang Zhu	Rhizoma Atractylodis	1.42	Regulate Middle Warmer; Strengthen Spleen
Group 4			
Qian Hu	Radix Peucedani	2.84	Open Lung Qi; Eliminate
Jie Geng	Radix Platycodi Grandiflori	2.13	Phlegm; Stop cough
Group 5			
Gan Cao	Radix Glycyrrhizae Uralensis	1.42	Harmonize other herbs

Group 6

Hong Cha	Black tea	45.39	Regulate the strength of the diaphoretic medicines; Stop headache; Clear OPI in the head, as well as the Lower Warmer (diuretic property)

Notes: 1. Use this to treat "shui tu bu fu," poor digestion due to problems with travelling or moving to a new location.

2. It is not recommended to use this with a patient who has Wind-Heat syndrome with symptoms such as high grade fever, swollen and sore throat, yellow tongue coat; dark urine.

3. When a patient uses this medicine, it will be most effective if the patient takes the medicine while it is still very hot. After taking it, the patient should be covered with a blanket to induce sweat, soon after taking it. If the patient takes the medicine when the tea is cold, or if the patient stays outside and catches Wind-Cold again, then the medicine will not be as effective.

1.3 桑 菊 饮 片

Sang	**Ju**	**Yin**	**Pian**
Mulberry leaf	Chrysanthemum	drink	tablets

Source: Treatise on Differentiation and Treatment of Seasonal Febrile Diseases, by Wu Tang, 1798.

Function:
1. Dispel Wind-Heat in Upper Warmer
2. Open Stagnant Lung Qi, Stop cough

Application:
1. Use to treat seasonal febrile disorders due to Wind-Heat. Use in the acute condition. Symptoms: Cough, headache, some fever (but not high fever), sore throat, slight thirst, dry mouth.

2. Some Western medicine disease applications (in the early stages) include the following: Flu, bronchitis, tonsillitis, pharyngitis, conjunctivitis, or other illnesses with fever, thirst, and cough.

Contraindication: Use only in cases where an Excess syndrome is present; do not use where a Deficiency syndrome is present.

Dose: 4-8 tablets, 2 or 3 times a day. A large quantity of fluids (juices, water, etc.) should also be taken when using this formula.

Sang Ju Yin Pian is produced by the Tientsin Drug Manufactory as uncoated 0.6 gram tablets, 8 tablets per vial.

Pinyin Name	Pharmaceutical Name	Percent	TCM Function
Sang Ye	Folium Mori Albae	19.84	Expel Wind-Heat in Lung
Ju Hua	Flos Chrysanthemi Morifolii	7.95	Expel Wind-Heat in Lung
Lian Qiao	Fructus Forsythiae Suspensae	11.90	Clear Heat
Xing Ren	Semen Pruni Armeniacae	15.87	These two herbs together Open Lung
Jie Geng	Radix Platycodi Grandiflori	15.87	Qi; Stop cough; Clear throat
Lu Gen	Rhizoma Phragmitis Communis	15.87	Clear Heat, Stop thirst
Gan Cao	Radix Glycyrrhizae Uralensis	6.35	Harmonize other herbs
Bo He	Herba menthae	6.30	Expel Wind-Heat

Note: 1. The Patent Medicine, Sang Ju Gan Mao Pian, is another name for Sang Ju Yin Pian.

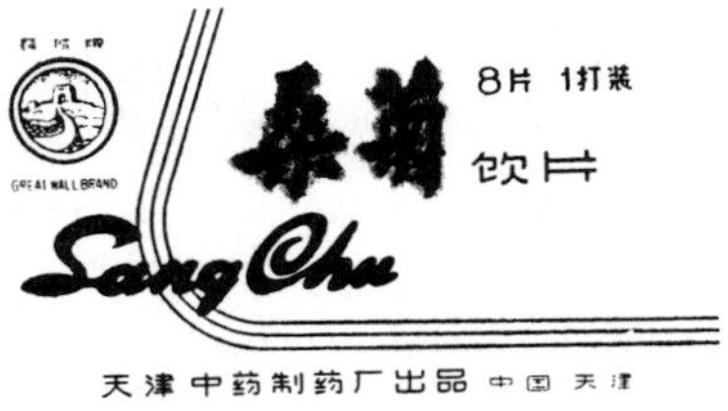

1.4 銀 翹 解 毒 片

銀	翹	解	毒	片
Yin	**Qiao**	**Jie**	**Du**	**Pian**
Lonicera	Forsythia	------detoxification------		tablets

Source: Wen Bing Tiao Bian, (More Discussion on Febrile Disease), Qing Dynasty, 1644-1911.

Function: 1. Expel Wind-Heat OPI in Spring/Summer

Application: 1. Use to treat early stage (Wei stage) of Four Stages of Seasonal Febrile Disease. Symptoms: Fever (although fever is not necessarily always present), possible aversion to wind, headache, thirst, cough and throat pain. The Tongue may be red with a white or yellowish coating. The Pulse is floating (compatible with Wind) and rapid (compatible with Heat).

2. Some Western medicine disease applications include the following: Common cold or flu, acute bronchitis, pneumonia, pharyngitis, otitis media, parotitis, measles, tonsillitis.

Dose: Adults: 3-5 coated tablets (or 2-4 uncoated tablets), 2 or 3 times a day with warm water.

Yin Qiao Jie Du Pian is produced by a number of manufactories in various formats. The Tientsin Drug Manufactory and the Beijing Tung Jen Tang pharmacy produce the formula as both uncoated tablets (8 per vial), and as coated tablets (20 tablets per bottle). Beijing Tung Jen Tang also produces bottles with 100 coated tablets, and the Tientsin Drug Manufactory also produces bottles with 60 and 120 coated tablets. The Tientsin Drug Manufactory produces two forms of Yin Qiao Jie Du Pian, with and without caffeine. The Yin Qiao formula from Beijing Tung Jen Tang contains no caffeine. The formulas used by the various manufactories are changed from time to time. It is suggested that the practitioner always read the label regarding the contents of each bottle.

A formula similar to this formula is also available in liquid, tincture form as "Prime Response," in the Jade Pharmacy product line, available through Crane Enterprises, Plymouth, MA, etc. See page 343.

Pinyin Name	Pharmaceutical Name	Percent	TCM Function
Jin Yin Hua	Flos Lonicerae Japonicae	17.76	Clear Heat; Detoxify Fire Poison, Expel some Wind
Lian Qiao	Fructus Forsythiae Suspensae	17.76	Clear Heat; Detoxify Fire Poison
Niu Bang Zi	Fructus Arctii Lappae	10.66	Detoxify Fire Poison
Jie Geng	Radix Platycodi Grandiflori	10.66	Soothe throat; Open Lung Qi
Bo He	Herba Menthae	10.66	Clear Wind-Heat
Lu Gen	Rhizoma Phragmitis Communis	8.88	Clear Heat; Promote Salivation; Stop thirst
Gan Cao	Radix Glycyrrhizae Uralensis	8.88	Clear Heat
Dan Zhu Ye	Herba Lophatheri Gracilis	7.10	Clear Heat; Stop thirst
Jing Jie	Herba seu Flos Schizonepetae Tenuifoliae	7.10	Expel Wind; Expel Fire Poison

Notes: 1. Yin Qiao Jie Du Pian is a very popular and commonly used medicine throughout China for the early stage of a common cold or flu.

2. The Patent Medicine, Gan Mao Ling Pian, is similar to Yin Qiao Jie Du Pian, used to treat Wind-Heat OPI. Gan Mao Ling Pian is produced in southern China (Guangzhou) and may contain herbs which are not commonly listed in Chinese herbal medicine texts.

SUPERIOR 60 TABS.

A GOOD REMEDY FOR COLDS

YINCHIAO TABLET

長城牌

GREAT WALL BRAND

TIENTSIN DRUG MANUFACTORY
TIANJIN, CHINA

精制

感冒良药

银翘

解毒片

長城牌

GREAT WALL BRAND

中国 天津
天津中药制药厰

北京銀翹

Superior Quality PEKING
YIN CHIAO CHIEH TU PIEN

BEIJING TUNG JEN TANG
BEIJING, CHINA

北京銀翹

Superior Quality PEKING
YIN CHIAO CHIEH TU PIEN

中國 北京
北京同仁堂

HIGH
STRENGTH
YINQIAO
TABLETS

THE UNITED PHARMACEUTICAL MANUFACTORY
KWANGCHOW, CHINA

銀翹片
感冒良藥

廣州聯合製药廠
中國 廣州

3. There are two additional Patent Medicines which are modifications of the Yin Qiao Jie Du Pian formula, these include the following:

羚	翘	解	毒	片
Ling	**Qiao**	**Jie**	**Du**	**Pian**
Antelope horn	Forsythiae	-----detoxification-----		tablets

Ling Qiao Jie Du Pian differs from Yin Qiao Jie Du Pian by the addition of one ingredient, Ling Yang Jiao (Cornu Antelopis). The Ling Yang Jiao has a more powerful Cold Property than any of the other ingredients in the Yin Qiao Jie Du Pian formula. Therefore, the Ling Qiao Jie Du Pian formula Clears more Heat. In addition, the Ling Yang Jiao gets into the Liver and Lung channels, it is especially effective in Clearing Lung Heat. The effect of Ling Qiao Jie Du Pian is stronger than that of Yin Qiao Jie Du Pian because it Clears more Lung Heat. It is especially useful to treat a patient in the early stage of Wind-Heat syndrome with cough and phlegm. In Shanghai, the name used for this formula is Ling Yang (Antelope) Gan Mao (Flu) Pian. Dose: 4 tablets, every 4 hours

ANTELOPE HORN AND FRUCTUS
FORSYTHIAE FEBRIFRUGAL TABLETS

羚翘解毒片

犀	羚	解	毒	片
Xi	**Ling**	**Jie**	**Du**	**Pian**
Rhinoceros horn	Antelope horn	-----detoxification-----		tablets

See #1.7, Xi Ling Jie Du Pian. Xi Ling Jie Du Pian differs from Yin Qiao Jie Du Pian by the addition of three ingredients, Xi Jiao (Cornu Rhinoceri), Ling Yang Jiao (Cornu Antelopis) and Bing Pian (Borneol). The Xi Jiao (Cornu Rhinoceri) has a very Cold Property and gets into the Heart channel. The Ling Yang Jiao (Cornu Antelopis) Clears Heat and gets into the Liver and Lung channels. The Bing Pian (Borneol) Clears Heat. Therefore, the effect of Xi Ling Jie Du Pian is stronger than that of Yin Qiao Jie Du Pian because it Clears more Heart Heat and Lung Heat. It is especially good to use to treat a patient with some fever in the early stage of Wind-Heat Syndrome with cough and phlegm.

4. The antelope and rhinoceros are considered endangered species. It is illegal to import antelope horn or rhinoceros horn into the U.S.; substitutions are often made (Dharmananda S: Prescriptions on Silk and Paper: The History and Development of Chinese Patent Medicines. Portland, Oregon, Institute for Traditional Medicine and Preventive Health Care, 1989.

   The horn of water buffalo is often substituted for Cornu Rhinoceri; and goat horn is often substituted for Cornu Antelopis. (Bensky D and Gamble A: Chinese Herbal Medicine MATERIA MEDICA, Seattle, Eastland Press, 1986, p. 95 and p. 603.)

1.5 感 冒 退 热 冲 剂

Gan	Mao	Tui	Re	Chun	Ji
---common cold, flu---		---eliminate fever---		-crystalline form-	

Function: 1. Expel Wind-Heat
2. Reduce inflammation

Application: 1. Use to eliminate fever due to Wind-Heat. It is used, for example, in cases of tonsillitis accompanied by fever, as well as in cases of acute or chronic tracheitis, with symptoms such as sore throat, headache, cough and sputum.

Viral infections sometimes lead to an underlying bacterial infection. In the early stage of a viral infection clear sputum and nasal discharge are present. Later, if the viral infection has led to an underlying bacterial infection, yellow sputum and nasal discharge are present. This medicine is used in the later stage, where Heat signs are present.

Dose: This is a mild formula, and is best used with mild cases or only with children. It can also be used prophylactically after exposure.

Dissolve 1 small bag of crystals in warm water before use. Use 1 bag, 3 times a day. If the patient's fever rises above 38° C (approximately 100° F), use 2 bags, 4 times a day.

Gan Mao Tui Re Chun Ji is produced by the Shanghai Chinese Medicine Works as "Ganmao Tuire Chongji." The four herbal ingredients are mixed with sugar in each plastic bag. Because this medicine absorbs moisture readily, it should be stored in a dry, cool area.

Pinyin Name	Pharmaceutical Name	Percent	TCM Function
Da Qing Ye	Folium Daqingye	33.33	Clear Heat; Detoxify Fire Poison; Clear Blood Heat; Clear skin rash due to Heat
Ban Lan Gen	Radix Isatidis seu Baphicacanthi	33.33	Clear Heat; Detoxify Fore Poison; Clear Blood Heat; Soothe throat
Cao He Che	Rhizoma Bistortae	16.67	Clear Heat; Detoxify Fire Poison
Lian Qiao	Fructus Forsythiae Suspensae	16.67	Clear Heat; Detoxify Fire Poison

Note: 1. This formula contains 4 herbs, each of which has the same general function as broad spectrum antibiotics (in TCM terms, Clear Heat, Detoxify Fire poison). Here they are used to treat the Wind-Heat syndrome, although none has the specific property to rid Wind. These 4 have proved to be useful, however, in treating Wind-Heat syndrome over many years of experience. This medicine is not appropriate to use with Wind-Cold syndromes. Because this medicine contains 4 herbs used to Clear Heat and Detoxify Fire Poison, it is appropriate to use it with other disorders where Heat is present such as carbuncles or sores (use internally).

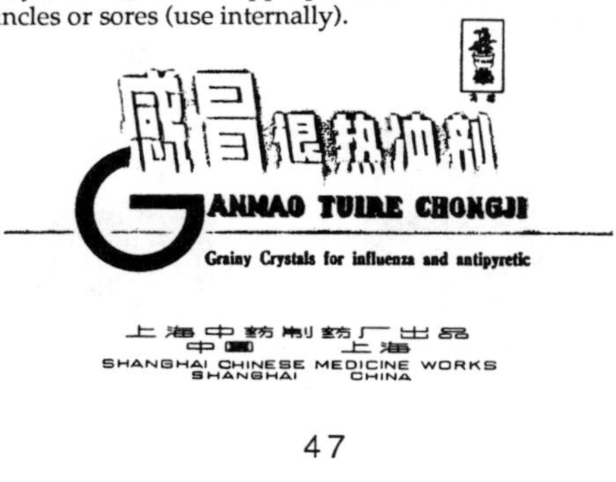
感冒退热冲剂
GANMAO TUIRE CHONGJI
Grainy Crystals for influenza and antipyretic
上海中药制药厂出品
中国 上海
SHANGHAI CHINESE MEDICINE WORKS
SHANGHAI CHINA

1.6 羚 羊 傷 風 靈

Ling	Yang	Shang	Feng	Ling
-------Antelope horn-------		--------common cold-------		effective

Function: 1. Expel Wind-Heat

Application: 1. Use to treat common cold or flu caused by a virus where fever is present from the beginning of the disease and there are no chills at first (vs. a common cold or flu caused by Wind-Cold, where chills are present at first). Additional symptoms of Wind-Heat: Throat pain, headache, cough, sputum, tonsillitis, bronchitis.

2. Additional Western medicine disease applications include acute bronchitis. Chronic bronchitis cases may have acute flare-ups; this formula is appropriate to use in the acute flare-up stage where Heat signs are present.

Dose: 4 tablets, 2 times a day. In serious cases, use 6-8 tablets, 3 times a day.

Ling Yang Shang Feng Ling is produced by the Tian Jin Drug Manufactory in bottles of 24 coated tablets.

Pinyin Name	Pharmaceutical Name	Percent	TCM Function
Ling Yang Jiao	Cornu Antelopis	0.54	Clear Lung Heat; Stop cough, Decrease phlegm
Tian Hua Fen	Radix Trichosanthis	3.7	Clear Lung Heat; Eliminate phlegm; Promote Body Fluids; Stop thirst
Lian Qiao	Fructus Forsythiae Suspensae	22.5	Clear Heat; Detoxify Fire Poison
Dan Zhu Ye	Herba Lophatheri Gracilis	11.3	Clear Heat; Tranquilize Heart Spirit
Jing Jie	Herba seu Flos Schizonepetae Tenuifoliae	11.28	Expel OPI Wind
Ge Gen	Radix Puerariae	3.7	Raise body fluids to reduce stiff neck
Gan Cao	Radix Glycyrrhizae Uralensis	9.4	Clear Heat; Stop cough
Jin Yin Hua	Flos Lonicerae Japonicae	22.5	Clear Heat; Detoxify Fire Poison
Niu Bang Zi	Fructus Arctii Lappae	15	Clear Wind-Heat; Detoxify Fire Poison; Soothe throat
Bo He	Herba Menthae	0.08	Clear Wind-Heat; Stop headache

Note: 1. The Ling Yang Shang Feng Ling formula is a modification of the standard formula, Yin Qiao Jie Du Pian. The function of this formula is similar to another modification of Yin Qiao Jie Du Pian called Ling Qiao Jie Du Pian. Ling Yang Shang Feng Ling, the present formula, is more effective in treating stiffness (especially neck stiffness) whereas Ling Qiao Jie Du Pian is more effective in treating the Heat which causes throat pain.

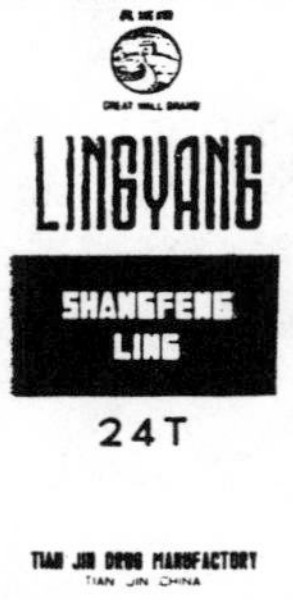

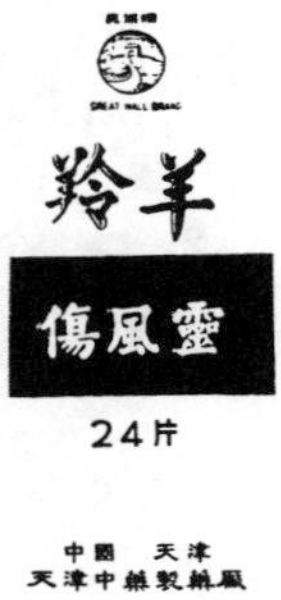

1.7 犀 羚 解 毒 片

犀	羚	解	毒	片
Xi	**Ling**	**Jie**	**Du**	**Pian**
Rhinoceros horn	Antelope horn	-----detoxification-----		tablets

Function: 1. Expel Wind-Heat
2. Detoxify Fire Poison

Application: 1. Use to treat common cold or flu caused by a virus where fever is present from the beginning of the disease and there are no chills at first (vs. a common cold or flu caused by Wind-Cold, where chills are present at first). Use this to treat the upper half of the body which has been affected by Wind-Heat with symptoms such as high fever and sore throat.

2. Additional Western medicine disease applications include the treatment of children's measles only after a large amount of the rash has appeared, it is red in color and fever is present.

Dose: 4 tablets every 4 hours. Take before a meal if the patient has a flu. In severe cases use 6-8 pills every 4 hours.

Xi Ling Jie Du Pian is produced as "Rhinoceros & Antelope Horn Febrifugal Tablets, " by the Shantung Native Produce Branch, Tsingtao, China, in vials containing 12 tablets.

Pinyin Name	Pharmaceutical Name	Percent	TCM Function
Lian Qiao	Fructus Forsythiae Suspensae	14.6	Clear Heat; Detoxify Fire Poison
Dan Dou Chi	Semen Sojai Preparatae	14.6	Expel Wind-Heat
Niu Bang Zi	Fructus Arctii Lappae	11	Clear Wind-Heat; Promote eruption of rash in the treatment of measles
Bo He	Herba Menthae	11	Clear Wind-Heat; Stop headache; Promote eruption of rash in the treatment of measles
Bing Pian	Borneol	0.7	Clear Heat; Stop pain; Open Orifices
Xi Jiao	Cornu Rhinoceri	0.2	Clear Blood Heat; Clear Heat in the Heart; Detoxify Fire Poison
Jing Jie	Herba seu Flos Schizonepetae Tenuifoliae	14.6	Expel OPI Wind
Jin Yin Hua	Flos Lonicerae Japonicae	11	Clear Heat; Detoxify Fire Poison
Dan Zhu Ye	Herba Lophatheri Gracilis	11	Clear Heat; Discharge Heat through urination
Gan Cao	Radix Glycyrrhizae Uralensis	9.4	Clear Heat; Stop cough
Ling Yang Jiao	Cornu Antelopis	0.3	Clear Lung Heat; Extinguish Liver Wind

Notes: 1. This formula is one of the most important modifications of the standard formula, Yin Qiao San. Xi Jiao and Ling Yang Jiao are the two most important herbal medicines which have been added here to the Yin Qiao San formula. These two herbs have a Cold property. Therefore, this formula, Xi Ling Jie Du Wan, is able to eliminate more Heat which has affected the Heart and Liver than Yin Qiao San. The Heart and Liver symptoms include high grade fever, dark red rash and agitation. This formula is also better to Clear Heat in the Lung than Yin Qiao San. This formula, therefore, is used in cases with pus-like sputum. In these cases it is necessary to use an increased dosage.

2. A similar Patent Medicine, Zhen Zhu Niu Huang Xi Jiao Jie Du Pian, uses additional strong Cold property herbs such as Niu Huang, Bing Pian, Zhi Zi and Zhen Zhu to Clear Excess Wind-Heat. Therefore, Zhen Zhu Niu Huang Xi Jiao Jie Du Pian is stronger in Clearing Heat than Xi Ling Jie Du Pian and is used with patients with more Heat and more intense symptoms. Do not use with pregnant women. The dose is 2 tablets, 2 times a day.

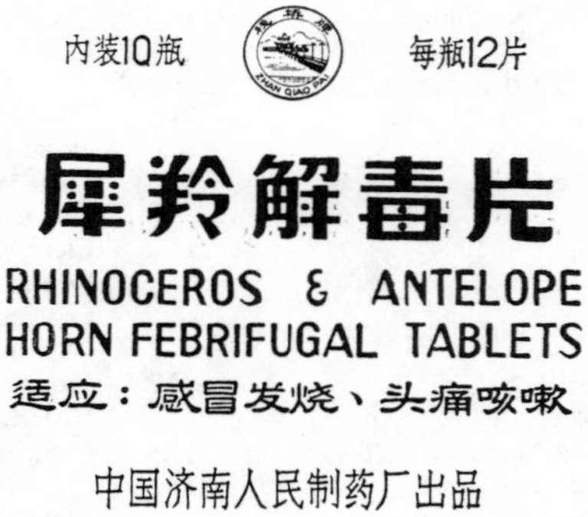

1.8 感 冒 丹

Gan	Mao	Dan
----common cold or flu----		pills

Source: Shih Chin-Mo, 20th century Chinese physician.

Function: 1. Expel Wind-Heat; Reduce fever
2. Stop cough; Relieve chest congestion

Application: 1. Use to treat Wind-Heat syndrome due to OPI. Symptoms: Fever, (with slight chills), headache, swollen or sore throat, cough, runny nose, red eyes, skin rash or skin erruptions, fatigue. If the Wind-Heat has affected the Spleen/Stomach, nausea and vomiting may also be present.

2. Some Western medicine disease applications include the following: (Note, the patient must have the above-mentioned Wind-Heat symptoms in order to use this herbal formula.) Influenza, measles, acute conjunctivitis, tonsillitis, pharyngitis, ear pain due to a flu, nasal infection.

Dose: 20 pills, 2 times a day.

Gan Mao Dan is produced as "Kanmaotan" by the Beijing Tung Jen Tang pharmacy in bottles of 200 pills.

The ingredients are listed below in 6 separate groups according to their function.

Pinyin Name	Pharmaceutical Name	Percent	TCM Function
Group 1			
Jin Yin Hua	Flos Lonicerae Japonicae	5	Clear Heat; Detoxify Fire
Lian Qiao	Fructus Forsythiae Suspensae	5	Poison
Group 2			
Zhi Zi	Fructus Gardeniae Jasminoidis	7	Clear Excess Heat; Reduce
Lu Gen	Rhizoma Phragmitis Communis	10	Fever; Clear Heat in Qi Stage
Group 3			
Chi Shao	Radix Paeoniae Rubra	16	Clear Heat; Clear Heat in
Bai Mao Gen	Rhizoma Imperatae Cylindricae	10	Blood Stage
Group 4			
Dan Dou Chi	Semen Sojae Preparatum	14	Expel Wind-Heat; Induce
Bo He	Herba Menthae	3	slight sweat; Reduce fever
Sang Ye	Folium Mori Albae	10	
Jing Jie	Herba seu Flos Schizonepetae Tenuifoliae	5	

<u>Group 5</u>			
Zi Yuan	Radix Asteris Tatarici	5	Stop cough; Eliminate phlegm
Jie Geng	Radix Platycodi Grandiflori	5	
<u>Group 6</u>			
Chen Pi	Pericarpium Citri Reticulatae	5	Strengthen Spleen; Regulate Stomach; Stop nausea and vomiting

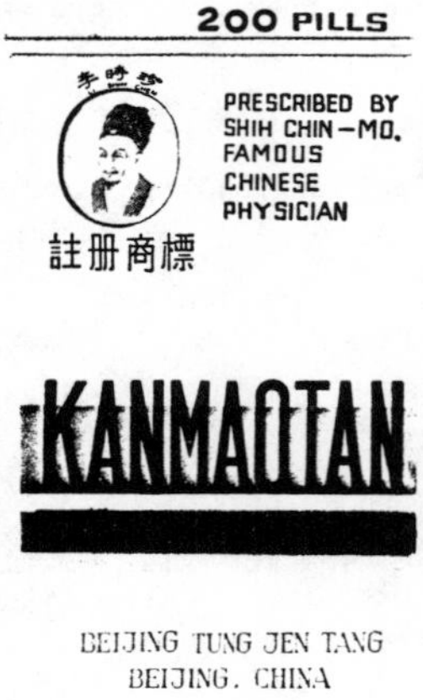

200 PILLS
PRESCRIBED BY SHIH CHIN-MO. FAMOUS CHINESE PHYSICIAN
註册商標
KANMAOTAN
BEIJING TUNG JEN TANG
BEIJING, CHINA

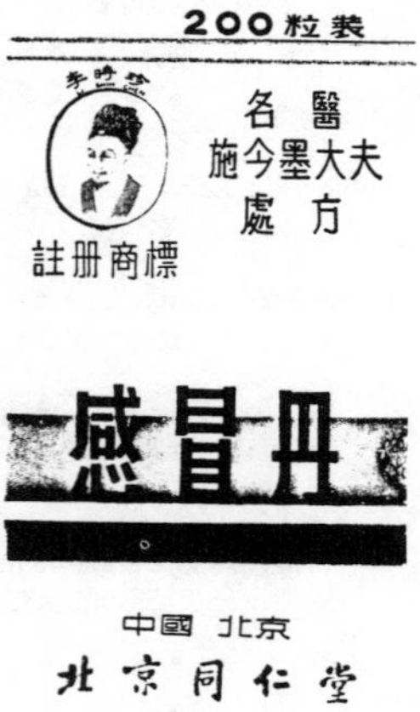

1.9 鼻 淵 丸

Bi	**Yuan**	**Wan**
nose	nasal sinusitis	pills

Function: 1. Expel Wind-Heat
2. Open nasal passages, relieve stuffy nose
3. Stop pain

Application: 1. Use to treat acute or chronic rhinitis, nasal sinusitis. Symptoms: Runny nose with yellowish, thick discharge and bad odor (bacterial infection).

2. Use to treat stuffy nose or obstruction in the nose.

3. Use to remove nasal polyps; remove blood stasis.

Contraindication: Due to the very slight toxic effect of Cang Er Zi, do not exceed recommended dosage of this formula. This formula is not recommended for use with children.

Dose: Adults: 12 pills, 3 times a day. Not recommended for use with children.

Bi Yuan Wan is produced by the Min-Kang Drug Manufactory, I-Chang, China, in bottles of 100 coated tablets.

Pinyin Name	Pharmaceutical Name	Percent	TCM Function
Cang Er Zi	Fructus Xanthii	72.1	Open nasal passages; Expel Wind; Stop headache
Xin Yi Hua	Flos Liliflorae Magnoliae	13.8	Open nasal passages; Expel Wind
Qian Cao Gen	Radix Rubiae Cordifoliae	4.7	Clear Blood Heat; Stop bleeding; Promote blood circulation; Remove Blood Stagnation
Jin Yin Hua	Flos Loanicerae Japonicae	4.7	Clear Heat in the Upper Warmer; Reduce inflammation; Detoxify Fire Poison
Ju Hua	Flos Chrysanthemi Morifolii	4.7	Clear Wind-Heat; Stop headache; Brighten the eyes

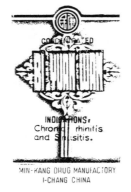

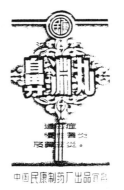

1.10 鼻 炎 片

鼻	炎	片
Bi	**Yan**	**Pian**
nose	inflammation	tablets

Function: 1. Expel Wind-Heat
2. Open nasal passages
3. Decrease swelling

Application: 1. Use to treat acute or chronic rhinitis, nasal sinusitis. Symptoms: Runny nose with large amounts of yellowish, thick discharge with foul-smelling odor (bacterial infection).

2. Use to treat stuffy nose. In a chronic case, the patient may also have dizziness and headache, especially in the forehead.

3. Use to treat hay fever or other allergies with rhinitis.

Contraindication: This formula contains a small amount of the very slightly toxic Cang Er Zi. Therefore, it is important not to exceed the recommended dosage

Dose: Adults: 3-4 tablets, 3 times a day, taken with warm water after meals.
Children 5-10 Years: Use a half-dose. Children over 10 Years: Use a regular dose.

Bi Yan Pian is produced by the Chung Lien Drug Works, Hangzhou, China, in bottles of 100 coated tablets.

Pinyin Name	Pharmaceutical Name	Percent	TCM Function
Cang Er Zi	Fructus Xanthii	22.5	Open nasal passages; Expel Wind
Xin Yi Hua	Flos Liliflorae Magnoliae	22.5	Open nasal passages, Expel Wind
Gan Cao	Radix Glycyrrhizae Uralensis	6.5	Clear Heat; Harmonize other herbs; Decrease toxic effect of Cang Er Zi
Huang Bai	Cortex Phellodendri	6.5	Clear Heat; Detoxify Fire Poison
Jie Geng	Radix Platycodi Grandiflori	4.15	Expel wind; Soothe nasopharynx; Discharge pus
Wu Wei Zi	Fructus Schisandrae Chinensis	4.15	Nourish Kidney; Collect Lung Qi; Stop cough
Lian Qiao	Fructus Forsythiae Suspensae	6.5	Clear Heat; Detoxify Fire Poison
Bai Zhi	Radix Angelicae	6.5	Expel Wind; Stop headache; Discharge pus; Open nasal passages
Zhi Mu	Radix Anemarrhenae Asphodeloidis	4.15	Clear Heat
Ye Ju Hua	Flos Chrysanthemi Indici	4.15	Clear Heat; Detoxify Fire Poison; Decrease swelling
Fang Feng	Radix Ledebouriellae Sesloidis	4.15	Expel Wind; Stop headache
Jing Jie	Herba seu Flos Schizonepetae Tenuifoliae	4.15	Expel Wind; Open Orifices; Open nasal passages

Notes: 1. This is a very common, very effective formula used to clear stuffy or runny nose associated with common cold or flu accompanied by Heat signs. It has no side effects such as drowsiness or dry mouth which are frequently observed with antihistamines commonly used for stuffy or runny nose.

2. This formula contains many Cold property herbs that have antibiotic effects - e.g. Huang Bai, Lian Qiao, Ye Ju Hua, etc. Therefore, this formula may be better for the patient with a large amount of pus-like nasal discharge which is caused by a bacterial infection.

3. In 1980, this formula was awarded a "High Quality (Silver Medal) Seal" from a National Pharmaceutical Exhibition in China. A copy of this Silver Medal Seal is usually imprinted on the box.

4. The Patent Medicine, Bi Tong Pian, has a similar function to Bi Yan Pian.

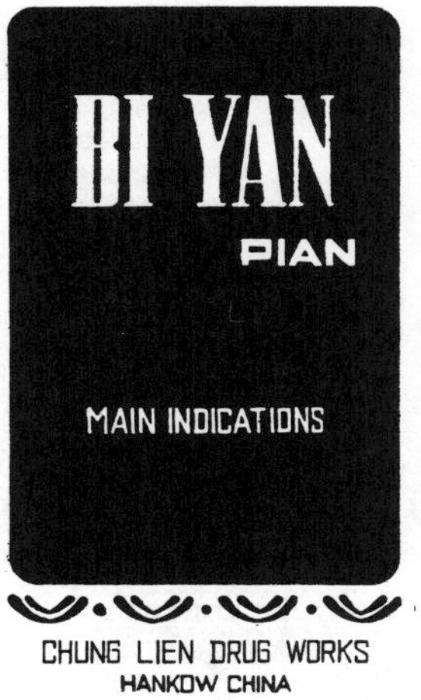

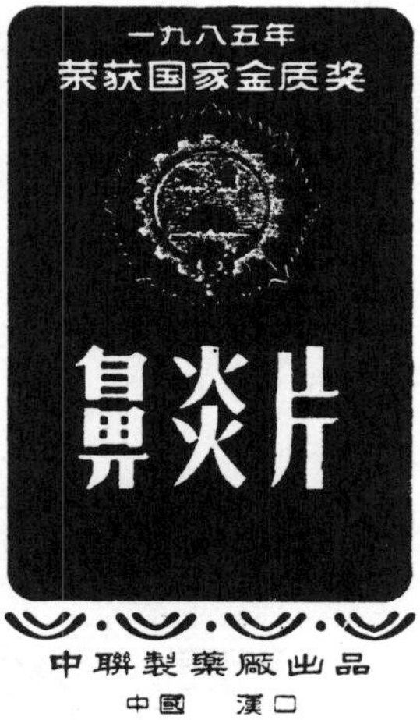

1.11 重 感 靈

Zhong	Gan	Ling
serious	common cold, flu	effective

Function: 1. Expel Wind-Heat
2. Clear Heat, reduce inflammation

Application: 1. Use to treat the flu. Symptoms: High fever, headache, soreness, pain in the limbs, throat pain, cough (all symptoms of Wind-Heat in the Upper Warmer). The patient may have slight chills; if strong chills are present, do not use this formula.

Contraindication: Do not use if the patient is very cold.

Dose: Adults: 4-6 tablets, 3 times a day. Children: 1-3 tablets, 3 times a day.

Zhong Gan Ling is produced by the Meizhou City Pharmaceutical Manufactory, Guangdong, China, in bottles of 48 coated tablets.

Pinyin Name	Pharmaceutical Name	Percent	TCM Function
Qing Hao	Herba Artemisiae Apiaceae	7	Clear Heat
Ban Lan Gen	Radix Isatidis seu Baphicacanthi	14	Clear Heat; Detoxify Fire Poison; Cool Blood Heat; Soothe throat
Mao Dong Qing	Radix Ilicis Pubescentis	27	Clear Heat; Detoxify Fire Poison; Increase blood circulation; Dredge blood vessels; Decrease blood pressure
Shi Gao	Gypsum	4	Clear Heat; Detoxify Fire Poison
Qiang Huo	Rhizoma et Radix Notopterygii	3	Expel Wind-Cold; Stop pain
Ge Gen	Radix Puerariae	27	Expel Wind; Bring fluids up to loosen stiff neck
Mao Bian Cao	Herba Verbenae	18	Clear Heat; Detoxify Fire Poison

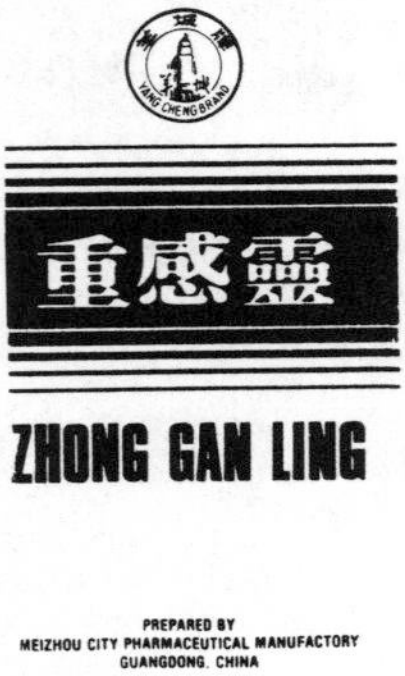

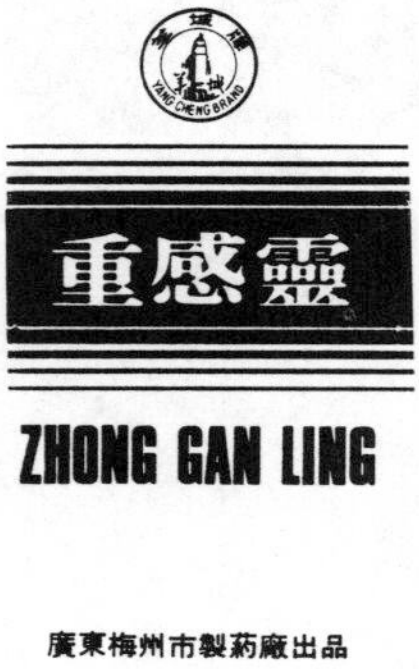

1.12 鼻 敏 感 丸

Bi	Min	Gan	Wan
nose	----------allergy----------		pills

Function:
1. Expel Wind, Eliminate inflammation
2. Stop Headache due to OPI Wind
3. Reduce asthma due to allergy

Application:
1. Use to treat a common cold or flu, especially in cases with nasal symptoms such as runny, stuffy nose. Additional symptoms: Headache and dizziness.

2. Use to treat rhinitis and acute or chronic sinusitis.

3. Some Western medicine disease applications include the following: Allergic rhinitis, chronic rhinitis and nasal sinusitis with symptoms such as stuffy nose, runny nose, sneezing, cough or asthma due to allergy. This is also used to treat acute or chronic bronchitis.

Dose: 2 or 3 pills, 3 times a day. In chronic cases, 30 days contitutes one course of treatment. For milder chronic cases, use for 2 or 3 courses. For severe chronic cases, use for several courses.

Bi Min Gan Wan is produced as "Pe Min Kan Wan" by the Fo Shan United Drug Manufactory in bottles of 50 coated tablets.

The major ingredients are listed below; the percent of each ingredient was not available. Additional ingredients and amounts were also not available

Pinyin Name	Pharmaceutical Name	TCM Function
Cang Er	Xanthium Sibiricum	Clear stuffy nose; Expel Wind; Stop pain
Huo Xiang	Herba Agastaches seu Pogostemi	Expel OPI Wind, Eliminate Dampness
Xiong Dan Zhi	Fel Ursi	Clear Heat; Detoxify Fire Poison
Niu Huang	Calculus Bovis	Clear Heat; Detoxify Fire Poison
Ye Ju Hua	Flos Chrysanthemi Indici	Clear Heat; Detoxify Fire Poison
Bai Zhi	Radix Angelicae	Expel OPI Wind-Cold; Stop headache; Clear stuffy nose
Xin Yi	Flos Magnoliae Liliflorae	Expel Wind-Cold; Clear stuffy nose

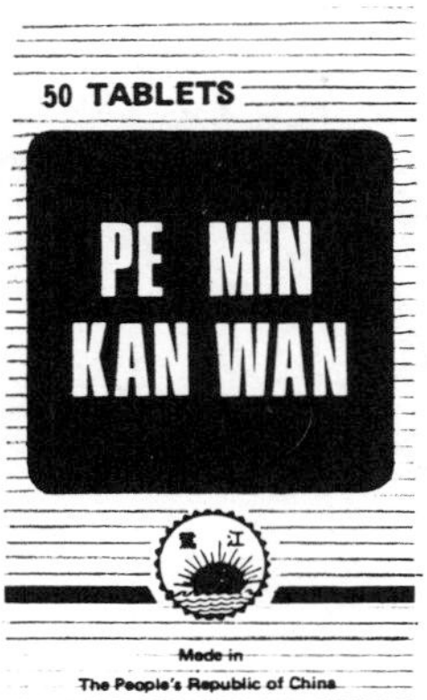

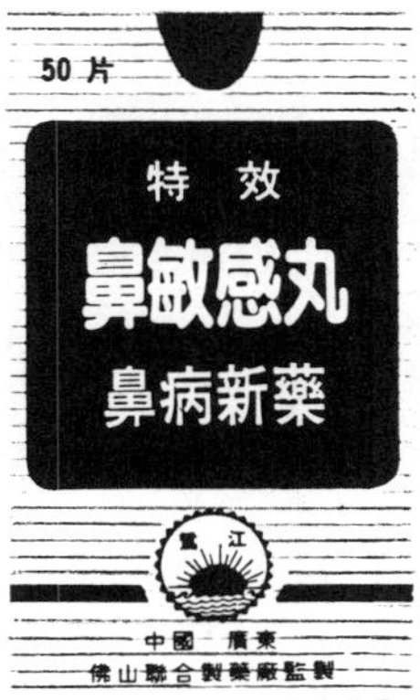

Chapter 2. Expel Summer Heat

2.1 藿 香 正 氣 丸

Huo	**Xiang**	**Zheng**	**Qi**	**Wan**
---------Agastaches---------		regulate	Qi	pills

Source: Tai Ping Hui Min He Ji Ju Fang, (Formulas of The People's Welfare Pharmacy), 1151 A.D., Song Dynasty, 960-1279.

Function:
1. Expel OPI Wind-Cold, Eliminate Dampness
2. Regulate Qi in the Middle Warmer

Application:

1. Use to treat OPI Wind-Cold plus Dampness during any of the four seasons, but primarily in the summertime, when the humidity is high and Dampness is present. Symptoms: Fever, chills, headache, distension in the Middle Warmer, abdominal pain, nausea, vomiting, diarrhea with gurgling and a lot of gas. The Tongue coat is white and greasy.

2. Use to treat gastric disorders caused by the seasonal factor of Dampness, where the Dampness symptoms predominate more than the Wind-Cold symptoms. Symptoms: Diarrhea may be the predominant symptom, although other symptoms may also be present such as fever, vomiting and little or no appetite.

3. Some Western medicine disease applications include acute gastroenteritis.

Contraindication: If the patient has no Dampness, and more signs of Heat such as dry mouth, thirst, yellow Tongue coat and fever without chills, do not use this formula.

Dose: There are two forms of packaging, pills in a bottle and tablets in a vial. For the pills, the dose is 10 pills, 3 times a day. For the tablets, the dose is 4-8 tablets, 3 times a day.

Huo Xiang Zheng Qi Wan is produced as "Lophanthus Antifebrile Pills" by the Lanzhou Chinese Medicine Works, Lanzhou, China, in bottles of 100 pills and vials of 12 tablets.

Pinyin Name	Pharmaceutical Name	Percent	TCM Function
Huo Xiang	Herba Agastaches seu Pogostemi	12	Expel Wind-Cold; Eliminate Dampness; Regulate the Middle Warmer;
Bai Zhi	Radix Angelicae	12	Expel Wind-Cold
Da Fu Pi	Pericarpium Arecae Catechu	12	Move Stuck Qi; Dispel Dampness
Zi Su Ye	Folium Perillae	12	Expel Wind-Cold; Regulate the Middle Warmer
Fu Ling	Sclerotium Poria Cocos	12	Strengthen Spleen/Stomach; Eliminate Dampness
Bai Zhu	Rhizoma Atractylodis Macrocephalae	8	Tonify Spleen; Reduce Dampness
Hou Po	Cortex Magnoliae Officinalis	8	Move Stuck Qi; Reduce Dampness
Jie Geng	Radix Platycodi Grandiflori	6	Open Lung Qi
Chen Pi	Pericarpium Citri Reticulatae	6	Regulate Middle Warmer Qi; Dry Dampness
Gan Cao	Radix Glycyrrhizae Uralensis	12	Harmonize other herbs

Note: 1. Another Patent Medicine, Ping Wei Pian, is similar in function to Huo Xiang Zheng Qi Wan. Ping Wei Pian was originally labelled Ping Wei San (i.e. it was originally in a powder form). There are 4 ingredients in Ping Wei Pian which have a function similar to Huo Xiang Zheng Qi Wan. Both formulas are able to Eliminate Dampness and Strengthen Spleen Qi. Ping Wei Pian, however, has a greater effect to Dry Dampness, Strengthen Spleen Qi, Remove Qi Stagnation and Regulate Stomach Qi. Thus, Ping Wei Pian is especially good to treat symptoms due to Dampness in the humid summer season with symptoms such as abdominal distension, poor appetite, nausea or vomiting, fatigue and feeling of heaviness in the limbs. Huo Xiang Zheng Qi Wan is used to treat these symptoms plus diarrhea.

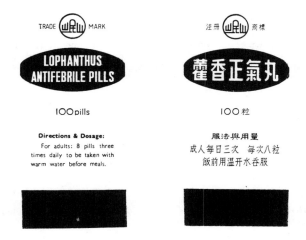

2.2 神 麯 茶

Shen	Qu	Cha
---Massa Fermentata---		tea

Function: 1. Expel Wind-Cold
2. Regulate Stomach/Spleen

Application: 1. Use to treat OPI Wind-Cold during the summertime when the humidity is high. There are three reasons why this medicine is used in the summertime to Expel Wind-Cold: 1. It contains some diaphoretic medicines. 2. It contains some Clear Summer Heat medicines. 3. It contains several medicines which Strengthen the Spleen and Eliminate Dampness due to a Seasonal Factor. Symptoms: Fever and slight chills; the body feels heavy and achy; there is poor appetite, abdominal distension, nausea, vomiting, diarrhea.

2. Use to treat "shui tu bu fu," digestive problems due to poor adjustment to travelling or moving. Symptoms include poor appetite, weight loss, nausea, poor digestion and diarrhea.

3. Use to treat nausea and vomiting due to drunken hangover.

Dose: Adults: Place one block of the dried herbal medicine into 8 oz. of water and cook the water down to 6 oz. Drink the liquid when cooled to a warm temperature; discard the remaining debris. Do this twice a day. If the patient has chills, use 3 grams of freshly chopped ginger root in the water with the herbal medicine block to be cooked down.
Children: Decrease the dose proportionately.

Shen Qu Cha is produced by the United Pharmaceutical Manufactory as blocks of tea; there are 8 blocks per box.

The herbs are listed below in 5 groups according to their function.

Pinyin Name	Pharmaceutical Name	Percent	TCM Function
Group 1			
Qing Hao	Herba Artemisiae Apiaceae	4.7	Clear Heat
Huang Qin	Radix Scutellariae Baicalensis	4.7	
Group 2			
Xiang Ru	Herba Elsholtziae Splendentis	4.7	Expel Wind-Cold; diaphoretic
Qiang Huo	Rhizoma et Radix Notopterygii	4.7	
Du Huo	Radix Duhuo	4.7	
Group 3			
Hou Po	Cortex Magnoliae Officinalis	4.7	Move Stuck Qi; Eliminate Dampness; Disperse Food Mass
Qing Pi	Pericarpium Citri Reticulatae Viride	4.7	
Cao Guo	Fructus Amomi Tsao-ko	4.7	
Mu Gua	Fructus Chaenomelis Lagenariae	4.7	
Group 4			
Jie Geng	Radix Platycodi Grandiflori	4.7	Open Lung Energy; Eliminate Phlegm

<u>Group 5</u>			
Shan Yao	Radix Dioscoreae Oppositae	5.0	Strengthen Spleen; improve appetite; Regulate Stomach function
Fu Ling	Sclerotium Poriae Cocos	5.0	
Gan Cao	Radix Glycyrrhizae Uralensis	5.0	
Chu	Fermented wheat flour	38.0	

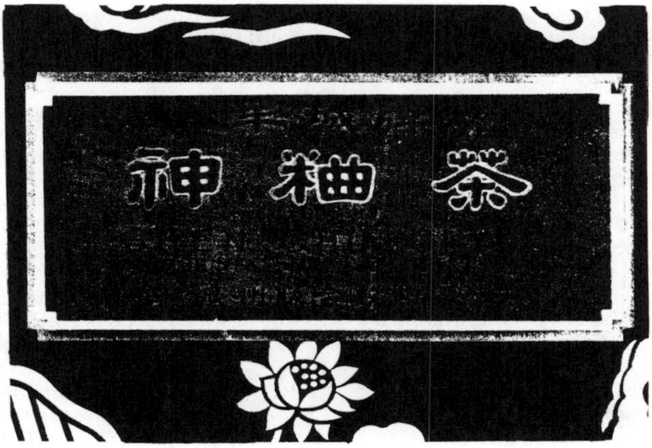

2.3 人 丹

人	丹
Ren	**Dan**
benevolence	pills

Function: 1. Clear Summer Heat; Detoxify Heat Poison and Clear Summer Dampness; (Open Orifices and Wake up the Spirit)
2. Regulate Spleen/Stomach function

Application: 1. Use to treat problems caused by hot, humid weather such as sunstroke.
Symptoms: Dizziness, vomiting, diarrhea, abdominal pain, unconsciousness. This formula is commonly used during the summertime.

2. Use to treat motion sickness (car-sickness, sea-sickness, etc.). Take this a half-hour before boarding to help prevent motion sickness. Can also use it after becoming sick.

3. Use to treat "shui tu bu fu" (poor adjustment to the climate of a new location).
Symptoms: Nausea, dizziness, poor appetite, diarrhea and tiredness, all associated with travel or moving to a new location.

Dose: Adults: 30 to 60 small pills each time. Children: 10 small pills for children age 5.
This is a very mild medicine and adults can take 40 or 50 pills at a time without any side effects. The best way to take the pills is to put 2 or 3 pills in the mouth at a time, let them dissolve, then take some more.

Ren Dan is produced by the United Pharmaceutical Manufactory, Guanzhou, China, with 320 small, silver-colored pills per package.

Pinyin Name	Pharmaceutical Name	Percent	TCM Function
Gan Cao	Radix Glycyrrhizae Uralensis	45	Harmonize other herbs; Treat halitosis
Ding Xiang	Flos Caryophylli	2	Warm the Middle Warmer; Stop pain from stomach ache
Bo He	Herba Menthae	4	Expel Summer Heat; Dispel Dampness
Bing Pian	Borneol	2	Clear Heat; Wake-up the Spirit and Brain; Clear Orifices; Detoxify Heat Poison
Jie Geng	Radix Platycodi Grandiflori	40	Open Lung Qi; Benefit the throat
Er Cha	Acacia seu Uncaria	4	Drain Dampness; Clear Heat; Detoxify Heat Poison
Sha Ren	Fructus seu Semen Amomi	1	Regulate Middle Warmer Qi; Strengthen Spleen; Dry Dampness; Stop Vomiting
Zhang Nao	Camphora	2	Open Orifices; Awaken the Spirit

Notes: 1. This is a very commonly used herbal medicine in China during the summertime. People often carry it with them when going on a trip, visiting the beach, working in a field or hot factory, watching a parade, etc. - i.e. any prolonged activity in the hot sunshine.

2. Different cities and counties produce Ren Dan with slightly different formulas.

3. Another Patent Medicine called "Ji Zhong Shui" is similar to Ren Dan and # 2.4, Liu Shen Shui. Ji Zhong Shui is produced in liquid form. The liquid form is effective faster than the pill form because it is directly absorbed from the stomach. Ji Zhong Shui is used for gastric disorders due to exhaustion or improper eating during the hot summer season or when travelling. The dose is one-half to one bottle, each time. If the symptoms do not subside, a second dose may be taken after four hours.

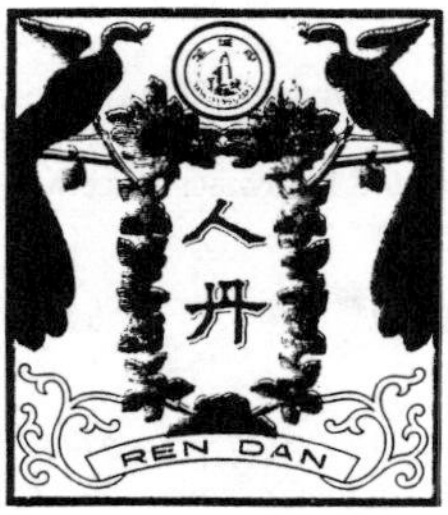

2.4 六 神 水

六	神	水
Liu	**Shen**	**Shui**
six	spirit	water

Source: From experience; produced at the United Pharmaceutical Manufactory, Guangzhou, China.

Function: 1. Expel Summer Heat and Warm the Middle Warmer.

Application: 1. Use in emergency conditions to treat the symptoms of sunstroke caused by Summer Heat, especially during the summertime when high humidity is present. The symptoms of sunstroke include dizziness, vomiting and/or abdominal pain.

2. Use to treat other intestinal disorders during the summertime including diarrhea, abdominal pain, nausea, vomiting.

Contraindication: Do not use with pregnant women.

Dose: Adults: Use one-half of a vial of the liquid diluted in warm water; repeat the dose in 2-3 hours, if necessary. After taking this medicine, additional prepared formulae are also sometimes used, such as #2.1 Huo Xiang Zheng Qi Wan (for slight chills or slight fever, nausea or diarrhea) or #11.4 Xiang Sha Liu Jun Wan (there are no fever or chills, but fatigue and digestive problems are the prominant symptoms with nausea, no appetite, stomach distension, diarrhea).

Children: Decrease the dose proportionately. Do not use with infants.

Liu Shen Shui is produced by the United Pharmaceutical Manufactory, Guangzhou, China in small vials (approximately 2cc per vial); 12 vials per box.

Pinyin Name	Pharmaceutical Name	Percent	TCM Function
Zhang Nao	Camphora	26.32	Open Orifices; Wake-up consciousness
Da Huang	Rhizoma Rhei	21.05	Clear Heat
Sheng Jiang	Rhizoma Zingiberis Officinalis Recens	26.32	Expel Exogenous Evil; Warm the Middle Warmer; Stop Vomiting
Rou Gui	Cortex Cinnamomi Cassiae	10.53	Replace Yang Qi; Warm the Middle Warmer
La Jiao	Chili Pepper	5.26%	Warm the Middle Warmer
Bo He Yu	Herba Menthae oil	25cc per liter	Clear Heat; Expel Wind-Heat; Move Stuck Qi
	Alcohol (70% Solution) to fill to 1 liter		

Note: 1. There is another Patent Medicine, Shi Di Shui, commonly used in Northern China. This has similar contents to Liu Shen Shui, and a similar function and application. Shi Di Shui and Ren Dan are the most popular Patent Medicines to prevent sunstroke. Shi Di Shui and Liu Shen Shui are stronger than Ren Dan, because they are liquid. Shi Di Shui, Liu Shen Shui or Ren Dan are taken as soon as slight discomfort is felt, thus preventing sunstroke. Families commonly carry Shi Di Shui or Ren Dan when going on trips into the countryside. Shi Di Shui or Ren Dan are commonly given to factory workers who work in non-air conditioned factories in the summertime to prevent sunstroke.

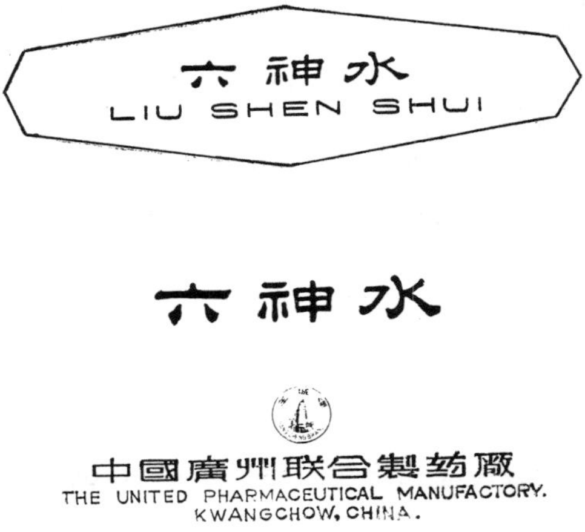

2.5 康 寧 丸

Kang	Ning	Wan
healthy	peaceful	pills

Function: 1. Regulate the Middle Warmer; Improve Digestion
2. Expel Wind-Cold during the Summertime

Application: 1. Use to treat gastric disorders due to Summertime Wind-Cold and Dampness.
Symptoms: Abdominal pain, nausea, vomiting, diarrhea, regurgitation and hyperacidity in the stomach, abdominal distension, poor appetite; some Wind-Cold symptoms may also be present such as low-grade fever, slight chills and headache.

2. Some Western medicine disease applications include the following: (Note, the patient must have the above-mentioned symptoms, in order to use this formula.) Gastroenteritis (bacterial or viral), motion sickness with gastric symptoms (nausea, vomiting, etc.) If the patient has a history of motion sickness, this can be taken 30 minutes to one hour before travelling. This medicine is also effective if used after the motion sickness has developed.

Dose: The pills are available in either a small package or a small vial.
Adults: 1 or 2 packages or vials, 3 times a day.
Children under 3 Years: Use a half-dose (half to one package, 3 times a day).
When using this medicine with children, the pills may be broken up and mixed with water.

Kang Ning Wan is produced as "Pill Curing" by the United Pharmaceutical Manufactory, Guangzhou, China, The pills are available in either a small package or a small vial (10 vials per box).

The ingredients are listed below in 5 separate groups according to function.

Pinyin Name	Pharmaceutical Name	Percent	TCM Function
Group 1			
Tian Ma	Rhizoma Gastrodiae Elatae	3.6	Expel Wind; Stop headache;
Bai Zhi	Radix Angelicae	7.2	Stop body-aches
Group 2			
Ju Hua	Flos Chrysanthemi Morifolii	3.7	Expel Wind-Heat; Reduce fever;
Bo He	Herba Menthae	3.2	Stop headache
Ge Gen	Radix Puerariae	7.2	
Tian Hua Fen	Radix Trichosanthis	5.5	
Group 3			
Cang Zhu	Rhizoma Atractylodis	7.2	Tonify Spleen; Eliminate Dampness
Yi Mi	Semen Coicis Lachryma-jobi	9.0	
Fu Ling	Sclerotium Poriae Cocos	15.5	
Group 4			
Mu Xiang	Radix Saussureae seu Vladimiriae	7.2	Regulate Middle Warmer Qi;
Hou Po	Cortex Magnoliae Officinalis	7.2	Remove Middle Warmer Qi Stagnation;
Ju Hong	Pericarpium Citri Erythrocarpae	3.6	Stop nausea and vomiting; Dry Dampness
Huo Xiang	Herba Agastaches seu Pogostemi	7.2	

<u>Group 5</u>			
Shen Qu	Massa Fermentata	7.2	Strengthen Spleen; Regulate digestion;
Gu Ya	Fructus Oryzae Sativae Germinantus	5.5	Disperse food mass

<u>Notes</u>: 1. This is a popular and commonly used medicine in China, both at home and when travelling. The name, "healthy and peaceful" reflects the idea that after using this medicine, the patient will feel "healthy and peaceful." This is especially useful to have while travelling where the food and water may contribute to gastric disorders.

2. There is a similar Patent Medicine, Bao Ji Wan, (Po Chai Pills) produced in Hong Kong. It has 15 ingredients which are almost the same as the formula listed above, except the Bao Ji Wan formula uses Chi Shi Zhi (Halloysitum Rubrum, 3.5%), instead of Tian Ma. The function of Chi Shi Zhi is to Warm the Middle Warmer and Stop diarrhea. Thus, the Bao Ji Wan formula is used to treat the same applications as the Kang Ning Wan formula, but it is especially useful to treat diarrhea. The Kang Ning Wan formula is especially useful to treat OPI and Stop headache and body-aches (the function of Tian Ma). The dose for Bao Ji Wan is the following: 1 or 2 vials of the pills, 4 times a day. For children under 3 years of age, use half the dose and mash the pills into a powder.

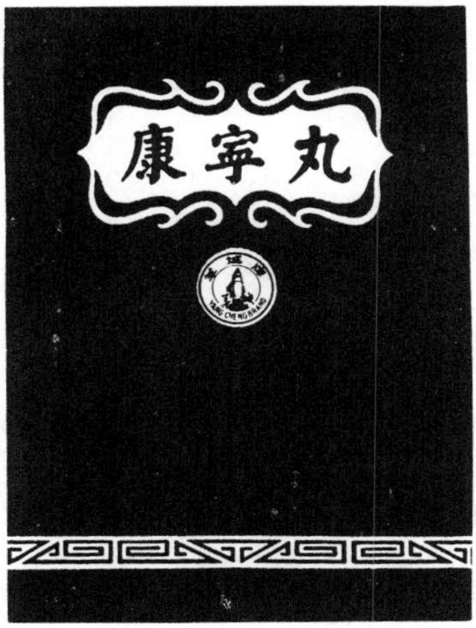

Chapter 3. Stop Cough, Eliminate Phlegm, Treat Asthma

3.1 川 贝 精 片

Chuan Bei Jing Pian

--------Fritillaria-------- extract tablets

Function: 1. Stop cough; Eliminate Phlegm; Moisten Lung

Application: 1. Use to treat acute or chronic cough with abundant expectoration
2. Some Western medicine disease applications include acute or chronic bronchitis and asthma.

Dose: Adults: 3-6 tablets, 3 times a day, taken with warm water.

Chuan Bei Jing Pian is produced as "Fritillaria Extract Sugar- Coated Tablets " by the Handan Pharmaceutical Works in bottles of 60 coated tablets.

Pinyin Name	Pharmaceutical Name	Percent	TCM Function
Chuan Bei	Bulbus Fritillariae Cirrhosae	21	Moisten Lung; Clear Heat; Stop cough; Eliminate phlegm
Yuan Zhi	Radix Polygalae Tenuifoliae	20	Eliminate phlegm
Wu Wei Zi	Fructus Shisandrae Chinensis	17	Stop cough, Stop asthma
Jie Geng	Radix Platycodi Grandiflori	15	Eliminate phlegm
Chen Pi	Pericarpium Citri Reticulatae	15	Eliminate phlegm
Gan Cao	Radix Glycyrrhizae Uralensis	12	Harmonize other herbs. Here, also moisten the Lung; Stop cough

Note: 1. When cough and phlegm are present due to OPI, another diaphoretic medicine should be added such as 1.3, Sang Ju Gan Mao Pian (Wind-Heat) or 1.1, Chuan Xiong Cha Tiao Wan (Wind-Cold).

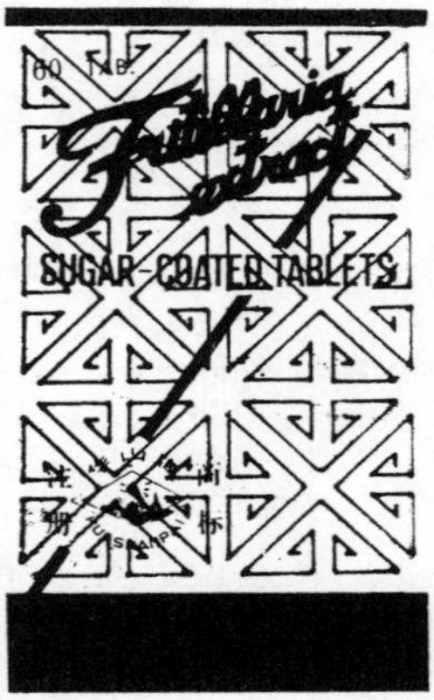

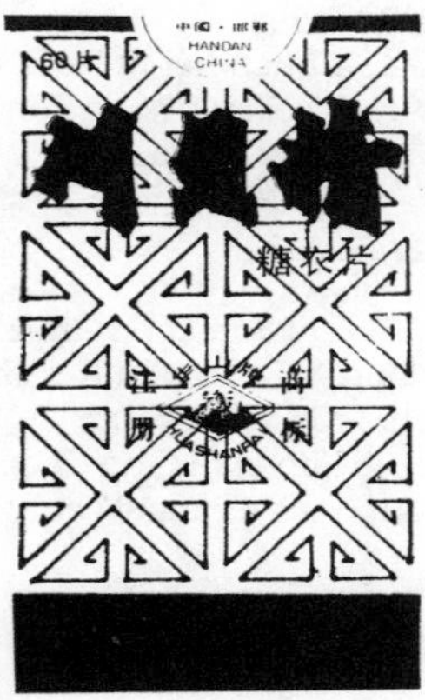

3.2 川 貝 枇 杷 露

川	貝	枇	杷	露
Chuan	**Bei**	**Pi**	**Pa**	**Lu**
---------Fritillaria--------		----------Loquat---------		distilled liquid

Function: 1. Clear Lung Heat; Stop cough; Eliminate Phlegm

Application: 1. Use to treat cough due to Wind-Heat or Exogenous Heat accumulation in the Lung.
Symptoms: Cough with thicker white or yellow sputum; feeling of dryness in the throat with thirst. Sore throat may or may not be present.

Dose: 10 to 15 cc. each time; 3 or 4 times a day. Children less than 12 Years: Use half-dose.
Children less than 5 Years: Use one-third dose.

Chuan Bei Pi Pa Lu is produced as "Fritillary and Loquat Leaf Mixture" by the Peking Chinese Drug Manufactory, Beijing, China, in 150 ml bottles.

Pinyin Name	Pharmaceutical Name	Percent	TCM Function
Chuan Bei Mu	Bulbus Fritillariae Cirrhosae	1	Clear Lung Heat; Moisten Dryness; Stop cough
Pi Pa Ye	Folium Eriobotryae Japonicae	26.2	Clear Lung Heat; EliminatePhlegm; Lower Adverse Rising Qi
Bai Bu	Radix Stemonae	4.7	Clear Lung Heat; Stop cough
Bo He Nao	Extract Herba Menthae	0.04	Expel Wind-Heat

Flavoring (Apricot Seeds) and sugar up to 100%

Note: 1. Another name for this Patent Medicine is Chuan Bei Pi Pa Tang Jiang. (Tang means sugar; Jiang means liquid.)

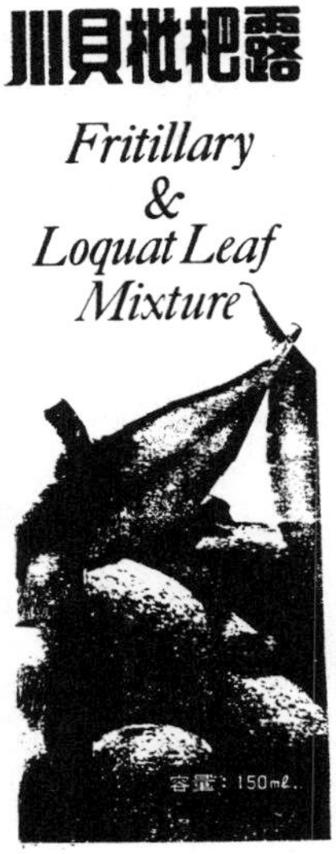

3.3 麻 杏 止 咳 片

麻	杏	止	咳	片
Ma	**Xing**	**Zhi**	**Ke**	**Pian**
Ephedra	apricot	stop	cough	tablets

Source: This formula is a modification of the formula, Ma Xing Shi Gan Tang , which is one of the most popular formulas for cough and asthma from the classical Chinese Medicine text, Shang Han Lun, by Zhang Zhongjing, 219 A.D., Han Dynasty.

Function:
1. Stop cough
2. Calm asthma
3. Clear Lung Heat
4. Eliminate sputum

Application:
1. Use to treat cough caused by Lung Heat due to OPI Heat

2. Use to treat asthma associated with Lung Heat

3. It is primarily used to treat acute bronchitis, but can also be used to treat chronic bronchitis, if the patient presents with Heat signs (yellow sputum). Chronic bronchitis cases have occasional acute bronchitis-like flare-ups where Heat signs are present. This formula will Clear the Heat and reduce the fever.

4. Some Western medicine disease applications include the following: (Note, the cases must present with Heat signs.) Pneumonia, flu, bronchitis.

Contraindication: If the patient has high blood pressure, use this carefully and use only the normal dose. The formula contains Ma Huang, Chinese Ephedra, which can increase blood pressure.

Dose: 4 tablets, 2 or 3 times a day.

Ma Xing Zhi Ke Pian is produced as "Ma Hsing Chih Ke Pien, Hsiang Yang Brand" by the Siping Pharmaceutical Works in bottles of 80 coated tablets.

Pinyin Name	Pharmaceutical Name	Percent	TCM Function
Ma Huang	Herba Ephedrae	5	Stop asthma; Open Lung Energy
Gan Cao	Radix Glycyrrhizae Uralensis	12	Stop cough; Clear Heat; Reduce phlegm
Xing Ren	Semen Pruni Armeniacae	15	Stop cough; Calm asthma
Jie Geng	Radix Platycodi Grandiflori	22	Clear Heat; Reduce phlegm
Chen Pi	Pericarpium Citri Reticulatae	12	Lower Adverse Rising Qi; Reduce phlegm
Shi Gao	Gypsum	12	Clear Heat; Disperse Fire
Hua Shi	Talcum	11	Clear Heat; Discharge Dampness
Feng Mi	Honey	11	Moisten Lung; Stop cough

Note: Case Report A medical student had had a loud, severe cough with some yellow sputum for 4 weeks, as a result of having had the flu. Two courses of antibiotics had been used, but with no effect; probably because the condition was most likely due to a virus. Although pneumonia was suspected, the x-ray showed no fluid accumulation in the lungs. This Patent Medicine, Ma Xing Zhi Ke Pian was combined with #3.5, Jie Geng Wan, and within 8 hours after the first dose, there was a marked reduction in the cough. She continued to use these two Patent Medicines, and the cough disappeared after 4 days.

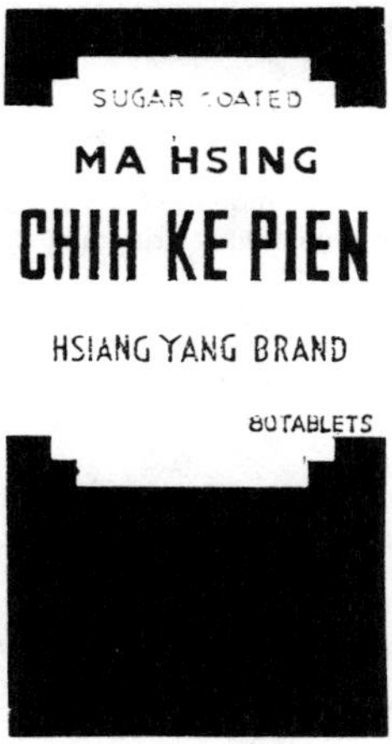

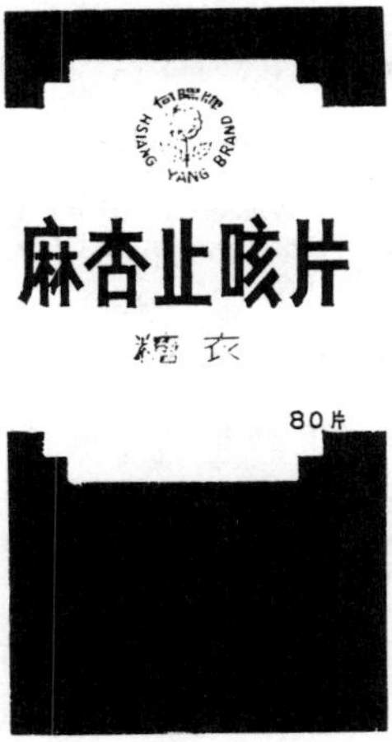

3.4 清 肺 抑 火 片

Qing	**Fei**	**Yi**	**Huo**	**Pian**
clear	Lung	eliminate	fire	pills

Source: Shou Shi Bao Yuan (Longevity and Health), Ming Dynasty, 1368-1644

Function:
1. Clear Lung Heat; Reduce Rising Fire
2. Stop cough
3. Promote increase in body fluids

Application:
1. Use to treat cough with abundant thick yellow sputum due to Lung Heat

2. Use to treat swollen, painful sore throat; mouth or nose sore; toothache or boil

3. Use to treat constipation due to Heat in the Large Intestine (reddish urine may also be present)

4. Use to stop bleeding from the nose or swollen gums due to Excess Heat

5. Some Western medicine disease applications include the following: (Note, Heat signs must be present.) Acute flare-ups in chronic bronchitis; acute tracheitis; pulmonary abscess; pneumonia

Contraindication: Do not use with pregnant women.
Do not use in cases where the cough is due to OPI Wind-Cold or Def. Lung Yin; this formula is only used for cases with Excess Lung Heat

Dose: 4 tablets, 2 times a day, taken with warm water. For more serious cases with high fever, the dose may be doubled. There are no harmful herbs in this formula, thus it may be taken as long as necessary.

Qing Fei Yi Huo is produced as "Ching Fei Yi Huo Pien" by the Tientsin Drug Manufactory in vials of 8 uncoated tablets.

Pinyin Name	Pharmaceutical Name	Percent	TCM Function
Huang Qin	Radix Scutellariae Baicalensis	21	Clear Lung Heat
Zhi Zi	Fructus Gardeniae Jasminoidis	12	Clear Heat
Da Huang	Rhizoma Rhea	18	Clear Heat; Purgative
Qian Hu	Radix Peucedani	7	Stop cough
Ku Shen	Radix Sophorae Flavescentis	9	Clear Damp Heat
Tian Hua Fen	Radix Trichosanthis	12	Clear Heat for sore throat
Jie Geng	Radix Platycodi Grandiflori	12	Clear Heat for sore throat
Zhi Mu	Radix Anemarrhenae Asphodeloidis	9	Moisten Lung

Note: 1. The Patent Medicine, Niu Huang Jie Du Pian, #7.8, is frequently used to Clear Heat with OPI syndromes. It is used to treat whole body Heat as well as mouth or nose sores, constipation and Lung Heat. Niu Huang Jie Du Pian cannot, however, stop cough or eliminate sputum.

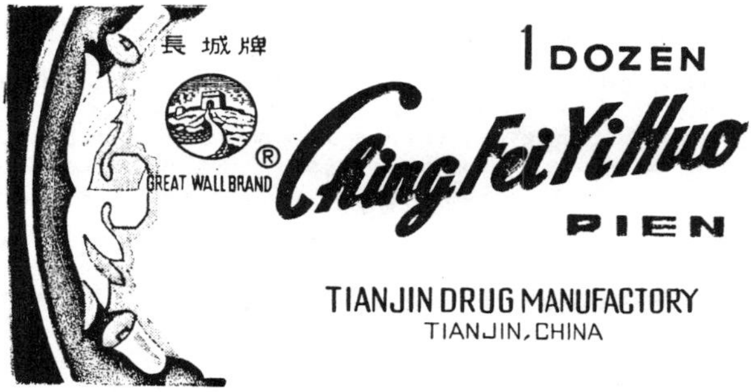
長城牌
1 DOZEN
GREAT WALL BRAND
Ching Fei Yi Huo
PIEN
TIANJIN DRUG MANUFACTORY
TIANJIN, CHINA

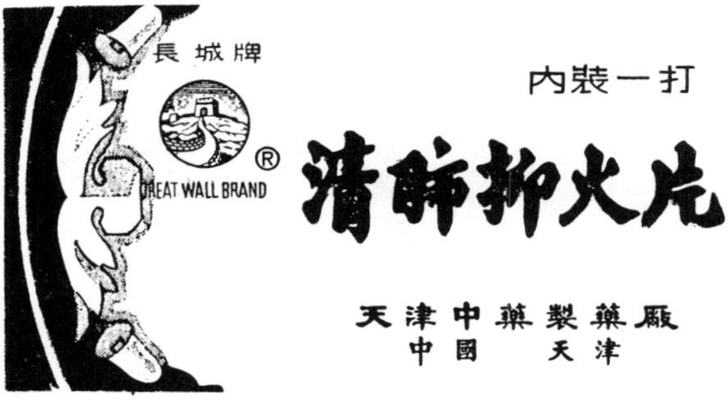
長城牌
内裝一打
GREAT WALL BRAND
清肺抑火片
天津中藥製藥廠
中國 天津

3.5 桔 梗 丸

Jie	**Geng**	**Wan**
--------Platycodon---------		pills

Source: Jin Gui Yao Lue, (Synopsis of the Golden Chamber) Zhang Zhongjing, 219 A.D., Han Dynasty.

Function: 1. Open Lung Energy; Decrease phlegm; Discharge pus from pulmonary abscess

Application: 1. Use to open Lung Energy, expectorate sputum, stop cough. May be used with either Wind-Heat OPI or Wind-Cold OPI. The primary ingredient, Jie Geng, eliminates sputum and discharges pus form the Lung.

2. Use to treat pumonary abscess with yellow, foul-smelling sputum.

3. Use to treat chronic bronchitis with yellow sputum.

4. Use to treat sore throat or tonsillitis

Dose: 5 to 10 pills, 3 times a day taken with warm water

Jie Geng Wan is produced as "Jie Geng Wan (Platycodon Pills)" by the Lanzhou Chinese Medicine Works, Lanzhou, China, in bottles of 100 pills.

Pinyin Name	Pharmaceutical Name	Percent	TCM Function
Jie Geng	Radix Platycodi Grandiflori	90	Open Lung Energy; Decrease phlegm; Discharge pus from pulmonary abscess
Gan Cao	Radix Glycyrrhizae Uralensis	10	Stop cough

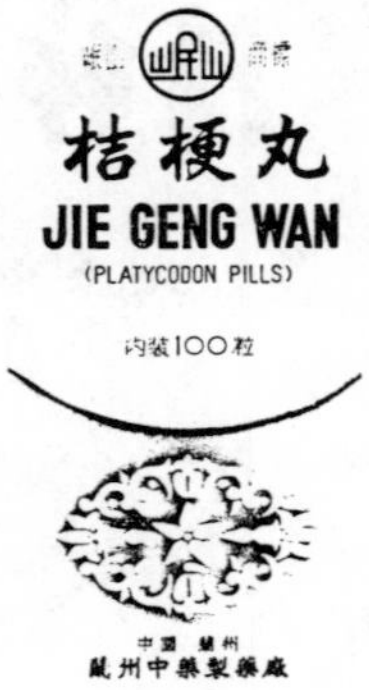

3.6 清 氣 化 痰 丸

清	氣	化	痰	丸
Qing	**Qi**	**Hua**	**Tan**	**Wan**
clear	Lung Energy	eliminate	sputum	pills

Source: Jing Yue's Complete Works, Zhang Jingyue, 1624, A.D.

Function:
1. Clear Lung Heat
2. Stop cough
3. Eliminate sputum
4. Calm asthma

Application: 1. Use to treat cough that is strong and loud associated with Phlegm Heat. Additional symptoms include sputum that is thick and sticky; the patient has a feeling of fullness in the chest; the coughing is so severe that it can even cause vomiting. The Tongue is reddish with a yellow fur. The Pulse is slippery (compatible with sputum and mucous) and rapid (compatible with Heat).

2. Some Western medicine disease applications include pneumonia or chronic bronchitis where there are signs of Heat in the Lung.

Contraindication: Do not use in cases where the cough is due to OPI Wind-Cold and the patient has chills. Do not use in cases where the cough is due to Def. Lung Yin and the patient has a dry cough with no phlegm.

Dose: 6 pills, 3 times a day, taken with warm water.

Qing Qi Hua Tan Wan is produced as "Pinellia Expectorant Pills" by the Lanzhou Fo Ci Pharmaceutical Factory, Lanzhou, China, in bottles of 200.

Pinyin Name	Pharmaceutical Name	Percent	TCM Function
Ban Xia	Rhizoma Pinelliae Ternatae (processed with ginger)	16.7	Reduce phlegm
Tian Nan Xing	Rhizoma Arisaematis (processed with bile)	16.7	Clear Lung Heat; Reduce phlegm
Zhi Shi	Fructus Citri seu Ponciri Immaturus	11.1	Lower Adverse Rising Qi
Huang Qin	Radix Scutellariae Baicalensis	11.1	Clear Lung Heat
Ju Hong	Pericarpium Citri Erythrocarpae	11.1	Reduce phlegm; Lower Adverse Rising Qi
Gua Lou	Fructus Trichosanthis	11.1	Clear Lung Heat; Reduce phlegm
Xing Ren	Semen Pruni Armeniacae	11.1	Stop cough; Calm the asthma
Fu Ling	Sclerotium Poriae Cocos	11.1	Strengthen Spleen to remove the source of Dampness; Eliminate phlegm

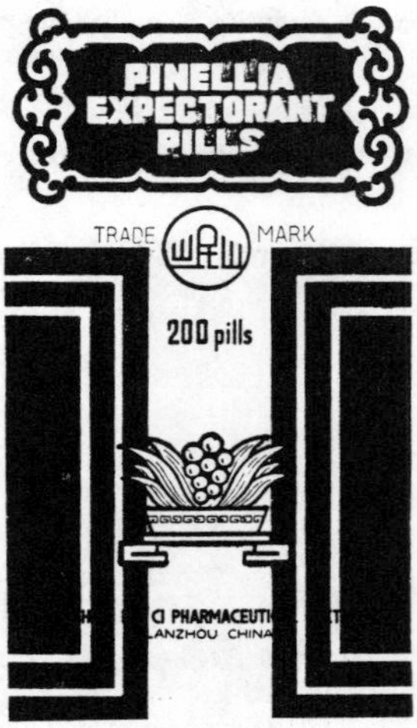
PINELLIA EXPECTORANT PILLS
TRADE MARK
200 pills
CHINA

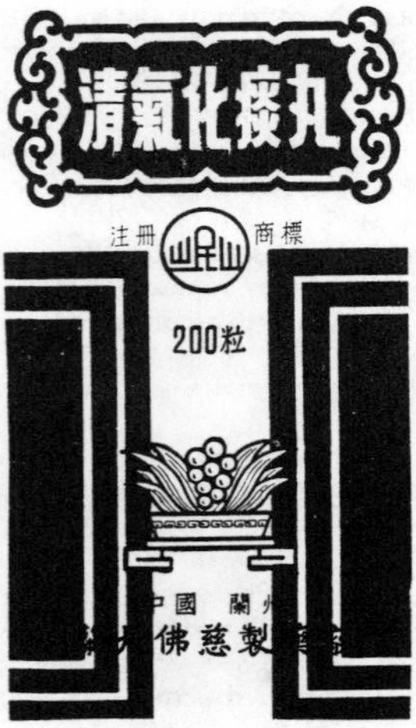
清氣化痰丸
注冊 商標
200粒
佛慈製

3.7 喘 咳 靈

Chuan	**Ke**	**Ling**
asthma	cough	effective

Function: 1. Clear Lung Heat and Regulate Lung Qi

Application: 1. Use to treat bronchitis with excess sputum

2. Use to treat cough due to common cold or flu.

3. Use to treat pulmonary abscess

Contraindication: Do not use in a case where the cough is due to Def. Lung Yin (dry cough with no phlegm). Use only in a case where the patient has a lot of Lung Heat.

Dose: 4 tablets, 3 times a day, taken with warm water.

Chuan Ke Ling is produced by the Fu Sung Pharmaceutical Works, Kirin, China, in bottles of 100 tablets.

Pinyin Name	Pharmaceutical Name	Percent	TCM Function
Jie Geng	Radix Platycodi Grandiflori	35	Open Lung Qi; Eliminate phlegm; Discharge pus
Xing Ren	Semen Pruni Armeniacae	25	Stop cough; Calm asthma
Gan Cao	Radix Glycyrrhizae Uralensis	30	Stop cough; Clear Lung Heat
Niu Dan	Fel Bovus	10	Clear Heat

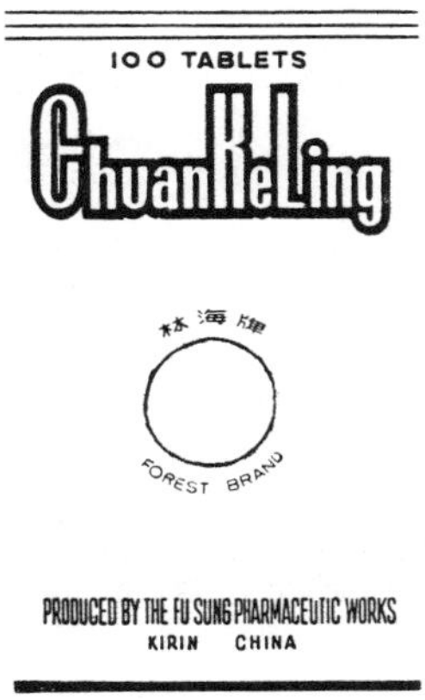

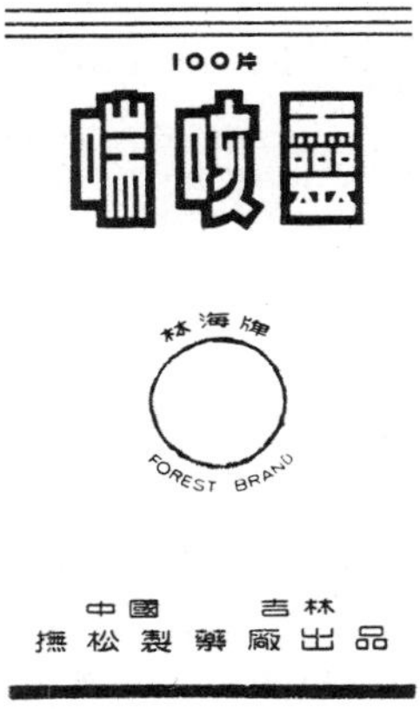

3.8 蛇 膽 陳 皮 散

She	Dan	Chen	Pi	San
snake	gall bladder	------tangerine peel-----		powder

Function: 1. Dispel External Wind and Eliminate phlegm in cases with cough and asthma
2. Tranquilize Heart Disharmonies which have led to mania, uneasiness, hysteria or epilepsy

Application: 1. Use to treat Wind-Heat OPI which has affected the Lung. Symptoms: High grade fever, cough with expectoration, sputum, asthma, problems breathing, chest fullness; chronic cough with stubborn phlegm (white or yellow); and chronic tracheitis with cough, sputum, asthma.

2. Some Western medicine disease applications include the following: Acute pneumonia, acute bronchitis, and whooping cough.

3. Use to treat Heart Disharmonies which have led to mania, uneasiness, hysteria (in Excess condition, only) or to epilepsy including grand mal or petit mal seizures; even very small ones (in Excess condition, only). This herbal medicine may be taken with other seizure medications such as phenobarbitol or dilantin.

Contraindication: Do not use this formula with patients who have a Def. syndrome; use only with patients who have an Excess syndrome.

Dose: This formula is in the form of powder in a small vial; each vial contains 0.6 grams of powder.
Adults: 0.6 grams, 2 times a day (Swallow powder with warm water)
Children: 0.3 grams, 2 times a day (Swallow powder with warm water)

She Dan Chen Pi Mo is produced by the United Pharmaceutical Manufactory, Guangzhou, China in vials containing 0.6 grams of the powder.

Pinyin Name	Pharmaceutical Name	Percent	TCM Function
She Dan	Agkistrodon Acutus	0.13	Clear Heat
Chen Pi	Pericarpium Citri Reticulatae	61.65	Reduce phlegm
Di Long Tan	Lumbricus (Carbonized)	12.33	Stop spasm when combined with
Jiang Can	Bombyx Batryticatus	12.33	Jiang Can
Zhu Sha	Cinnabaris	12.33	Tranquilize and Calm the Spirit
Hu Po	Succinum	1.23	Tranquilize and Calm the Spirit

Notes: 1. The name, "She Dan Chen Pi Mo" is used for more than one Patent Medicine. The formula listed here is the standard formula with 6 ingredients. Other formulas, such as "San She Dan Chen Pi Mo" (United Pharmaceutical Manufactory, Canton) have only 2 ingredients (She Dan and Chen Pi). The function of these 2 ingredients is to Eliminate phlegm and Lower Adverse Rising Lung Qi (Stop asthma). These 2 ingredients also have the function to Expel Wind and Strengthen Stomach (reduce nausea). San She Dan Chen Pi Mo is therefore used to treat both chronic cough with phlegm, and nausea and regurgitation.

2. Another Patent Medicine, "She Dan Chuan Bei San" has only 2 ingredients (She Dan and Chuan Bei Mu). The function of this formula is to Clear Heat, Stop cough and Reduce phlegm. The application of this formula is to treat cough and phlegm caused by Phlegm Heat as seen in cases with the flu, acute bronchitis or acute tracheitis.

3. "San She Dan Chuan Bei Gao" is a syrup similar to She Dan Chen Pi Mo. "San She Dan Chuan Bei Ye" is a liquid similar to She Dan Chen Pi Mo. These Patent Medicines are effective to stop cough, eliminate phlegm, and stop asthma. She Dan Chen Pi Mo has herbs to treat the Lungs as well as herbs to calm the Spirit and stop spasms. San She Dan Chuan Bei Gao and San She Dan Chuan Bei Ye have herbs only to affect the Lungs.

4. The results from a clinical study conducted with She Dan Chen Pi Mo in the treatment of whooping cough in children are presented below. Source: <u>Jiang Su Zhong Yi</u> (<u>Journal of Traditional Chinese Medicine</u>), 1965, Vol. 12, p. 39. A total of 59 children with whooping cough were treated with She Dan Chen Pi Mo. The amounts listed below were divided into 3 doses per day:

Children under 1 year used a total of 1 vial per day.

Children age 1 to 5 years used a total of 1 and 1/2 vials per day.

Children age 6 to 10 years used a total of 2 vials per day.

Children age 11 to 15 years used a total of 3 vials per day.

The most common treatment period lasted from 7 to 10 days. The shortest treatment period lasted 4 days; the longest treatment period, 16 days. In 42/59 cases there was complete recovery; in 14 cases there was obvious improvement and in 3 cases there was no change.

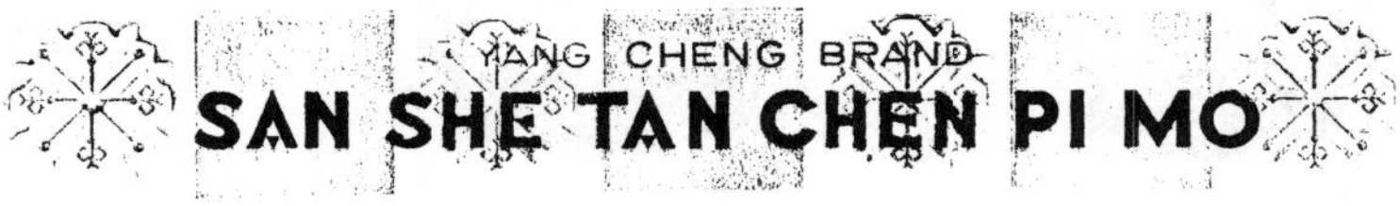

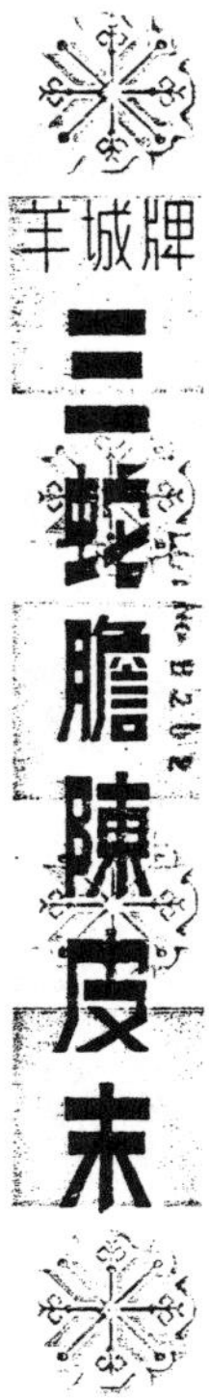

3.9 海 藻 精

Hai **Zao** **Jing**

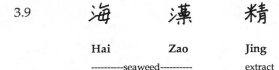

----------seaweed---------- extract

Function: 1. Reduce and help to remove nodes.

Application: 1. Use to treat simple goiter (due to inadequate dietary intake of iodine).

2. Use to treat chronic lymphadenitis in the neck (must be chronic); this includes scrofula (tuberculosis in the neck)

3. Use to prevent and treat hypertension and atherosclerosis

4. Use as an anticoagulant to help prevent and treat blood clots.

Dose: 2 pills, 3 times a day.

Hai Zao Jing is produced as "Haiodin" by the Lanzhou Fo Ci Pharmaceutical Factory, Lanzhou, China, in bottles of 50 pills.

Pinyin Name	Pharmaceutical Name	Percent	TCM Function
Hai Zao	Herba Sargassii	60	Remove Nodular Phlegm Accumulation
Kun Bu	Thallus Algae	40	Remove Nodular Phlegm Accumulation

Note: 1. Both of the above-listed contents contain high amounts of iodine.

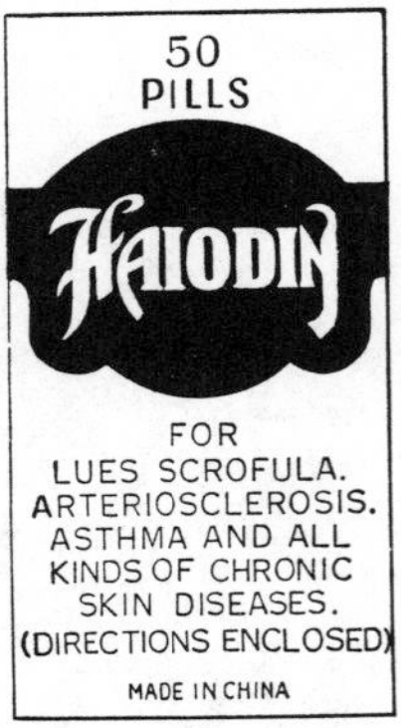

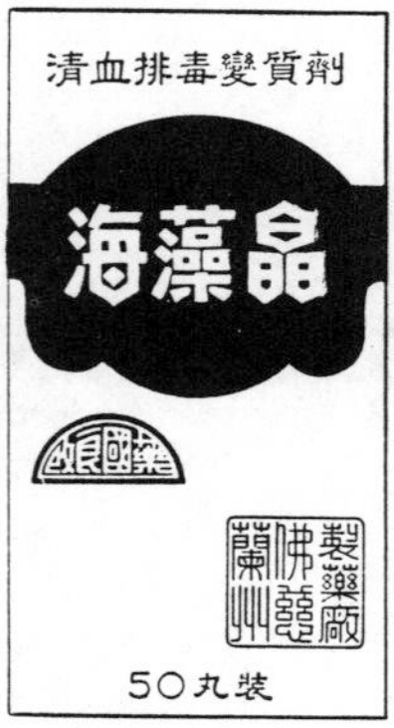

3.10 二 陳 丸

Er	**Chen**	**Wan**
two	older-medicine	pills

Source: Tai Ping Hui Min He Ji Ju Fang, (Formulas of The People's Welfare Pharmacy), 1151 A.D., Song Dynasty, 960-1279.

Function: 1. Dry Dampness; Decrease phlegm caused by Dampness
2. Regulate Qi in the Middle Warmer

Application: 1. Use to treat cough with excess phlegm where there is a sensation of chest fullness with nausea and possible vomiting. There is abundant white expectoration where the sputum is thin (not thick). The Tongue has a thick, white and greasy coat. The Pulse is slippery.

2. Use to treat abdominal distension with digestive problems and possible vomiting. This may be due to OPI in the fall associated with Autumn Dampness.

3. Use to treat dizziness or palpitations caused by Dampness retention.

4. Some Western medicine disease applications include the following: Chronic bronchitis with excess sputum and gastric problems (poor appetite or excess stomach acid); gastroenteritis with cough or phlegm.

Dose: Small Pills: 7 or 8 pills, 3 times a day, taken with warm water.

Honey Pills: 2 pills, 2 times a day, taken with warm water.

Er Chen Wan is produced as "Er Chen Wan (Pinellia-Pachyma Compound Pills)" by the Lanzhou Chinese Medicine Works, Lanzhou, China, in bottles of 200. The honey pill form is not readily available in the U.S.

Pinyin Name	Pharmaceutical Name	Percent	TCM Function
Ban Xia	Rhizoma Pinelliae Ternatae (processed with ginger)	44.45	Dry Dampness; Reduce phlegm; Stop vomiting; Lower the Stomach Qi
Chen Pi	Pericarpium Citri Reticulatae	11.11	Regulate the Middle Warmer Qi; Dry Dampness
Fu Ling	Sclerotium Poriae Cocos	22.22	Strengthen Spleen; Rid Dampness through urination
Gan Cao	Radix Glycyrrhizae	22.22	Harmonize other herbs

Note: 1. The name "two older medicines" refers to the Ban Xia and the Chen Pi. The older these two herbs are, the more effective the formula will be.

TRADE MARK

二陳丸

ERH CHEN WAN

(Pinellia-Pachyma Compound Pills)

200 pills

LANCHOW CHINESE MEDICINE WORKS
LANCHOW CHINA

岷山 商標

二陳丸

ERH CHEN WAN

(Pinellia-Pachyma Compound Pills)

200粒

中國 蘭州
蘭州中藥製藥廠

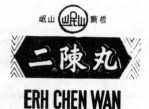

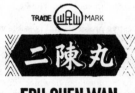

3.11 苏 籽 降 氣 丸

Su	**Zi**	**Jiang**	**Qi**	**Wan**
-------Perilla seed-------		lower	Qi	pills

Source: Tai Ping Hui Min He Ji Ju Fang, (Formulas of The People's Welfare Pharmacy), 1151 A.D., Song Dynasty, 960-1279.

Function:
1. Eliminate Phlegm
2. Lower Adverse Rising Qi

Application:
1. Use to treat Cold Phlegm Accumulation in the Lung, which has caused asthma, shortness of breath, and cough. The phlegm is white and foamy.

2. Use to treat Def. Kidney Yang which has failed to support the Lung Qi, resulting in asthma, shortness of breath and cough. The phlegm is white and foamy.

3. Some Western medicine disease applications include the following: (Note, the patient must have the symptoms listed above.) Chronic bronchitis and emphysema.

Contraindications: Do not use with patients who have Lung Heat, with yellow phlegm, and fever. This formula contains many ingredients that have Dry, Warm Properties.

Dose: 3 grams, 3 times aday, taken on an empty stomach.

Su Zi Jiang Qi Wan is available in small bags, each bag contains 18 grams; 10 bags per box.

The contents are listed below in 5 groups, according to function.

Pinyin Name	Pharmaceutical Name	Percent	TCM Function
Group 1			
Su Zi	Fructus Perillae Frutescentis	10.6	Lower Adverse Rising Qi;
Ban Xia	Rhizoma Pinelliae Ternatae	10.6	Eliminate phlegm; Stop asthma
Hou Po	Cortex Magnoliae Officinalis	10.6	
Qian Hu	Radix Peucedani	10.6	
Chen Pi	Pericarpium Citri Reticulatae	10.6	
Group 2			
Chen Xiang	Lignum Aquilariae	7.6	Warm the Kidney Yang; Stop asthma
Group 3			
Dang Gui	Radix Angelicae Sinensis	7.6	Nourish Blood; Reduce Dryness
Group 4			
Sheng Jiang	Rhizoma Zingiberis Officinalis Recens	10.6	Warm the Middle Warmer;
Da Zao	Fructus Zizyphi Jujubae	10.6	Regulate Stomach Qi
Group 5			
Gan Cao	Radix Glycyrrhizae Uralensis	10.6	Moisten Lung; Stop cough; Eliminate phlegm; Harmonize other herbs

3.12 养阴清肺糖浆

养	阴	清	肺	糖	浆
Yang	**Yin**	**Qing**	**Fei**	**Tang**	**Jiang**
nourish	Yin	clear	Lung	sweet	syrup

Source: Chong Lou Yu Yao (Key to Enter the Magic Building), Cheng Nei-jin, 1836.

Function:
1. Clear Def. Yin type of Lung Heat; Nourish the Lung
2. Stop chronic cough or cough at end-stage of OPI; Eliminate phelgm
3. Soothe throat

Application:
1. Use to treat dry cough or cough with little phlegm and possibly some blood. This formula will nourish Def. Lung Yin.
2. Use to treat dryness, thirst and pain in the throat
3. Use to treat hoarseness due to Def. Lung Yin or following an OPI
4. Some Western medicine disease applications include the following: (Note, the patient must have the above-mentioned Def. Lung Yin signs.) Tonsillitis, pharyngitis, chronic dry cough (as seen with tuberculosis or lung cancer patients), diphtheria.

Dose: Adults: 20 cc, 2 times a day or 4 tsp., 2 times a day. Children: Use half-dose.

Yang Yin Qing Fei Tang Jiang is produced as "Yangyin Chingfei Tang Chiang" by the Tientsin Drug Manufactory, Tientsin, China, in 120 cc bottles.

Pinyin Name	Pharmaceutical Name	Percent	TCM Function
Mu Dan Pi	Cortex Moutan Radicis	10.52	Clear Blood Heat; Reduce Infection
Zhe Bei Mu	Bulbus Fritillariae Thunbergii	10.52	Clear Heat; Moisten Lung; Stop cough; Eliminate phelgm
Bai Shao	Radix Paeoniae Lactiflorae	10.52	Nourish Yin; Moisten body fluid
Yuan Shen	Radix Scrophulariae Ningpoensis	21.04	Nourish Yin; Moisten body fluid; Decrease inflammation
Sheng Di Huang	Radix Rehmanniae Glutinosae (Uncooked)	26.31	Nourish Yin; Clear Heat; Decrease inflammation
Mai Men Dong	Tuber Ophiopogonis Japonici	15.78	Nourish Yin; Clear Lung Heat; Moisten Lung
Gan Cao	Radix Glycyrrhizae Uralensis	5.27	Harmonize other herbs; Clear Heat; Moisten Lung
Bo He	Herba Menthae	0.04	Open Lung Qi; Soothe throat

長城牌

GREATWALL BRAND

YANGYIN
CHINGFEI

TANG CHIANG

TIENTSIN DRUG MANUFACTORY
TIENTSIN, CHINA

長城牌

GREATWALL BRAND

养阴清肺

糖浆

中国 天津
天津中药制药厂

3.13 利 肺

Li **Fei**

benefit Lung

Function: 1. Benefit Lung; Calm asthma due to Def. Lung Yin
2. Stop chronic cough due to Def. Lung Yin

Application: 1. Use to treat Def. Lung Yin chronic cough without mucous (Internal Heat has dried out the mucous).

2. Use to treat asthma due to weak Def. Lung Qi. (Do not use with asthma due to Heat and Dampness where there is Lung Heat and the patient has problems breathing.)

3. Use to treat coughing with blood in cases with Def. Lung Yin (night sweats may also be present).

4. Some Western medicine disease applications include the following: (Note, the patient must have the above-mentioned Def. Lung Yin signs.) Chronic dry cough (as seen with tuberculosis or lung cancer patients).

Dose: Adults: 4-6 tablets, 3 times a day, taken with warm water within a half-hour after meals.

Li Fei is produced as "Sugar-coated Pulmonary Tonic Tablets" by the Hebei Branch of the China National Native Produce & Animal Import & Export Corp. in bottles of 60 coated tablets.

Pinyin Name	Pharmaceutical Name	Percent	TCM Function
Dong Chong Xia Cao	Cordyceps Sinensis	5	Strengthen Lung Qi; Stop cough
Ge Jie	Gecko	5	Strengthen Lung
Bai He	Bulbus Lilii	8	Strengthen Lung Yin; Clear Lung Heat; Moisten Lung; Stop cough
Wu Wei Zi	Fructus Schisandrae Chinensis	13	Stop cough; Moisten Lung
Bai Ji	Rhizoma Aletillae Striatae	27	Stop bleeding
Bai Bu	Radix Stemonae	15	Stop cough; Clear Lung Heat
Mu Li	Concha Ostreae	11	Strengthen Yin; Eliminate Yang; Stop sweat
Pi Pa Ye	Folium Eriobotryae Japonicae	10	Clear Lung Heat; Stop cough; Eliminate phlegm
Gan Cao	Radix Glycyrrhizae Uralensis	6	Stop cough; Clear Heat

Note: 1. There are nine herbs to Nourish and Tonify the Lung in this formula. In TCM when treating Lung disorders, two major types of herbs are used: 1) herbs to Clear Lung Heat or 2) herbs to Nourish and Tonify the Lung. When Clearing Lung Heat, the formula such as that in #3.4, Qing Fei Yi Huo Pian, is used; a formula which will treat cough, sputum or asthma due to Lung Heat. When Tonifying the Lung, the formula listed here with #3.13, Li Fei, is commonly used; a formula which will treat cough, sputum or asthma due to Def. Lung Yin.

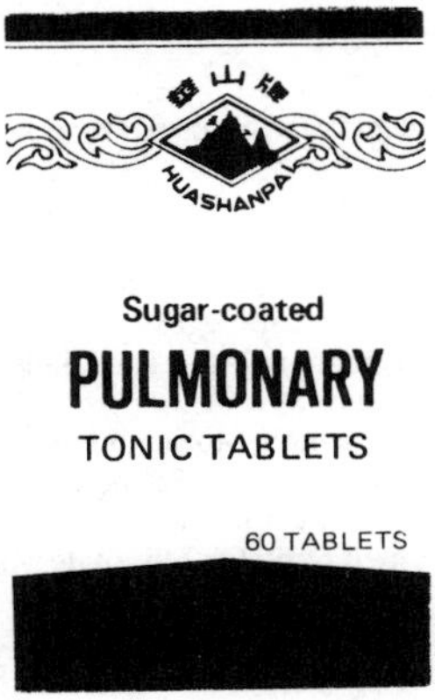

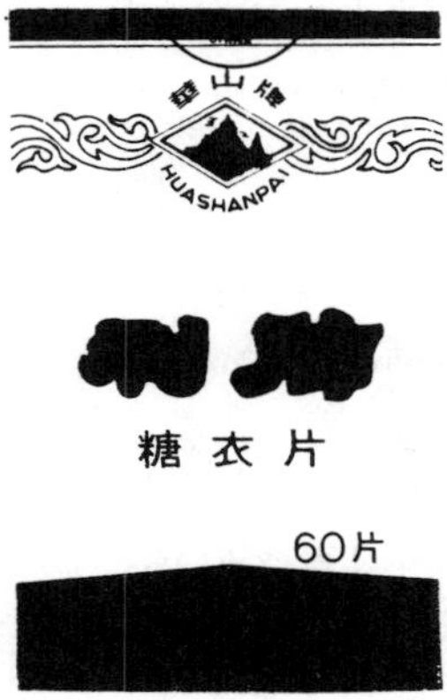

3.14 川 貝 枇 杷 膏

Chuan	Bei	Pi	Pa	Gao
---------Fritillaria---------		----------Loquat----------		syrup

Source: Wen Re Lun (Treatise on Seasonal Febrile Diseases), Ye Gui, 1746, A.D.

Function:
1. Moisten Lung
2. Clear Lung Heat, Stop cough
3. Calm asthma (Lower Adverse Rising Lung Qi)

Application: 1. Use to Nourish Lung Yin in cases where there is a dry cough, but no phlegm or only a little phlegm. The Def. Yin has lead to Internal Heat and a low-grade fever may be present as well as mouth and throat dryness. This condition is often seen with a smoker's cough. Smoking makes it easy for bacteria to grow in the Lung, thus, the Lung does not have good protection. This formula can be used over a long period of time, e.g. with smokers.

2. Use to treat acute or chronic cough caused by Lung Heat; difficult expectoration of sputum and throat pain may be present.

Dose: Adults: 10 cc (1 Tablespoon), 3 times a day. Can be diluted in water or tea, etc.
Children: Half-dose, 3 times a day.

Chuan Bei Pi Pa Gao is produced as "Natural Herb Loquat Flavored Syrup" by the Nin Jiom Manufactory, Hong Kong , in 10 fluid ounce bottles. The percent of each ingredient is not available.

Pinyin Name	Pharmaceutical Name	TCM Function
Pi Pa Ye	Folium Eriobotryae Japonicae	Stop cough; Eliminate phlegm
Bei Mu	Bulbus Fritillariae	Clear Lung Heat; Moisten Lung; Stop cough; Eliminate phlegm
Sha Shen	Radix Glehniae Littoralis	Strengthen Yin; Clear Lung Heat; Moisten Lung; Stop cough
Wu Wei Zi	Fructus Schisandrae Chinensis	Stop cough; Moisten Lung
Chen Pi	Pericarpium Citri Reticulatae	Lower Adverse Rising Lung Qi; Eliminate phlegm
Jie Geng	Radix Platycodi Grandiflori	Open Lung Qi; Eliminate phlegm
Ban Xia	Rhizoma Pinelliae Ternatae	Eliminate phlegm
Bo He	Herba Menthae	Expel Wind-Heat; Clear Lung Heat
Kuan Dong Hua	Flos Tussilagi Farfarae	Stop cough; Lower Adverse Rising Lung Qi
Xing Ren	Semen Pruni Armeniacae	Moisten Lung; Stop cough
Feng Mi	Honey	Moisten Lung; Stop cough

Note: 1. Chuan Bei Pi Pa Gao is a very popular and commonly used cough medicine; it has a pleasant taste when diluted.

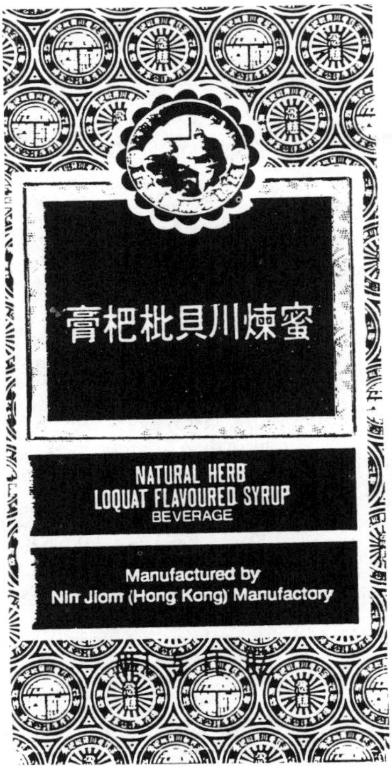

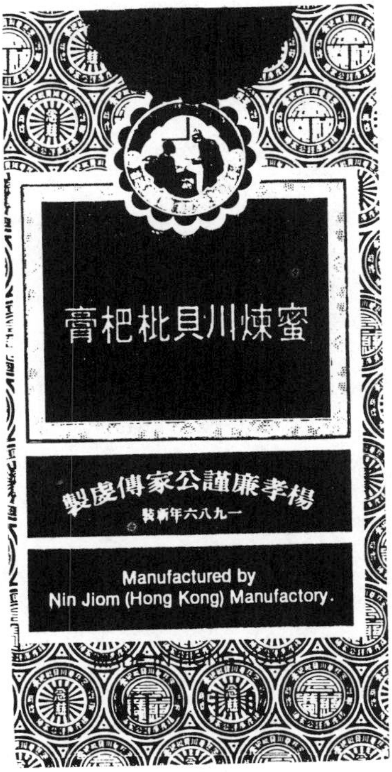

3.15 八仙長壽丸

八	仙	長	壽	丸
Ba	**Xian**	**Chang**	**Shou**	**Wan**
eight	immortals	long	life	pills

Function: 1. Treat Def. Lung Yin or Def. Kidney Yin
2. Collect Lung Yin and Strengthen Kidney Qi with astringents

Application: 1. Use to treat chronic cough due to Def. Kidney Yin. Symptoms: Dry cough, lumbago, dizziness, vertigo, tinnitus, deafness, night sweats, thirst, Heat in the 5 Centers; spermatorrhea. The Tongue is reddish with no moss or only a little moss. The Pulse is thin and rapid.

Dose: 8 pills, 3 times a day

Ba Xian Chang Shou Wan is produced as "Baxian Longevity Pills" by the Lanzhou Chinese Medicine Works, Lanzhou, China, in bottles of 200.

Pinyin Name	Pharmaceutical Name	Percent	TCM Function
Shou Di	Radix Rehmanniae Glutinosae Conquitae	26.66	Nourish Yin; Strengthen Kidney; Tonify Blood
Shan Zhu Yu	Fructus Corni Officinalis	13.33	Nourish Liver; Nourish Kidney; Stop spermatorrhea
Shan Yao	Radix Dioscoreae Oppositae	13.33	Strengthen Spleen and Kidney; Stop spermatorrhea
Dan Pi	Cortex Moutan Radicis	10.00	Clear Blood Heat; Reduce Liver Fire
Ze Xie	Rhizoma Alismatis Plantago-aquaticae	10.00	Clear Heat in Kidney; Promote urination (diuretic-like)
Fu Ling	Sclerotium Poriae Cocos	10.00	Strengthen Spleen; Promote urination; Discharge Dampness
Mai Dong	Tuber Ophiopogonis Japonici	10.00	Clear Lung Heat; Moisten Lung; Strengthen body fluid; Nourish Yin
Wu Wei Zi	Fructus Schisandrae Chinensis	6.68	Strengthen Kidney; Astringent for Lung; Strengthen Lung Qi

Note: 1. This same Patent Medicine has a another name, Mai Wei Di Huang Wan. The formula is based on the formula for Liu Wei Di Huang Wan, #13.19, plus 2 other herbs, Mai Dong and Wu Wei Zi.

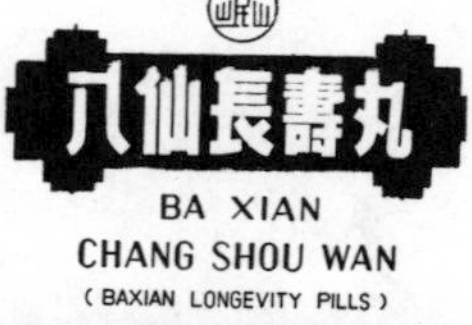

[redacted]

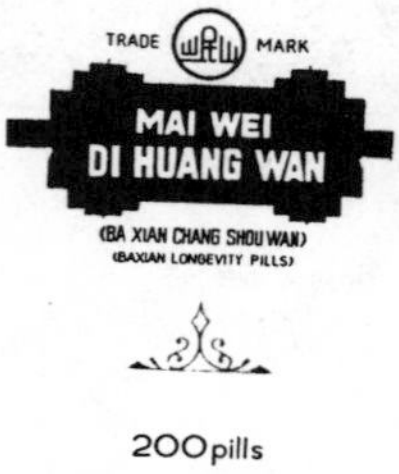

[redacted]

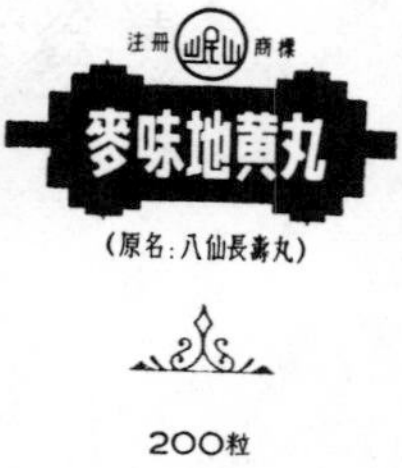

[redacted]

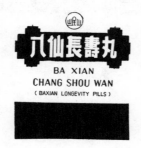

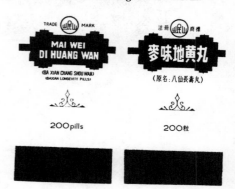

3.16 秋 梨 膏

秋	梨	膏
Qiu	**Li**	**Gao**
autumn	pear	syrup

Source: Yi Xue Cong Zhong Lu, (Medicine for the Large General Population), Qing Dynasty, 1644 - 1911.

Function: 1. Stop cough; Eliminate phlegm
2. Nourish Lung Yin; Promote body fluid

Application: 1. Use to treat cough, phlegm, asthma, especially for the patient who has sputum with blood due to damaged body fluid and Lung Dryness due to Deficient Yin.

2. Use to treat throat dryness with frequent thirst and hoarseness.

3. Some Western Medicine Applications include the following: Dry cough associated with tuberculosis, chronic bronchitis or other lung disease.

Dose: 15 grams twice a day.

Qiu Li Gao is produced by many manufactories in China and they have similar ingredients and function. It is commonly available in 12-ounce bottles.

Pinyin Name	Pharmaceutical Name	Percent	TCM Function
Qiu Li	Pears harvested in the fall	95.23	Clear Lung Heat; Stop cough; Moisten Lung; Nourish Lung; Stop thirst
Mai Men Dong	Tuber Ophiopogonis Japonici	.095	Nourish Lung Yin; Decrease Lung Dryness; Eliminate phlegm; Stop cough
Zhe Bei Mu	Bulbus Fritillariae Thunbergii	.095	Clear Lung Heat; Stop cough; Stop Cough; Eliminate phlegm
Ou	Fresh Lotus Rhizoma	.19	Increase Body Fluid; Stop thirst; Stop bleeding
Qing Luo Bo	Green Turnip	.095	Regulate Lung Qi; Stop cough; Eliminate phlegm

Note: 1. In this formula, the only pears which can be used are those which are harvested in the fall. If they are picked earlier, they will not be ripe enough. It is important that the pears stay on the tree as long as possible, before picking. In addition, by picking the pears in the fall, they are believed to have absorbed the seasonal factor. These pears are then used to treat the Lung, which according to the Five Element Theory, belongs to the autumn season.

In Beijing, China, there is a special factory, Tong San Yi, on the street Qian Men Da Jie, which is becoming famous because it is the leading producer of Qiu Li Gao. Qiu Li Gao is the only Patent Medicine which this factory produces. Traditionally, this store produced two kinds of Qiu Li Gao: 1) Ling Bei Qiu Li Gao, where the major ingredients are Fu Ling, Chuan Bei Mu and Qiu Li, plus honey; and 2) Yen Wo Qiu Li Gao, where the major ingredients are birds' nest and the pears, plus honey. The first one is used to treat chronic cough due to Lung Dryness; the second one is used as a Tonic to strengthen the Lung and general health in older people. Both can be used over a long period of time as a medicinal beverage to promote health. Qiu Li Gao is usually available in a large bottle similar to a wine bottle.

3.17 止 咳 定 喘 丸

Zhi	**Sou**	**Ding**	**Chuan**	**Wan**
stop	cough	stop	asthma	pills

Source: Shang Han Lun, 219, A.D.

Function:
1. Open Lung Qi; Disperse Lung Heat
2. Stop cough and asthma

Application:
1. Use to treat cough and asthma due to Lung Heat from OPI. Symptoms: Cough with thick yellow expectoration (abundant or small amount), asthma, shortness of breath, fever. This is the primary prescription to treat Lung Heat, with or without sweating.

2. Some Western medicine disease applications include the following: (Note, the patient must have signs of Lung Heat.) Acute or chronic bronchitis, acute pneumonia, acute or chronic tracheitis, pneumonia with children's measles.

Contraindication: If the patient has high blood pressure, use this carefully and use only the normal dose. The formula contains Ma Huang, Chinese Ephedra, which can increase blood pressure.

Dose: 10 small pills, 2 times a day, taken with warm water.

Zhi Sou Ding Chuan Wan is produced by the Tientsin Drug Manufactory in bottles of 150 pills.

Pinyin Name	Pharmaceutical Name	Percent	TCM Function
Ma Huang	Herba Ephedrae	1	Expel Wind-Cold; Open Lung Energy; Stop asthma
Xing Ren	Semen Pruni Armeniacae	19	Lower Adverse Rising Qi; Stop cough; Stop asthma
Shi Gao	Gypsum	15	Clear Lung Heat and Stomach Heat
Gan Cao	Radix Glycyrrhizae Uralensis	25	Harmonize other herbs; Clear Heat; Stop cough
	Subsidiary substances to 100%		

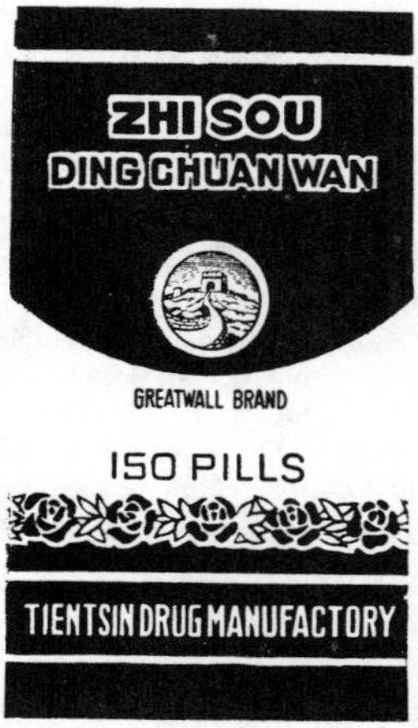

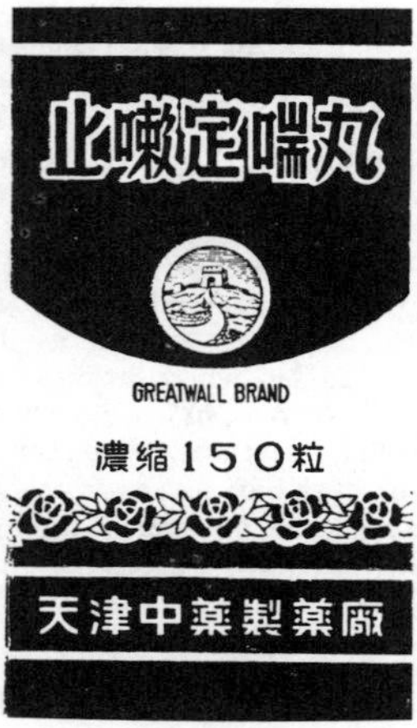

3.18 氣 管 炎 咳 嗽 痰 喘 丸

Qi	Guan	Yan	Ke	Sou	Tan	Chuan	Wan
------------bronchitis------------			--------cough--------		phlegm	asthma	pills

Function: 1. Reduce phlegm and cough; Calm asthma

Application: 1. Use to treat chronic bronchitis and bronchiectasis (especially in the elderly patient).
Symptoms: Abundant expectoration of thin, white phlegm.

Dose: Adults: 20 pills, 2 times a day, taken with warm water.

Qi Guan Yan Ke Sou Tan Chuan Wan is produced as "Chi Kuan Yen Wan" by the Beijing Tung Jen Tang pharmacy in bottles of 200 pills.

Pinyin Name	Pharmaceutical Name	Percent	TCM Function
Qian Hu	Radix Peucedani	4	Lower Adverse Rising Lung Qi; Eliminate phlegm
Xing Ren	Semen Pruni Armeniacae	6	Reduce cough; Calm asthma
Yuan Zhi	Radix Polygalae Tenuifoliae	4	Reduce phlegm
Sang Ye	Folium Mori Albae	8	Expel Wind; Open Lung Energy; Clear Lung Heat
Chuan Bei Mu	Bulbus Fritillariae Cirrhosae	6	Moisten Lung; Stop cough; Reduce phlegm
Ju Hong	Pericarpium Citri Erythrocarpae	2	Reduce thin white phlegm
Pi Pa Ye	Folium Eriobotryae Japonicae	28	Stop cough; Reduce phlegm
Kuan Dong Hua	Flos Tussilagi Farfarae	2	Lower Adverse Rising Lung Qi; Stop cough; Reduce phlegm
Dang Shen	Radix Codonopsis Pilosulae	16	Lower Adverse Rising Lung Qi; Stop cough; Reduce phlegm
Ma Dou Ling	Fructus Aristolochiae	2	Stop cough; Stop asthma; Clear Lung Heat
Wu Wei Zi	Fructus Schisandrae Chinensis	2	Stop cough; Calm asthma
Sheng Jiang	Rhizoma Zingiberis Officinalis Recens	8	Regulate Ying and Wei
Da Zao	Fructus Zizyphi Jujubae	12	Regulate Ying and Wei

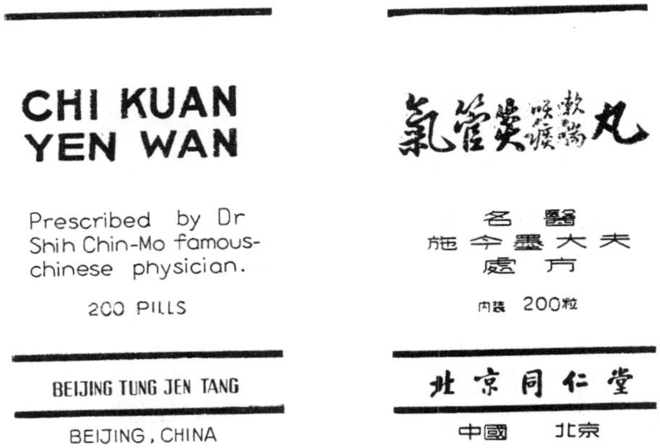
CHI KUAN YEN WAN
Prescribed by Dr Shih Chin-Mo famous-chinese physician.
200 PILLS
BEIJING TUNG JEN TANG
BEIJING, CHINA
氣管炎咳嗽痰喘丸
名醫
施今墨大夫
處方
内装 200粒
北京同仁堂
中國 北京

3.19 消 咳 喘

消	咳	喘
Xiao	**Ke**	**Chuan**
disappear	cough	asthma

Function: 1. Stop cough and reduce expectoration of sputum
2. Calm asthma

Application: 1. Use to treat cough with a lot of sputum due to common cold or flu.

2. Use to increase the body's resistance to disease.

3. Some Western medicine disease applications include chronic tracheitis or bronchitis with a lot of sputum.

Dose: Adults: Liquid: 10 cc, 3 times a day Capsules: 2 capsules, 3 times a day, with warm water.
Children: Use half-dose

Xiao Ke Chuan is produced as "Hsiao Keh Chuan" by the Harbin Medicine Manufactory, Harbin, China, in liquid form (200 cc per bottle) and in capsule form (18 capsules per bottle).

Pinyin Name	Pharmaceutical Name	Percent	TCM Function
Man San Hung	Folium Rhododendri Daurici	100	Stop cough; Reduce phlegm; Calm asthma

Case Report: In December, 1990, a 9 year old boy was seen for the treatment of asthma. He had had recurrent bronchitis for several years. (He had been born 3 weeks pre-mature, with incomplete development of the respiratory system.) When first seen for herbs, the boy was using inhalation aerosol treatments 2 or 3 times a day. His asthma was accompanied by a very productive cough with light yellow, or mostly white sputum (probably associated with some Lung Heat). He was given this patent medicine, #3.19, Xiao Ke Chuan, and used a half-dose, e.g., 1 capsule, 3 times a day for 3 weeks. He then used the patent medicine #3.17, Zhi Sou Ding Chuan Wan, for two weeks. The boy returned for a follow-up visit in March, 1990, after having used the herbs for 5 weeks in December and January. He and his parents stated that after beginning the herbs in December, he no longer had asthma attacks requiring the inhalation aerosol treatments. He used no herbs in most of January or February, and as of March, he had only occasional problems breathing (once a week on Saturday, after a lot of running). He was now able control these minor breathing problems himself, by breathing deeply.

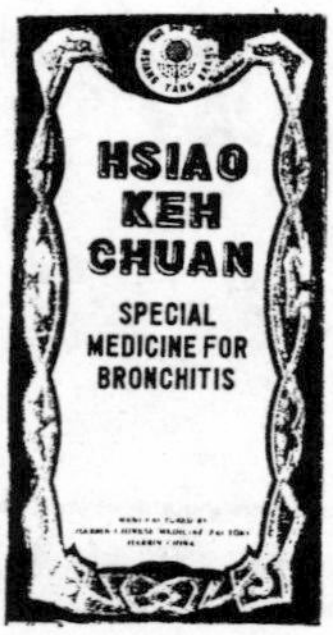

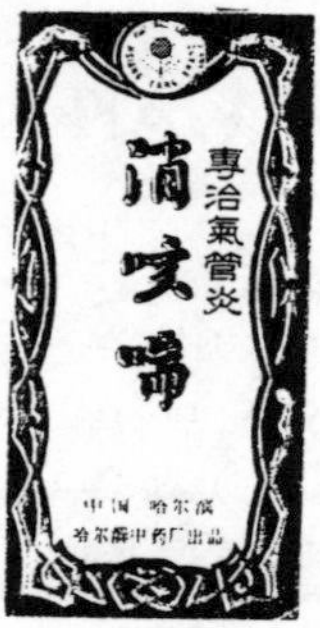

3.20 羅 漢 果 冲 剂

Luo	Han	Guo	Chong	Ji
-----smiling Buddha-----		fruit	powder for making a liquid medicine	

Function:
1. Clear Lung Heat
2. Nourish and moisten the Lung
3. Stop cough

Application:

1. Use to treat cough due to Lung Heat from Def. Lung Yin or weak Lung; sticky or bloody phlegm may be present. The Def. Lung Yin may be due to Dryness or Heat Evil.

2. Use as a summer beverage to eliminate Summer Heat and stop thirst. May be drunk either hot or cold.

3. Some Western medicine disease applications include treatment of a cough with sticky or bloody phlegm and dry, itchy throat associated with bronchitis, pharyngitis or tonsillitis.

4. Use to treat stubborn, chronic cough such as that associated with whooping cough or tuberculosis.

Dose: Dissolve 1 block in 1 cup, or 1 and 1/2 cups, of boiling water for each dose. Use one dose, 2 or 3 times a day.

Luo Han Guo Chong Ji is produced as "Lo Han Kuo Infusion" by the Luo Han Guo Products Manufactory, Kwangsi, China, with 12 blocks per package.

Pinyin Name	Pharmaceutical Name	Percent	TCM Function
Luo Han Guo	Fructus Mormordicae Grosvenori	95	Expel Summer Heat; Nourish Lung; Stop cough; Stop thirst
	Cane sugar	5	

Notes:

1. Luo Han Guo has a sweet taste and a Cooling property; Luo Han Guo fruit has a laxative effect.

2. The formula Luo Han Guo Zhi Ke Lung is similar to Luo Han Guo Chong Ji. Luo Han Guo Zhi Ke Lung is somewhat stronger than Luo Han Guo Chong Ji because it contains additonal herbs to Clear Lung Heat, Open Lung Qi, stop cough and eliminate phlegm.

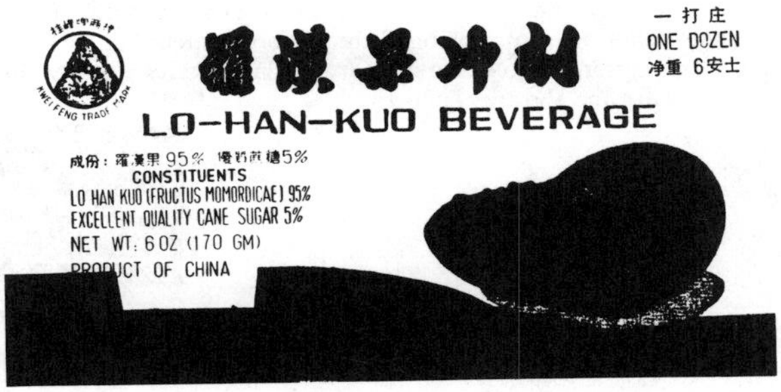

3.21 平 喘 丸

Ping	**Chuan**	**Wan**
relieve	dyspnea	pills

Function: 1. Stop cough; improve shortness of breath
2. Nourish Lung Yin

Application: 1. Use to treat chronic shortness of breath which has caused Def. Lung Qi and Def. Lung Yin. Symptoms: Shortness of breath which is worse in the evening, or when the patient has over-exerted himself, or when he has OPI; cough with thin white phlegm may be present.

2. Some Western medicine disease applications include the following: (The patient must have the above-mentioned symptoms in order to be able to use this herbal formula.) Chronic bronchitis and emphysema.

Dose: 10 pills, 3 times a day.

Ping Chuan Wan is produced by the Sing-Kyn Drug House, Guangzhou, China, in bottles of 120 pills.

The contents are listed below in 3 separate groups according to function.

Pinyin Name	Pharmaceutical Name	Percent	TCM Function
Group 1			
Dang Shen	Radix Codonopsis Pilosulae	15	Tonify Lung; Nourish Lung Yin
Ge Jie	Gecko	5	
Dong Chong Cao	Cordyceps Sinensis	5	
Group 2			
Xing Ren	Semen Pruni Armeniacae	15	Stop cough; Eliminate phlegm
Chen Pi	Pericarpium Citri Reticulatae	8	
Gan Cao	Radix Glycyrrhizae Uralensis	10	
Group 3			
Sang Bai Pi	Cortex Mori Albae Radicis	10	Calm asthma;
Bai Qian	Radix et Rhizoma Cynanchii Stautoni	8	Lower Adverse Rising Qi
Meng Shi	Phlogopitum	4	
Wu Zhi Mao Tao	Ficus Simplicissima Lour	10	
Man Hu Tui Zi	Elaeagnus Glabra Thunb	10	

Note: 1. The manufacturer has written in the flier that in their clinical experience, a single bottle can produce noticeable effects for a "general case;" three bottles can soothe cough and shortness of breath for patients suffering from prolonged chronic bronchitis. For chronic cases with asthma or with pulmonary emphysema, 3 to 4 courses of treatment (40 days a course) in succession will end the cough with sputum and shortness of breath.

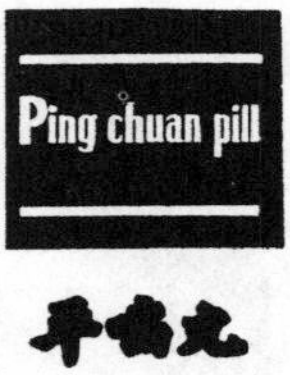

Chapter 4. Treat Muscular and Joint Pain due to Wind Dampness (Bi)

(Includes Patent Medicines used with arthritis, sports injuries, etc.)

4.1 腰 痛 片

Yao Tong Pian

---------lumbago---------- tablets

Function: 1. Strengthen Kidney; Promote Blood circulation

Application: 1. Use to treat lumbago caused by Def. KidneyYang or by chronic over-straining.

Dose: 6 tablets, 3 times a day.

Yao Tong Pian is produced in tablet form as "Anti-Lumbago Tablets" (100 tablets per bottle) and in honey pill form as "Yao Tong Wan" by the Hu Qing Yu Tang Medicine Factory, Hangzhou, China.

Pinyin Name	Pharmaceutical Name	Percent	TCM Function
Dang Gui	Radix Angelicae Sinensis	17.4	Tonify Blood; Promote Blood circulation
Du Zhong	Cortex Eucommiae Ulmoidis	17.4	Strengthen Kidney and Liver; Improve tendons and bones
Xu Duan	Radix Dipsaci	13.04	Strengthen Kidney and Liver; Improve tendons and bones; Reduce lumbago
Gou Ji	Rhizoma Cibotii Barometz	13.04	Strengthen Kidney and Liver; Strengthen lumbar
Bai Zhu	Rhizoma Atractylodis Macrocephalae	13.04	Strengthen Spleen; Tonify Qi
Bu Gu Zhi	Fructus Psoraleae Corylifoliae	13.04	Warm the Kidney Yang
Niu Xi	Radix Achyranthis Bidentatae	13.04	Promote Blood circulation; Strengthen Liver and Kidney

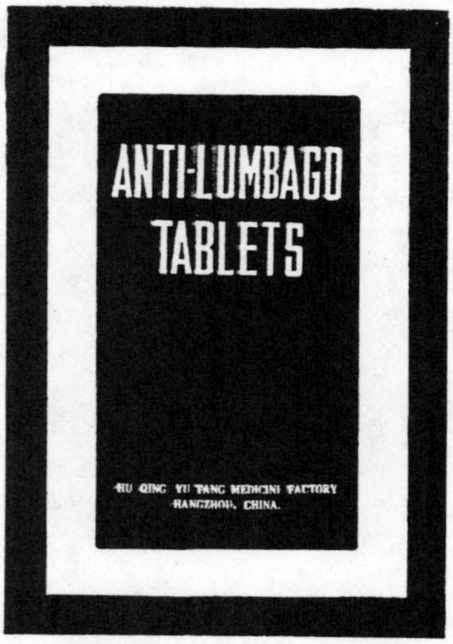

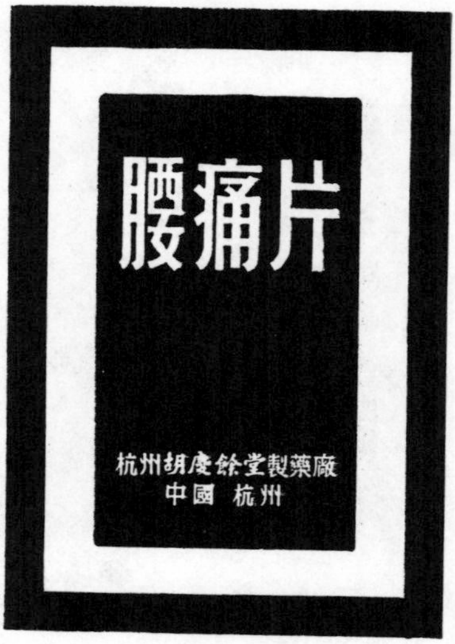

4.2 鷄 血 藤 浸 膏 片

Ji	Xue	Teng	Qin	Gao	Pian
---------Millettia reticulata---------			----liquid extract----		tablets

Function: 1. Nourish Blood; Promote Blood circulation

2. Clear Meridians

Appplication: 1. Use to treat Bi Syndrome (Joint pain due to a combination of Wind-Cold and Dampness). Symptoms: Numbness of limbs, stiff and painful joints, backache, weakness in the knees. Because this medicine has the two-fold effect to both Nourish and Move Blood, it is especially good for the older or weaker patients who have Def. Blood which has failed to Nourish the Meridians, thus causing dysfunction of the Meridians.

2. Use to treat amenorrhea or dysmenorrhea due to Def. Blood and/or Stagnation of Blood. The primary symptom is dizziness due to Def. Blood. It is common to combine this with other formulas used for gynecological disorders including Tonics, if necessary. This herb has the same effect as Dang Gui in Nourishing Blood, however, it is not as strong as Dang Gui.

3. This medicine has been observed to have the special effect to increase the white Blood cell count in cancer patients who, as a result of receiving chemotherapy or radiation for cancer, had lowered white Blood cell counts. Research in Shanghai with these cancer patients showed an increase in the WBC count following 3 or 4 days of treatment with this herbal medicine. Thus, the chemotherapy or radiation treatments were able to continue without prolonged interruption. (Shanghai Traditional Chinese Medicine Journal, No. 9, 1965, 16-17)

4. Use to treat aplastic anemia.

Dose: 4 tablets, 3 times a day

Ji Xue Teng Qin Cao Pian is produced as "Caulis Milletiae Tablets" by the Shanghai Native Medicine Works, Shanghai, China, in bottles of 100 coated tablets.

Pinyin Name	Pharmaceutical Name	Percent	TCM Function
Ji Xue Teng	Millettia reticulata Benth.	100	Nourish Blood; Promote Blood Circulation

Notes: 1. Case Report: A cancer patient was seeing Dr. Zhu in Boston, for weakness following surgery for breast cancer which had metastasized to the lung. At the time of a scheduled chemotherapy treatment within a series of chemotherapy treatments, she was told her WBC count was only 2,000, a level too low to receive more chemotherapy treatment. Dr. Zhu prepared an herbal formula containing this herbal medicine for her, and she used it for three days. After that time (less than one week), her WBC count had increased to 5,900, and the treatments were continued. She continued to take the herbal medicine and was able to continue the series of chemotherapy treatments without interruption. Her WBC count after two weeks on the herbal medicine had risen to 9,500, while continuing to receive the chemotherapy treatments.

2. Ji Xue Teng is mild and gentle. It can be taken for at least 2 or 3 months and has not been observed to produce any side effects. Even Def. Yin patients with signs of Empty Fire can take this medicine without any exacerbation of Empty Fire signs; it may help to relieve the condition.

3. Prof. Yang Qing Yao of the Shanghai Teacher's University, has recently conducted research on another product from China produced in pill form which is used with cancer patients receiving radiation therapy, to help increase the tolerance of the patient to the radiation therapy. The name of this product is Polysaccharide-peptide (PSP) extracted from the deep-layer cultivated mycelia of Coriolus versicolor.

Forty-one cases with moderate-to-advanced esophageal carcinoma (pathologically confirmed as squamous cell carcinoma) received a combination of PSP and radiation therapy at the Cancer Hospital, Shanghai Medical University, in 1986 and 1987. All patients had a minimum follow-up of 1 year. Results of patients treated by radiotherapy alone, as reported in 1978, were used as historical controls.

The survival rate at 1 year for cases with lesions 3-7 cm in length who used both PSP and radiation therapy was 71.4%. This was better than that observed in 1978, for cases treated with radiation therapy alone, 56.8%. Similarly, for upper and mid-thoracic cases, the use of PSP plus radiation therapy improved 1 year survivals as compared to controls (87.5% versus 50.4%). Other advantages of PSP combined with radiotherapy were that it increased the tolerance of the patient to the side-effects of radiation therapy. Patients receiving PSP during the course of the radiation treatments reported less anorexia, listlessness and asthenia. They were given two 0.5 gm capsules, 3 times a day, during the course of the radiation treatments. It was suggested that for patients with lesions longer than 7 cm, or with lesions situated in the lower esophagus, that the PSP be given for a longer period of time, in larger dosage, and before the radiation treatments begin.

The dosage of 3 gm per day did not show any toxicity. More information may be obtained from the report, "The Polysaccharide-Peptide of Coriolus Versicolor (Yun-Zhi)," from the Biology School, Shanghai Teacher's University, 10 Quilin Rd., Shanghai, PRC. The capsules may be ordered directly from Hong Kong, through Winsor Health Products, Ltd., Harbour Crystal Centre, Suite 1008, 100 Granville Rd., Tsim Sha Tsui East, Kowloon, H.K. Telephone: 3883128 FAX: 3666760

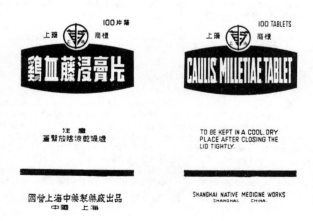

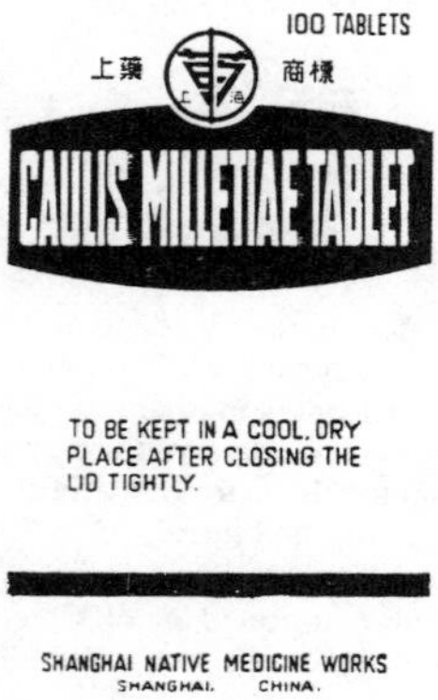

4.3 杜 仲 虎 骨 丸

杜	仲	虎	骨	丸
Du	**Zhong**	**Hu**	**Gu**	**Wan**
----------Eucommiae---------		tiger	bone	pills

Function: 1. Strengthen Liver and Kidney
2. Nourish Blood; Strengthen Qi
3. Promote Blood Circulation; Stop pain

Application: 1. Use to treat chronic Bi syndrome (pain in the joints due to Wind-Cold and Dampness). When Bi syndrome has been present for a long period of time, the Liver and Kidney are also damaged. Hence, when the Liver and Kidney are damaged, there is additional weakness in the lower back and the knees. This formula is designed to treat the Bi syndrome symptoms, as well as to Nourish the Liver and Kidney. Symptoms: Joint pain, lumbago, joint stiffness, fatigue, feeling of cold in the limbs, pale face, impotence, spermatorrhea.

2. Use to treat older patients with Def. Liver and Kidney condition which has produced a gradual onset of slowness in walking, feeling of numbness or almost paralysis of limbs, feeling of coldness in the body, dizziness.

Contraindication: Do not use with pregnant women. Also, do not eat beans or seafood while taking this Patent Medicine.

Dose: Adults: 8-12 pills, 3 times a day
Children 8 to 11 Years: 4-6 pills, 3 times a day Children 12 to 16 Years: 6-8 pills, 3 times a day.

Du Zhong Hu Gu Wan is produced as "Pilulae Corticis Eucommiae et Ossis Tigris" by the Guiyang Chinese Medicine Factory, Guiyang, China, in bottles of 100 pills.

The contents in this herbal formula are listed below in 4 groups according to function.

Pinyin Name	Pharmaceutical Name	Percent	TCM Function
Group 1			
Ren Shen	Radix Ginseng	6.2	Strengthen Spleen; Nourish Qi
Bai Zhu	Rhizoma Atractylodis Macrocephalae	3.8	
Group 2			
Dang Gui	Radix Angelicae Sinensis	6.0	Nourish Blood; Promote
Chuan Xiong	Radix Ligustici Wallichii	6.2	Blood circulation
Ji Xue Teng	Millettia reticulata Benth.	3.8	
San Qi	Radix Pseudoginseng	6.2	
Group 3			
Du Zhong	Cortex Eucommiae Ulmoidis	17.8	Strengthen Liver and Kidney;
Hu Gu	Os Tigris	6.8	Improve mobility of limbs
Mu Gua	Fructus Chaenomelis Lagenariae	5.5	
Yin Yang Huo	Herba Epimedii	3.8	

Group 4

Wu Shao She	Zaocys Dhumnades	6.8	Expel Wind-Cold, Dampness;
Lu Lu Tong	Fructus Liquidambaris Taiwanianae	5.5	Clear Meridians; Stop pain
Cang Zhu	Rhizoma Atractylodis	5.5	
Xun Gu Feng	Herba Aristolochiae Mollissimae	4.0	
Wei Ling Xian	Radix Clemetidis Chinensis	4.0	
Shi Nan Teng	Photinia serrulata Lindl.	4.0	
Sang Zhi	Ramulus Mori Albae	3.8	

Note: 1. This Patent Medicine is produced by several different manufactories under the same name; the ingredients may vary somewhat, but the general function is the same.

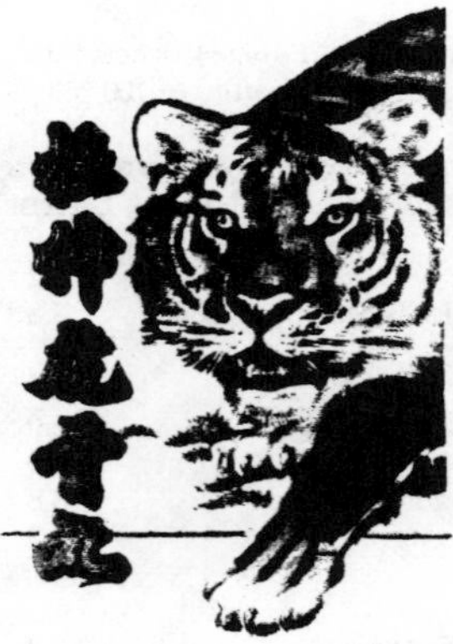

4.4

雲	南	風	濕	灵
Yun	**Nan**	**Feng**	**Shi**	**Ling**
-----Yunnan Province-----		wind	damp	very good
		-------rheumatism--------		

Function: 1. Expel Wind-Cold, Eliminate Dampness, Stop pain
2. Nourish Blood; Promote Blood Circulation

Application: 1. Use to treat Bi syndrome (joint pain due to combination of Wind-Cold and Dampness). Symptoms: Joint pain and stiffness, limb numbness, chronic swollen joints.

2. Some Western medicine disease applications include the following: Rheumatoid arthritis (Do not use in acute or flare-up stage with fever and redness around joints, etc.,this herbal formula contains some Warming herbs.); osteoarthritis; sports injury including sprains or strains.

Contraindication: Do not use with pregnant women. Do not use with women who are within three months, post-partum. Do not use with children under age 10. Also, do not use with pulmonary tuberculosis cases or cases with heart disease.

Dose: 1 capsule in the evening before going to bed, with or without food. Do not overdose.

Yun Nan Feng Shi Ling is produced as "Yunnan Rheumatilin" by the Gorjiu Pharmaceutical Factory, Gorjiu, Yunnan, China, in boxes of 20 capsules.

The percents for each ingredient are not available.

Pinyin Name	Pharmaceutical Name	TCM Function
Chuan Wu	Radix Aconiti	Expel Wind-Cold, Dampness
Tian Qi	Radix Pseudoginseng	Promote Blood circulation; Reduce Swelling; Stop pain
Bai Yun Shen	Radix Bai Yun Shen	Nourish Blood; Strengthen Qi; Reduce Swelling; Stop pain
Duan Jie Shen	Radix Duan Jie Shen	Clear Meridians; Regulate Blood circulation; Strengthen Kidney

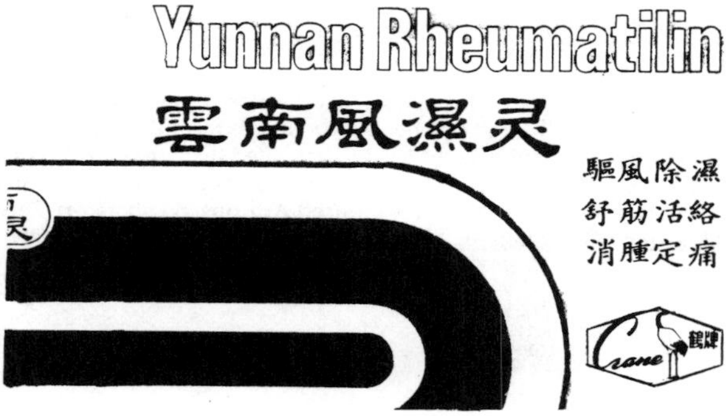

4.5 风 湿 消 痛 丸

Feng	Shi	Xiao	Tong	Wan
--------rheumatism-------		reduce	pain	pills

Function: 1. Expel Wind-Cold; Eliminate Dampness

2. Promote Blood circulation; Stop pain

3. Strengthen tendons and bones

Application: 1. Use to treat Bi syndrome (joint pain due to Wind-Cold, Dampness). Symptoms: Feeling of cold in the limbs, joint stiffness and joint pain; joints may be swollen. Especially used with chronic rheumatoid arthritis patients, or osteoarthritis patients or older persons with debility of legs and problems walking due to pain and stiffness in the joints. This formula is especially effective for joint pain and stiffness.

Contraindication: While taking this medicine, do not eat pig's liver, sheep's meat (mutton) or blood, or sweet potatoes.

Dose: 10 pills, 2 times a day, taken with water or wine after a meal. (It is not necessary to take with food, however.)

Feng Shi Xiao Tong Wan is produced as "Feng Shih Hsiao Tung Wan" by the Tientsin Drug Manufactory, Tientsin, China, in bottles of 120 pills.

Pinyin Name	Pharmaceutical Name	Percent	TCM Function
Xi Xian Cao	Herba Siegesbeckiae Orientalis	15	Treat Bi syndrome
Chou Wu Tong	Clerodendron trichotomum Thunb.	15	Treat Bi syndrome
Hu Gu	Os Tigris	15	Strengthen tendons and bones; Stop pain
Lu Jin	Nervus Cervi	10	Strengthen tendons
Hong Hua	Flos Carthami Tinctorii	10	Promote Blood circulation; Remove Blood Stagnation
Mu Gua	Fructus Chaenomelis Lagenariae	10	Strengthen tendons; Clear Meridians; Stop pain
Qiang Huo	Rhizoma et Radix Notopterygii	15	Expel Wind-Cold; Stop pain
	Plus subsidiary substances to 100%		

Notes: 1. The Feng Shi Xiao Tong Wan formula is a modification of another effective formula, Xi Tong Wan, which contains only the first two herbs listed in this formula. Xi Tong Wan has been tested in laboratory research with animals, which demonstrated that it has an effect in decreasing inflammation in cases of arthritis. ["The Treatment Effect of Guan Jie Ling (an herbal formula containing these two herbs) on Artificially Induced Arthritis in Laboratory Rats," Proceedings of the Annual Meeting of the Chinese Pharmacological Association, 1963, 328-329]

2. The original formula, Xi Tong Wan, contained two herbs which are not only effective in treating Bi syndrome, but also effective in treating hypertension, Xi Xian Cao and Chou Wu Tong. Thus, cases with Bi syndrome plus hypertension will especially benefit from taking this herbal formula, Feng Shi Xiao Tong Wan.

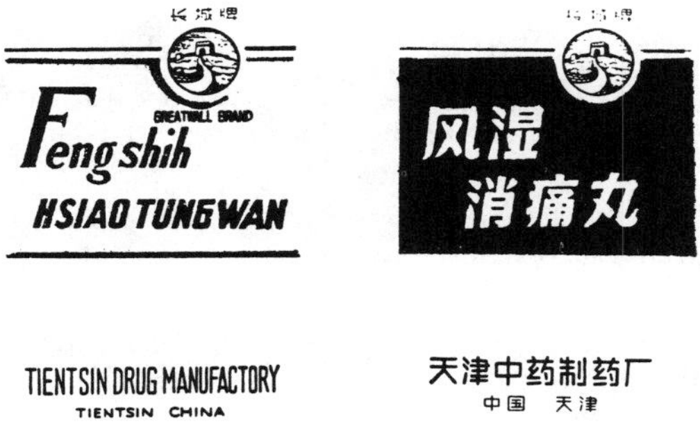

4.6 風濕片

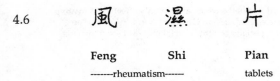

Feng	Shi	Pian
-------rheumatism------		tablets

Function: 1. Expel Wind, Cold, Dampness (Bi syndrome)

2. Promote Blood circulation; Soothe muscles and tendons, Stop pain

Application: 1. Use to treat Bi syndrome (Wind, Cold, Dampness in muscles or joints). This includes rheumatism, arthritis, and rheumatoid arthritis with symptoms such as limb numbness, joint pain, difficult walking. Also use to treat neuralgia in the arms and legs associated with Bi syndrome

Contraindication: Do not use with pregnant women. Do not use with patients who are hypertensive.

Dose: 2 tablets, once a day. If the pain is worse in the morning, the medicine should be taken early in the morning. Do not increase the dosage; do not overdose. The medicine should be taken with warm water or warm wine.

Feng Shi Pian is produced as "Hong She" by the Zhong Lian Drug Manufactory, Wuhan, China, in bottles of 24 tablets.

The contents are listed below in 4 groups according to function.

Pinyin Name	Pharmaceutical Name	Percent	TCM Function
Group 1			
Ma Huang	Herba Ephedrae	18.5	Expel Wind Cold; Warm the
Gui Zhi	Ramulus Cinnamomi Cassiae	18.5	Meridians; Clear Meridians;
Fang Feng	Radix Ledebouriellae Sesloidis	10.4	Stop pain, numbness, tremors
Du Huo	Radix Duhuo (Angelica pubescens Maxim.)	10.4	
Group 2			
Ma Qian Zi	Semen Strychnotis	18.5	Decrease swelling; Stop pain
Group 3			
Du Zhong	Cortex Eucommiae Ulmoidis	18.5	Nourish Liver, Kidney;
Niu Xi	Radix Achyranthis Bidentatae	2.6	Strengthen tendons and bones; Strengthen back and legs
Group 4			
Gan Cao	Radix Glycyrrhizae Uralensis	2.6	Harmonize other herbs; Decrease poisoning effect

Note: 1. This formula contains two herbs which need further comment because they have a strong effect:

1. Ma Huang This herb stimulates the cerebral cortex and can increase blood pressure. The side effects can include insomnia or excess sweating.

2. Ma Qian Zi This herb is a poisonous medicine which is able to stimulate the central nervous system; increase Blood circulation and strengthen breathing. It also increases blood pressure. If an overdose is used, it may cause serious poisoning effects with symptoms such as dizziness, nausea, numbness and seizures. Therefore, this medicine should not be used, if the patient has hypertension. The antidote for treatment of toxicity with Ma Qian Zi is barbiturates (Bensky & Gamble, 1986 p. 647).

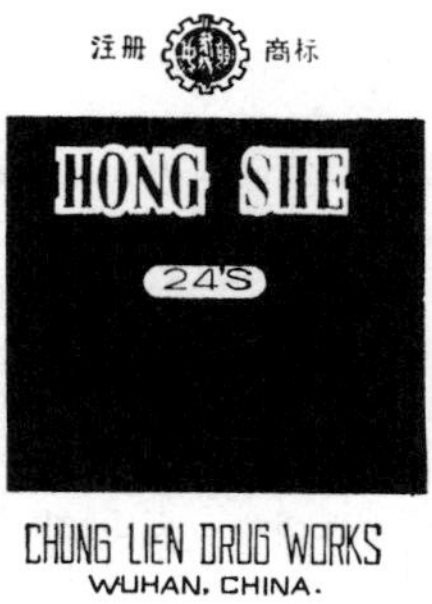
注册 商标
HONG SHE
24'S
CHUNG LIEN DRUG WORKS
WUHAN, CHINA.

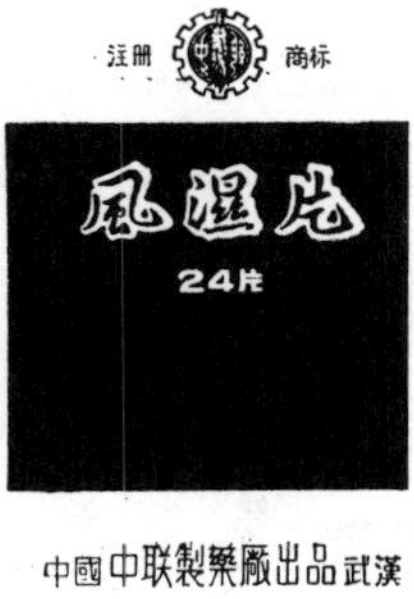
注册 商标
風濕片
24片
中國中联製藥廠出品武漢

4.7 小 活 络 丹

小	活	络	丹
Xiao	**Huo**	**Luo**	**Dan**
small	activate	Meridians	pill

Source: Tai Ping Hui Min He Ji Jiu Fang, (Formulas of the People's Welfare Pharmacy), Song Dynasty 960-1279.

Function: 1. Clear Meridians; Promote Blood circulation

2. Remove Wind-Cold Accumulation; Stop pain

Application: 1. Use to treat Stuck Meridian Circulation due to Wind-Cold Accumulation. Symptoms: Joint pain (sharp pain), stiff joints, limb numbness, aching anywhere in joints or muscles, rheumatism. If joints are red and swollen, and fever is present, do not use this formula; it contains some Hot herbs.

2. Use to treat sports injury or other traumatic injuries including those due to overexertion. This medicine is able to Promote Blood circulation and Remove Blood Stagnation, thus the pain is reduced and healing takes place sooner.

Contraindication: Do not use with pregnant women. Xiao Huo Luo Dan contains 6 ingredients, but 3 are toxic (Chuan Wu, Cao Wu, Dan Nan Xing), thus do not increase the dosage unless directed to do so by the physician,

Dose: 6 pills, 2 or 3 times a day, taken with warm water or wine.

Xiao Huo Luo Dan is produced by the Lanzhou Chinese Medicine Works, Lanzhou, China, in bottles of 100 pills.

Pinyin Name	Pharmaceutical Name	Percent	TCM Function
Chuan Wu	Radix Aconiti	21.25	Warm the Meridians; Stop pain
Cao Wu	Aconitum Kusnezoffii	21.25	Warm the Meridians; Stop pain
Dan Nan Xing	Pulvis Arisaemae cum Felle Bovis	21.25	Eliminate Wind-Phlegm; Treat limb numbness
Di Long	Lumbricus	21.25	Calm the Wind; Clear Meridians
Ru Xiang	Gummi Olibanum	7.5	Promote Blood circulation; Stop pain; Stop swelling; Promote tissue regeneration
Mo Yao	Myrrha	7.5	Promote Blood circulation; Stop pain; Stop swelling; Promote tissue regeneration

Note: 1. The name of this Patent Medicine, Xiao Huo Luo Dan, differs by only one Chinese character from another Patent Medicine, Da Huo Luo Dan, #6.2. The functions and applications of the two formulas are quite different. Both medicines can be used for joint or muscular pain due to Wind-Cold Accumulation in the Meridians, but Xiao Huo Luo Dan is used with a stronger patient with these symptoms. The Da Huo Luo Dan is used with patients who have Def. Qi and Def. Blood with these symptoms.

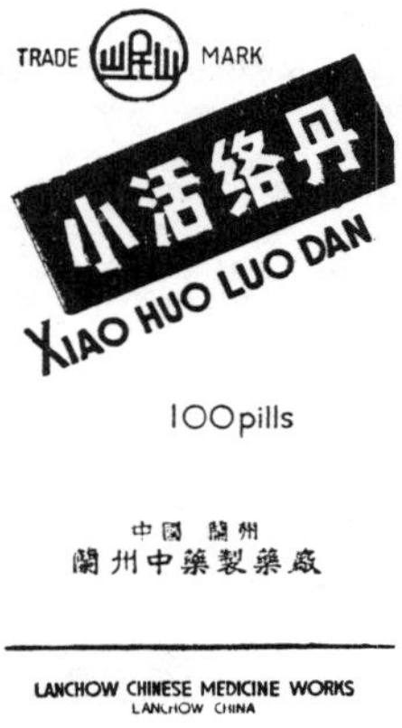

4.8 独 活 寄 生 丸

Du	Huo	Ji	Sheng	Wan
----------Angelica----------		----------Loranthus----------		pills

Source: Bei Ji Qien Jin Yao Fang, (A Thousand Golden Remedies for Emergencies), Tang Dynasty, 618-907.

Function: 1. Eliminate Wind-Dampness; Stop pain
2. Nourish Blood and Qi; Strengthen Liver and Kidney

Application: 1. Use to treat Bi syndrome in weaker patients with Def. Qi and Def. Blood.
Symptoms: Pain and coldness in the lumbar area or legs or joints (especially knee joints); tremor may be present (due to Def. Blood); joint stiffness and numbness; fatigue; feeling of cold (the patient likes the warmth). The Tongue may be pale, with a thin, white Tongue coat. The Pulse may be thin, weak or Empty.

2. Some Western medicine disease applications include the following: (Note, the patient must have the above-listed symptoms associated with Bi syndrome due to Def. Qi and Def. Blood, in order to use this.) Chronic Arthritis (rheumatoid or osteoarthritis); sciatica.

Dose: 6 pills, 2 or 3 times a day.

Du Huo Ji Sheng Wan is produced by the Min Kang Pharmaceutical Manufactory, Szechuan, China in bottles of 100 pills.

The contents are listed below in 6 groups which are arranged according to function.

Pinyin Name	Pharmaceutical Name	Percent	TCM Function
Group 1			
Du Huo	Radix Angelica pubescens Maxim	7.31	Expel Wind-Dampness;
Qin Jiao	Radix Gentianae Macrophyllae	7.31	Treat Bi syndrome; Stop pain
Fang Feng	Radix Ledebouriellae Sesloidis	7.31	
Group 2			
Xi Xin	Herba Asari cum Radice	7.31	Expel Wind-Cold; Eliminate Dampness; Stop pain
Group 3			
Du Zhong	Cortex Eucommiae Ulmoidis	7.31	Strengthen Liver and Kidney;
Niu Xi	Radix Achyranthis Bidentatae	7.31	Reinforce tendons and bones;
Sang Ji Sheng	Ramus Loranthi seu Visci	7.31	Eliminate Wind-Dampness
Group 4			
Dang Gui	Radix Angelicae Sinensis	4.88	Strengthen Blood;
Chuan Xiong	Radix Ligustici Wallichii	7.31	Promote Blood circulation
Shou Di Huang	Radix Rehmanniae Glutinosae Conquitae	4.88	
Bai Shao	Radix Paeoniae Lactiflorae	4.88	
Group 5			
Dang Shen	Radix Codonopsis Pilosulae	7.31	Tonify Qi; Strengthen Spleen
Fu Ling	Sclerotium Poriae Cocos	7.31	
Gan Cao	Radix Glycyrrhizae Uralensis	4.88	

Group 6

Rou Gui	Cortex Cinnamomi Cassiae	7.31	Dispel Cold; Stop pain

Notes: 1. This is a commonly used medicine in China for Bi syndrome, especially for cases with Def. Qi and Def. Blood. In TCM theory, Bi syndrome is a combination of Wind, Cold and Dampness. When these three factors affect the tendons and bones over a long period of time, the Liver (tendons) and Kidney (bones) are also affected. This will thus lead to the development of Def. Blood and Def. Qi. In this formula, the herbs in Groups 1 and 2 are the primary ingredients used to treat Bi syndrome; these herbs will help prevent progression of the Bi syndrome into weakening the Liver and Kidney. The herbs in Group 3 will Strengthen the Liver and Kidney to reinforce the tendons and bones. The herbs in Group 4 will Strengthen Blood, and the herbs in Group 5 will Strengthen Qi. Thus, the ingredients in this formula will treat both the symptoms associated with Bi syndrome, as well as the root cause.

2. Another Patent Medicine, Guan Jie Yan Wan is similar to Du Huo Ji Sheng Wan.

3. Another Patent Medicine, Te Xiao Yao Tong Ling , is also similar to Du Huo Ji Sheng Wan, however, Te Xiao Yao Tong Ling uses several Tonic medicines which Strengthen Kidney Yang. These Kidney Yang Tonics are not in Du Huo Ji Sheng Wan. Thus, Te Xiao Yao Tong Ling contains medicine to stop pain (treat Bi syndrome) plus Strengthen Kidney Yang; thus, this medicine is specially formulated to treat lumbago. Du Huo Ji Sheng Wan can be used to stop pain in a more general sense, and is not specific for the lumbar area, whereas Te Xiao Yao Tong Ling is more specific for the lumbar area. Note, the formula in #4.1, Yao Tong Pian, is designed to treat the patient with lumbago especially due to Deficient Kidney Yang. Te Xiao Yao Tong Ling is designed to treat the patient with lumbago due to both Deficient Kidney Yang and Bi syndrome.

4. A formula similar to this formula is also available in liquid, tincture form as "Meridian Circulation," in the Jade Pharmacy product line, available through Crane Enterprises, Plymouth, MA, etc. See bottom of page 343.

4.9 狗 皮 膏

Gou	**Pi**	**Gao**
dog	skin	plaster

Function: 1. Expel Wind-Cold
2. Promote Blood circulation; Stop pain; Relax tendons

Application: 1. Use to treat Bi syndrome due to Wind-Cold. Symptoms: Lumbago, leg pain, numbness.

2. Use to treat neuralgia or rheumatism; sports or other traumatic injury and sprains or strains with swelling and pain.

Contraindication: Do not use on the abdomen of pregnant women.

How to use the plaster: The plaster comes folded in half; the herbal medicines are inside the folded area. The plaster is quite hard, thus it must first be heated and softened. Use the steam from boiling water to warm and moisten the plaster on both sides, while it is still folded. After the plaster is softened, gently open it up. While it is still warm, but not too hot, place it on the affected area, with the herbs facing the chosen area.

If itching develops after applying the plaster, or the skin becomes red and a rash develops, the patient may have an allergy to the plaster and it should be removed. If there is no allergic reaction to the plaster, the plaster may be kept on the skin for up to one or two weeks. Keep the plaster dry. When ready to remove the plaster, gently peel the plaster off the skin. If any of the plaster remains on the skin, it may be removed with paint thinner. The plaster may be re-used a few times.

Go Pi Gou is produced as "Kou Pi Kao" by the Tientsin Drug Manufactory with one traditional plaster per envelope.

The contents are listed below in 5 groups which are arranged according to function.

Pinyin Name	Pharmaceutical Name	Percent	TCM Function
Group 1			
Tian Ma	Rhizoma Gastrodiae Elatae	10.53	Eliminate Wind-Cold and Dampness;
Xi Xin	Herba Asari cum Radice	10.53	Stop pain
Group 2			
Ru Xiang	Gummi Olibanum	5.26	Promote Blood circulation;
Mo Yao	Myrrha	5.26	Remove Blood Stagnation;
Xue Jie	Sanguis Draconis	5.26	Stop pain
Er Cha	Acacia seu Uncaria	5.26	
Chuan Shan Jia	Squama Manitis Pentadactylae	10.53	
Group 3			
Ding Xiang	Flos Caryophylli	5.25	Remove Stuck Qi; Stop pain
Group 4			
Du Zhong	Cortex Eucommiae Ulmoidis	10.53	Strengthen Liver and Kidney;
Niu Xi	Radix Achyranthis Bidentatae	10.53	Reinforce tendons and bones

Group 5			
Dang Gui	Radix Angelicae Sinensis	10.53	Tonify Blood; Promote Blood circulation
	Plus subsidiary substances to 100%		

Notes: 1. The original formula required placement of this plaster onto dog skin, because the dog skin has a Warm property. Thus, the dog skin would keep the skin warm and help to treat the Bi syndrome. Due to the shortage of dog skin now, however, some factories use either cloth or paper or sheep skin, instead of dog skin; the function is the same.

2. A new form of Gou Pi Gao is now available where the herbs are inside a cloth tape, and the tape is placed on the affected area.

3. Another plaster, She Xiang Zhui Feng Gao, is similar to Gou Pi Gao. She Xiang Zhui Feng Gao, however, contains musk; thus, do not use on pregnant women.

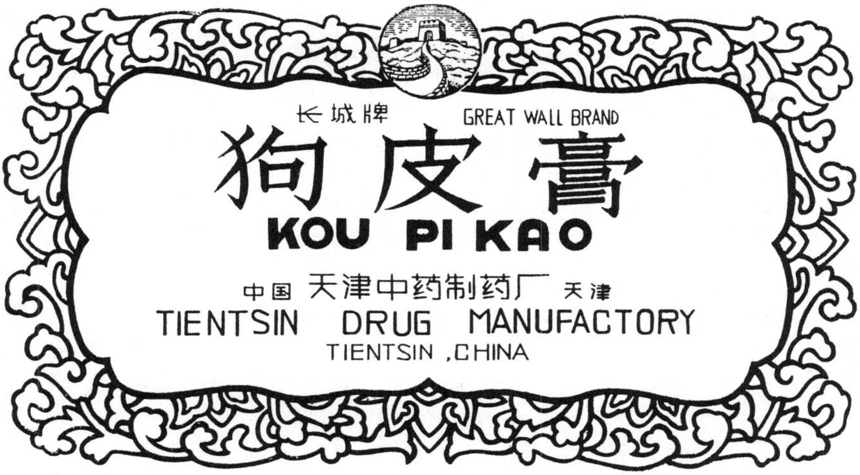

4.10 伤 湿 止 痛 膏

Shang	Shi	Zhi	Tong	Gao
attacked by Dampness		stop	pain	plaster

Function: 1. Expel Wind-Dampness

2. Promote Blood circulation; Stop pain

Application: 1. Use to treat Bi syndrome with muscle and joint pain, including arthritis (osteoarthritis or rheumatoid arthritis).

2. Use to treat sports injury or other traumatic injury to muscles and tendons including sprains and strains.

Contraindication: Do not apply to the skin of pregnant women. Do not apply the plaster to an open wound.

How to use the plaster: The affected area should be cleaned with gentle soap and warm water before applying the plaster; applying the plaster after a warm bath is even better. The herbal medicine is inside a cloth tape with adhesive backing which is available in plasters which are approximately 2" x 3." The plasters are attached to a piece of cellophane; two plasters per piece of cellophane. Peel the plaster off the cellophane and place on the affected area. Use two or more plasters, if necessary to cover the entire area.

The herbal medicine in the plaster is most effective for the first 8 to 12 hours. After that time, new plasters may be re-applied for as many days as necessary. Water does not affect the herbal medicine, therefore, the patient may wear the plasters while bathing or swimming.

If the patient has an allergic skin reaction to the adhesive tape or redness, itching or skin irritation appears, do not use it.

The plasters contain many aromatic ingredients, therefore it is important to keep the unused plasters in a tight container.

Shang Shi Zhi Tong Gao is produced by the Shanghai Chinese Medicine Works, Shanghai, China.

The ingredients are listed below in 3 separate groups according to function.

Pinyin Name	Pharmaceutical Name	Percent	TCM Function
Group 1			
Yun Xiang Qin Gao	Resina Liquidambaris (purified)	10.64	Eliminate Cold-Dampness
Group 2			
Bo He Nao	Menthol Crystals	8.51	Expel Wind-Heat;
Bing Pian	Borneol	8.51	Decrease swelling; Stop pain
Zhang Nao	Camphora	17.02	
Dong Qing Yu	Wintergreen oil	12.77	

Group 3

Fu Fang Ding Xiang Liu Qin Gao	Extractum Flos Caryophylli Liquidum Compositus	42.55	This liquid extract consists of 16 different herbal medicines which Promote Blood circulation; Stop pain; Expel Wind-Cold; Strengthen tendons and bones.

Note: 1. This is a popular and commonly used herbal plaster in China. It is convenient to use and the herbal medicines are released quickly; therefore, pain relief is rapid.

Shangshi **ZHITONG GAO**

中国上海中药制药厂出品
SHANGHAI CHINESE MEDICINE WORKS
SHANGHAI, CHINA

4.11 宝 珍 膏

Bao	Zhen	Gao
------------treasure-----------		plaster

Function: 1. Eliminate Wind-Dampness
2. Warm the Meridians; Remove Stagnation (Wind-Cold, Dampness)

Application: 1. Use to treat Bi syndrome due to Wind-Cold and Dampness Accumulation, including shoulder pain, back pain, aching muscles.

2. Use to treat sports injury or other traumatic injuries to muscles and tendons.

3. Use to treat neuralgia, rheumatism, arthritis (acute or chronic, osteoarthritis or rheumatoid arthritis).

Contraindication: Do not apply to the skin of pregnant women. Do not apply the plaster to an open wound.

How to use the plaster: The affected area should be cleaned with gentle soap and warm water before applying the plaster; applying the plaster after a warm bath is even better. The herbal medicine is inside a cloth tape with adhesive backing which is available in plasters which are approximately 2" x 3." The plasters are attached to a piece of cellophane; two plasters per piece of cellophane. Peel the plaster off the cellophane and place on the affected area. Use two or more plasters, if necessary to cover the entire area.

This herbal medicine plaster is effective for 4 or 5 days. After that time, new plasters may be re-applied for as many days as necessary. Water does not affect the herbal medicine, therefore, the patient may wear the plasters while bathing or swimming.

If the patient has an allergic skin reaction to the adhesive tape or redness, itching or skin irritation appears, do not use it.

The plasters contain many aromatic ingredients, therefore it is important to keep the unused plasters in a tight container.

Bao Zhen Gao is produced as "Shang Shi Bao Zhen Gao" by the Shanghai Medicine Works, Shanghai, China in boxes of 10 plasters.

The ingredients are listed below in 4 separate groups according to function.

Pinyin Name	Pharmaceutical Name	Percent	TCM Function
Group 1			
She Xiang	Secretio Moschus moschiferi	0.62	Warm the Meridians; Promote Blood circulation; Decrease swelling; Stop pain
Group 2			
Yun Xiang Qin Gao	Resina Liquidambaris (purified)	17.74	Eliminate Cold-Dampness
Group 3			
Bo He Nao	Menthol Crystals	7.1	Expel Wind-Heat; Decrease swelling;
Zhang Nao	Camphora	7.1	Stop pain
Dong Qing Yu	Wintergreen oil	14.2	

Group 4

Fu Fang Xi Xin Liu Qin Gao	Extractum Herba Asari Liquidum Compositus	53.25	This liquid extract consists of several different herbal medicines which Promote Blood circulation; Stop pain; Expel Wind-Cold

Note: 1. The major difference between this formula, #4.11, Bao Zhen Gao, and #4.10, Shang Shi Zhi Tong Gao, is that this formula contains She Xiang, Secretio Moschus, which provides strong action to Promote Qi and Blood circulation to Remove Stagnation. The She Xiang is also able to quickly penetrate into deep tissues, thus leading the other herbs into the deep tissues as well. This medicine is particularly good for neuralgia, arthritis and muscle pain.

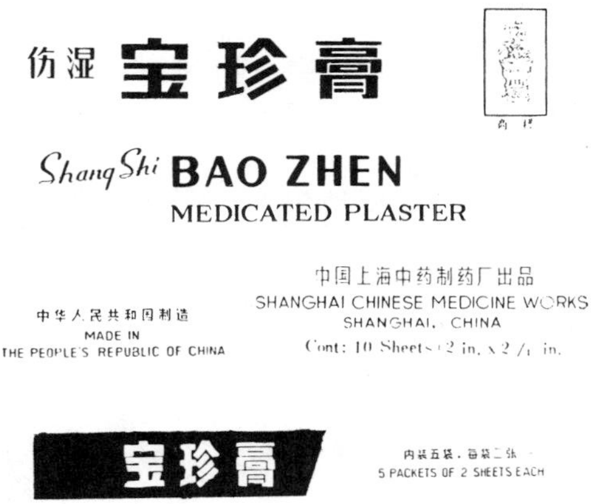
伤湿 宝珍膏
Shang Shi BAO ZHEN
MEDICATED PLASTER
中国上海中药制药厂出品
SHANGHAI CHINESE MEDICINE WORKS
SHANGHAI, CHINA
中华人民共和国制造
MADE IN
THE PEOPLE'S REPUBLIC OF CHINA
宝珍膏
内装五袋，每袋二张
5 PACKETS OF 2 SHEETS EACH

4.12 追风活血片

Zhui	Feng	Huo	Xue	Pian
eliminate	wind	promote circulation	Blood	tablets

Function: 1. Promote Blood circulation; Relax tendons
2. Eliminate Wind-Cold in the Meridians

Application: 1. Use to treat Bi syndrome due to Wind-Cold-Dampness. (In this case the Wind-Cold is stronger than the Dampness.) Symptoms: Feeling of cold and numbness in the limbs, weakness in the legs and lumbar area, rheumatism, chronic arthritis, joint or muscle pain. The pain may be sharp or travelling and there is more sharp pain than dull pain. (The dull pain would be associated with Dampness.)

2. Use to treat long-term sequelae following sports or traumatic injuries where there is aching in the tendons, muscles or joints; dysfunction may be present.

Contraindication: Do not use with pregnant women.

Dose: 4 tablets, 2 times a day

Zhui Feng Huo Xue Pian is produced as "Chui Feng Huohsueh" by the Siping Pharmaceutic Works, Kirin, China, in bottles of 80 coated tablets.

The ingredients are listed below in 3 separate groups according to function.

Pinyin Name	Pharmaceutical Name	Percent	TCM Function
Group 1			
Gui Zhi	Ramulus Cinnamomi Cassiae	6	Eliminate Wind-Cold; Warm the Meridian circulation; Stop pain
Du Huo	Angelica pubescens Maxim. or A.	6	
Ma Huang	Herba Ephedrae	5	
Fang Feng	Radix Ledebouriellae Sesloidis	8	
Di Feng	Cortex Illici Defebgpi	6	
Qiang Huo	Rhizoma et Radix Notopterygii	6	
Group 2			
Ru Xiang	Gummi Olibanum	8	Promote Blood circulation; Stop pain; Decrease inflammation and promote healing of injured tissues
Zi Ran Tong	Pyritum	5	
Mo Yao	Myrrha	8	
Group 3			
Du Zhong	Cortex Eucommiae Ulmoidis	12	Strengthen Liver and Kidney; Reinforce tendons and bones
Qian Nian Jian	Rhizoma Homalomenae Occultae	6	
Mu Gua	Fructus Chaenomelis Lagenariae	6	
Niu Xi	Radix Achyranthis Bidentatae	6	
Additional herbs:			
Gan Cao	Radix Glycyrrhizae Uralensis	5	Harmonize other herbs
Feng Mi	Honey	5	Used as medium

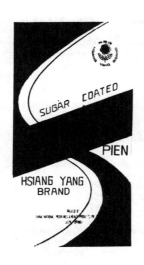

SUGAR COATED
PIEN
HSIANG YANG
BRAND

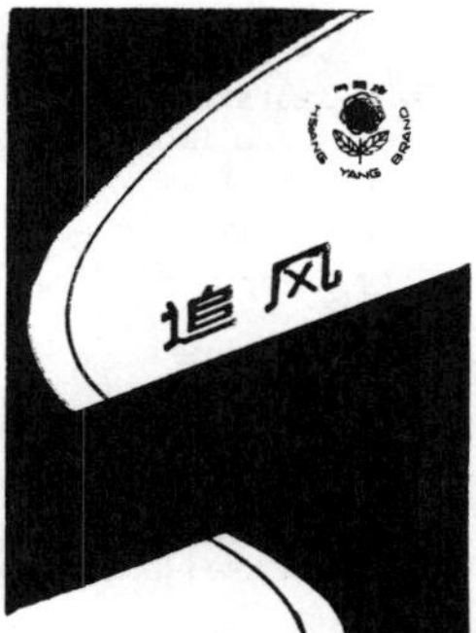
追风
中國醫藥保健品進出口
吉林省分公司

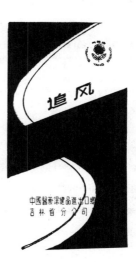

4.13 雲 香 精

雲	香	精
Yun	**Xiang**	**Jing**
cloud	fragrance	extract

Function: 1. Stop pain, decrease swelling

2. Regulate Stomach Qi

Application: 1. Use to treat Bi Syndrome (Wind, Cold, Dampness in muscles or joints). This includes rheumatism, arthritis, and rheumatoid arthritis.

2. Use to treat neuralgia due to Wind, Cold, Dampness.

3. Use to stop headache pain due to flu, common cold (Wind-Cold syndrome)

4. Use to treat stomach ache or abdominal pain due to improper eating (too much cold food), or common cold, flu (Wind-Cold syndrome). Also use to treat motion sickness.

5. Use to treat poor circulation in the extremities. Use to treat frostbite anywhere, including fingers, toes, nose, ear, etc.

6. Use to treat early stage of carbuncles or skin sores to help decrease inflammation and swelling.

Contraindication: Do not use internally with pregnant women.

Usage: The medicine can be used for external or internal use. Each bottle contains 30 cc.

External: Use with applications 1, 2, 3, 5 and 6. Use as a lotion, externally, with a cotton ball. Rub the lotion on the affected area. Each day, apply 2 or 3 times. It is not necessary to cover the area after use. The lotion is clear, with a water base.

Internal: Use with applications 3 and 4. Do not give internally to children less than 3 years of age. From age 3 to 7 years, use 1 cc; between 8 to 15 years, 1.5 cc; over age 16, use 2 cc. Mix the medicine with water before taking, in a ratio of 9 parts water to 1 part medicine. This medicine should be used for acute or emergency cases; therefore, it is usually used only once, but it may be repeated in another 4 hours. For a serious case, the dose of the medicine may be increased, but the dose must be less than double-dose. If the patient takes too much of this medicine and side effects are present, use the loose herb, Huang Lian (Rhizoma Coptidis, Cold Property), to make a tea to treat the side effects.

Yun Xiang Jing is produced by the Yulin Drug Manufactory, Kwangsi, China in 30 cc bottles.

There are 5 major ingredients which are listed below, according to function. The percentages are not included because they are not available from the manufacturer.

Pinyin Name	Pharmaceutical Name	TCM Function
Group 1		
Guo Jiang Long	(Not available)	Promote Blood Circulation;
Chuan Bi Feng	(Not available)	Decrease joint swelling; Stop pain; Eliminate rheumatism
Group 2		
Gui Zhi	Ramulus Cinnamomi Cassiae	Expel Wind Cold; Promote Blood circulation;
Xi Xin	Herba Asari cum Radice	Stop pain from Bi Syndrome
Group 3		
Bo He Nao	Herba Menthae Crystal	Stop pain; Decrease inflammation; Regulate Stomach Qi. When used externally, it will stop itching on the skin

Note: 1. The Patent Medicine, Bai Hua You, is similar to Yun Xiang Jing.

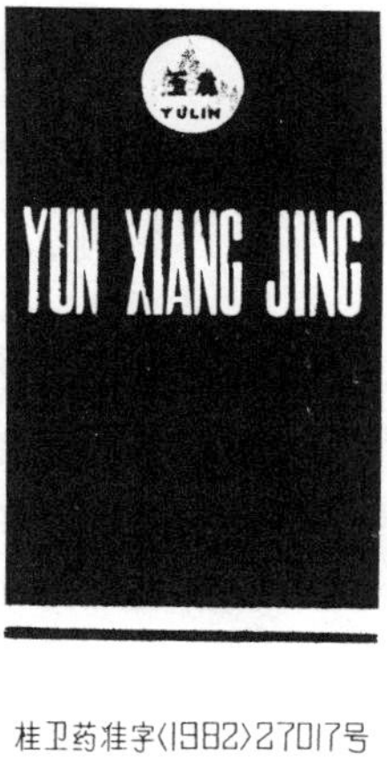

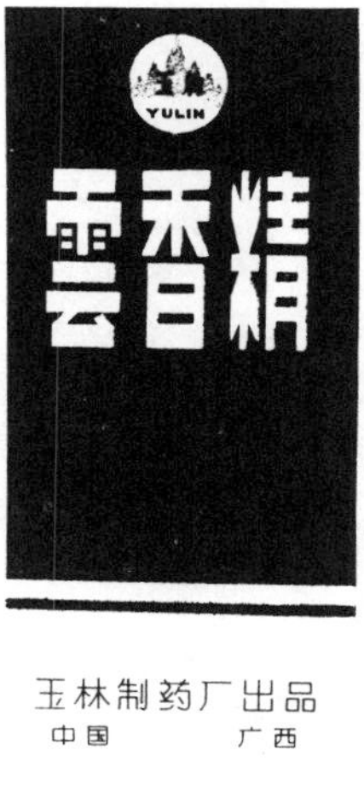

Chapter 5. Open Orifices

(Includes Patent Medicines used with High Fevers, Coma, etc.)

Section A. **Open Orifices with Cold Property Herbs**

Section B. **Open Orifices with Warm Property Herbs**

5.1 紫 雪 丹

Zi	**Xue**	**Dan**
purple	snow	crystals

Source: Tai Ping Hui Min He Ji Ju Fang, (Formulas of The People's Welfare Pharmacy), 1151 A.D., Song Dynasty, 960-1279.

Function:
1. Clear Heat, especially Heat in the Pericardium
2. Reduce spasm
3. Open Orifices (Waken patient from unconsciousness or coma)
4. Clear Fire Poison (Eliminate inflammation caused by infection)

Application: 1. Use to treat Heat Evil in the Pericardium, especially for children, but also for adults. This formula is particularly effective to Clear Heat and relieve coma and spasms due to Heat. The Heat may have been caused by infection, such as pneumonia, tonsillitis, dysentery or flu. Symptoms: The patient has Heat signs from the onset, including high-grade fever and no feeling of chilliness; thirst, constipation, dark yellow urine and uneasiness or unconsciousness may also be present.

2. Some Western medicine disease applications include the following: (Note, The above-mentioned Heat signs must be present.) Epidemic encephalitis (serious brain infection due to Heat Evil in the summer); cerebrospinal meningitis (may be viral) in winter or spring. (Even if this formula saves the patient's life, there may be some after-effects from the disease.) Children's measles with high-grade fever and dark purple rash on the skin. (Complications from this may be present such as pneumonia.)

Contraindication: Do not use with pregnant women.

Dose: Adults: 2 vials, 2 times a day.
Children less than 1 Year: one-half vial, 2 times a day.
Children more than 1 Year: 1 vial, 2 times a day.

Take with warm water. Be sure that the patient drinks all the medicine; the cinnabar sinks to the bottom.

Use this formula until the fever has returned to normal. If the fever has not been greatly reduced within 3 days, re-confirm the diagnosis or use another preparation to Clear Heat.

Zi Xue Dan is produced as "Tzuhsueh Tan" by the Guangzhou United Drug Manufactory, Guangzhou, China, in vials containing 0.8 grams.

Pinyin Name	Pharmaceutical Name	Percent	TCM Function
Hua Shi	Talcum	7.1	Clear Heat; Promote urination
Ding Xiang	Flos Caryophylli	0.7	Open Orifices; Move Qi
Shi Gao	Gypsum	7.1	Clear Heat; Reduce Fire Poison
Sheng Ma	Rhizoma Cimicifugae	7.1	Clear Heat; Reduce Fire Poison
Han Shui Shi	Calcitum	7.1	Clear Heat; Reduce Fire Poison
Xuan Shen	Radix Scrophulariae Ningpoensis	7.1	Clear Heat; Cool Blood; Reduce Fire Poison
Ci Shi	Magnetitum	14.3	Tranquilize Spirit; Calm the patient; Stop spasm
Gan Cao	Radix Glycyrrhizae Uralensis	5.7	Clear Heat; Detoxify

Gan Cao	Radix Glycyrrhizae Uralensis	5.7	Clear Heat; Detoxify
Ling Yang Jiao	Cornu Antelopis	3.6	Clear Heat; Stop spasm
Mang Xiao	Mirabilitum	14.3	Clear Heat in Intestines, move stool
Mu Xiang	Radix Saussureae seu Vladimiriae	3.6	Move Qi
Xiao Xi	Nitrum	14.3	Clear Heat; Remove Heat Stasis
Xi Jiao	Cornu Rhinoceri	3.6	Clear Heat; Open Orifices
She Xiang	Secretio Moschus moschiferi	0.8	Open Orifices
Chen Xiang	Lignum Aquilariae	3.6	Move Qi; Remove Stuck Qi and Heat Stasis
Zhu Sha	Cinnabaris	(Amount not specified)	Clear Heat, Tranquilize the Spirit

Notes: 1. This Patent Medicine is effective, but also expensive. It is considered to be one of the "Three Treasures" in Chinese medicine to Clear Heat in serious cases. The Three Treasures include 1) An Gong Niu Huang Wan, #5.2; 2) Zi Xue, #5.1; and 3) Ju Fang Zhi Bao Dan. All three of these have a similar effect in that they Clear Heat, Detoxify Fire Poison, Stop spasm and Open Orifices. All three are used to treat Seasonal Febrile Diseases with high-grade fever, unconsciousness and Phlegm Heat Retention.

The special function of each of these "Treasures" is as follows: An Gong Niu Huang Wan, #5.2, has the greatest Cold property strength. It has a strong effect to Clear Heat and Detoxify Fire Poison. It is used to treat high-grade fever with unconsciousness. In Zi Xue, #5.1, the Cold property strength is between that of An Gong Niu Huang Wan and Ju Fang Zhi Bao Dan. Zi Xue is used to Clear Heat and Stop spasm. It is used to treat spasm caused by high-grade fever. In Ju Fang Zhi Bao Dan, the Cold property strength is less than that in Zi Xue. The specialty for Ju Fang Zhi Bao Dan is to Open Orifices and Eliminate turbid Phlegm Retention. It is used to treat patients with spasm, seizures and/or coma.

3. The name, "Purple Snow," has the following origin: The color of the compound is purple, and the shape of the "crystal-like powder" is similar to frost, or snowflakes. It has an extreme Cold property, which is said to be "as cold as snow."

4. There are 2 alternate names for "Zi Xue." One is "Zi Xue San" which means "Purple Snow Powder." The other name is "Zi Xue Dan." The term "Dan" refers to a Patent Medicine form which contains mineral or metal ingredients.

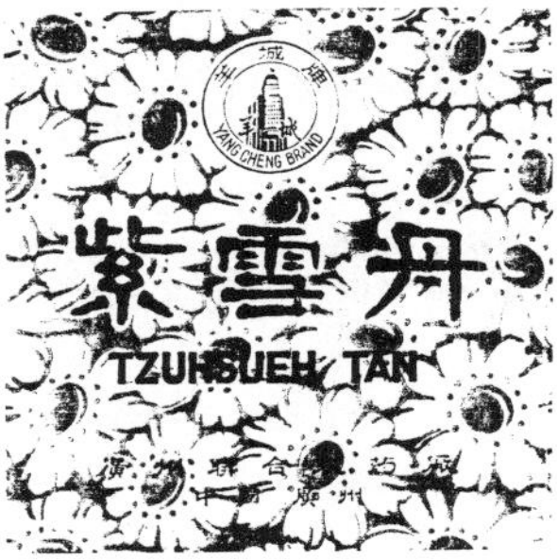

5.2 安 宮 牛 黃 丸

安	宮	牛	黃	丸
An	**Gong**	**Niu**	**Huang**	**Wan**
peaceful	Pericardium	cow	gallstone	pills

Source: Wen Bing Tiao Bian, (More Discussion of Febrile Diseases), Qing Dynasty, 1644-1911.

Function: 1. Clear Heat; Detoxify Fire Poison
2. Open Heart Orifices; Remove Phlegm Heat Accumulation

Application: 1. Use to treat Seasonal Febrile Disease with high-grade fever, unconsciousness, delirium and agitation due to blockage of Heart Orifices with Phlegm Heat Accumulation. The TCM diagnosis is Heat Evil attacks the Pericardium, causing Pericardium syndrome which is similar to Heart syndrome. Additional symptoms to those listed above, include a red Tongue with yellow or white, greasy coating (in the earlier stage, the Tongue coating is white; in the later stage, the Tongue coating is yellow, when the body fluid has been damaged); the Pulse is rapid and full.

2. Use to treat children's spasms due to high-grade fever.

3. Some Western medicine disease applications include the following: (Note: In order to use this with the disorders listed below, the patient must have signs of Phlegm Heat Accumulation.) Stroke (apoplexy); seizures; coma due to high-grade fever in acute epidemic diseases such as epidemic encephalitis B, bacillary dysentery; coma due to other serious infections, such as septicemia.

Contraindication: Do not use with pregnant women.

Dose: 1 pill orally, 1 or 2 times per day. For serious cases, 1 pill, 3 times a day. Each honey pill weighs 3 grams. This formula is also available in powder form.

If the patient has extra Phlegm as the primary symptom, an herbal tea should be prepared as the Yao Yin for taking this medicine. The Yao Yin should be made with Tian Zhu Huang (Concretio Silicea Bambusae, cooked 20 minutes) or Zhu Li (Succus Bambusae, fresh bamboo juice). Use 6 grams of the herb to make one cup of herbal tea.

If the patient has a high-grade fever as the primary symptom, a Yao Yin should be used to take the medicine made of Jin Yin Hua (Flos Lonicerae Japonicae, 10 grams per cup of herbal tea, cooked only 10 to 15 minutes) and Bo He (Herba Menthae, 6 grams per cup of herbal tea, cooked together with the Jin Yin Hua).

If the patient has constipation, another Yao Yin should be used. Dissolve the honey pill in warm water and mix with 10 grams of Da Huang (Rhizoma Rhei) powder. The patient should drink this liquid.

An Gong Niu Huang Wan is produced by the Beijing Tung Jen Tang pharmacy in boxes of 10 honey pills coated with gold powder.

The contents are listed below in 5 groups according to function.

Pinyin Name	Pharmaceutical Name	Percent	TCM Function
Group 1 (The major ingredients are in this group)			
Niu Huang	Calculus Bovis	11.11	Clear Heart Heat; Detoxify Fire Poison; Expel Phlegm Accumulation
Xi Jiao	Cornu Rhinoceri	11.11	Clear Heart Heat; Clear Heat in Blood Stage; Detoxify Fire Poison
She Xiang	Secretio Moschus moschiferi	2.78	Open Orifices; Waken the Patient from unconcsiousness
Group 2			
Huang Lian	Rhizoma Coptidis	11.11	Clear Heat;
Huang Qin	Radix Scutellariae Baicalensis	11.11	Detoxify Fire Poison
Zhi Zi	Fructus Jasminoidis Gardeniae	11.11	
Group 3			
Xiong Huang	Realgar	11.11	Detoxify Fire Poison; Expel Phlegm Accumulation
Group 4			
Bing Pian	Borneol	2.78	Fragrant Property to Open the
Yu Jin	Tuber Curcumae	11.11	Orifices; Remove Turbid Blockage of Heart Orifices
Group 5			
Zhu Sha	Cinnabaris	11.11	Calm the Spirit; Stop spasm;
Zhen Zhu	Magarita	5.56	Stop tremor

Notes: 1. The principle ingredient in this formula, Niu Huang (Calculus Bovis), has the special function to open the Heart Orifices, Clear Heat and Calm the Pericardium. Therefore, the name An Gong (Calm the Pericardium) Niu Huang (Calculus Bovis) Wan. In TCM the Heart controls the Spirit (consciousness). When a patient has a Seasonal Febrile Disease, there is always a high-grade fever, which can cause unconsciousness and delirium. Therefore, for this condition, a medicine which Clears Heat and Opens the Heart Orifices is always used.

2. This medicine may be coated with gold powder for two reasons. 1. The gold is a medicine which is heavy, therefore it will Calm the Spirit and Tranquilize. 2. The manufacturers prefer to use the gold in producing special medicines such as this one, to show that it is not a common, everyday, medicine. It is important that the patient take the entire honey pill, including the gold powder which is on the outside.

3. This Patent Medicine, An Gong Niu Huang Wan, is a modification of the formula, Wan Shi Niu Huang Qing Xin Wan. They have similar functions, although An Gong Niu Huang Wan is more effective.

4. During the "Cultural Revolution," 1967-1977, the name of this medicine was changed from An Gong Niu Huang Wan to Kang Re (Against Heat) Niu Huang Wan. The name was changed, because during that time, the term "Gong," meaning "Palace" of the Heart (Pericardium) was forbidden. The Red Guard believed that the term "Palace" was associated with Feudalism and therefore, it was removed from the title of the Patent Medicine.

5. This medicine is usually used only with a serious or emergency case. In China, the injection form is also available for intravenous use.

6. An Gong Niu Huang Wan is one of the Three Treasures for Seasonal Febrile Disease (An Gong Niu Huang Wan, 5.1, Zi Xue Dan and Ju Fang Zhi Bau Dan). See Notes under 5.1, Zi Xue Dan. This Patent Medicine is in the current Chinese Pharmacopoeia.

Case History: Clinical experience with an infant, of Dr. Mei Zhu, O.M.D., Beijing, China. Cited from his book, Clinical Experience with Chinese Herbal Medicines, In Preparation.

This Patent Medicine was used successfully to treat Thrush (infection of the oral mucous membrane by Candida albicans, characterized by superficial, confluent white patches on a red, moist, inflammatory surface). The powder form (0.3 grams, twice a day) was first used each time with water, then it was followed by the use of an herbal tea formula. (If the honey pill is used with an infant, use 1/3 honey pill each time.) The herbal tea formula consisisted of the following herbs: Sheng Di, 6 grams; Lu Gen, 20g; Zhu Ye, 6g; Jin Yin Hua, 10g; Gou Teng, 6g; Bo He, 3g; Shan Zha, 3g; Shen Qu, 3g; Sheng Shi Gao, 15g. This would make one cup of herbal tea, when cooked down after 20 minutes (the Sheng Shi Gao must be cooked for 10 mintues longer than the other ingredients, therefore it is put in before the other ingredients). This cup of herbal tea would be used for two doses in an infant.

5.3 万 氏 牛 黄 清 心 丸

Wan	Shi	Niu	Huang	Qing	Xin	Wan
name, Wan	family	cow	gallstone	Clear Heat	Hrt.syndrome	pills

Source: Do Zhen Shi Yi Xin Fa, by Wan Mi-zhai, Ming Dynasty (1368-1644); and Jing Yue Quan Shu, (Complete Works of Jing Yue), Ming Dynasty (1368-1644).

Function: 1. Clear Heat, Unblock obstructed Heart Orifices; Waken the patient from unconsciousness
2. Calm restlessness due to Heat
3. Waken the patient from unconsciousness where high fever has lead to coma

Application: 1. Use to treat Outside Heat Factor attacks the Pericardium. Symptoms: Unconsciousness, delirious speech, uneasiness with high fever.

2. Some Western medicine disease applications include the following: (Note, this formula may only be used when the above-mentioned Heat signs are present.) Acute stroke, encephalitis (may be viral); cerebrospinal meningitis (may be viral); infantile convulsions; serious pneumonia; high-grade fever caused by infection (> 39 C); kidney function failure leading to unconsciousness with fever; liver function failure leading to unconsciousness with fever; essential hypertension.

Contraindications: Do not use with pregnant women or patients with Def.Yin

Dose: Adults: One 3-gram honey pill 2 times a day Children less than 1 year: One-half pill 2 times a day

Wan Shi Niu Huang Qing Xin Wan is produced by the Beijing Tung Jen Tang pharmacy in honey pill form with 10 pills per box.

Pinyin Name	Pharmaceutical Name	Grams	TCM Function
Niu Huang	Calculus Bovis	10	Clear Heat, Open Heart Orifices
Zhi Zi	Fructus Gardeniae Jasminoidis	120	Clear Heat in Heart
Huang Lian	Rhizoma Coptidis	200	Clear Heat
Huang Qin	Radix Scutellariae Baicalensis	120	Clear Heat
Yu Jin	Tuber Curcumae	80	Eliminate Phlegm; Open Orifices
Zhu Sha	Cinnabaris	60	Tranquilize the Spirit

Note: 1. The effect of this formula is not as strong as the Three Treasures medicines, thus, this medicine is not used for the most serious, critical cases.

5.4 冠 心 苏 合 丸

冠	心	苏	合	丸
Guan	**Xin**	**Su**	**He**	**Wan**
coronary	Heart	----Styrax Liquidis----		pills

Function: 1. Open Heart Orifices and Move Stagnation in the Chest through aromatic property herbs
2. Regulate Qi and Stop pain

Application: 1. Use to treat symptoms related to coronary heart (coronary artery) disease due to Stagnation of Qi. Symptoms: Chest fullness, chest pain or pressure, angina. This formula may improve the EKG faster than #12.1, Fu Fang Dan Shen Pian. This formula will distend the arteries of the heart, thus improving the Blood supply to the heart muscle.

2. Use to improve Blood circulation in patients with cold in the extremities.

3. In China, many people use this formula to prevent, as well as to treat, angina. This formula will not interfere with other Western medicines used to treat heart disease.

Contraindication: This formula, Guan Xin Su He Wan, is used for coronary heart disease due to Stagnation of Qi associated with Cold Evil. Do not use this formula if the coronary heart disease is casued by another disharmony such as Stagnation of Blood with symptoms such as fixed, stabbing, strong, sharp pain (possibly worse at night); also palpitations may be present. The Tongue is dark purple and the Pulse is deep and choppy. If the coronary heart disease is due to Stagnation of Blood, use #12.1, Fu Fang Dan Shen Pian.

Dose: 2 capsules, 2 times a day.

Guan Xin Su He Wan is produced as "Guanxin Su Ho" by the Tianjin Drug Manufactory, Tianjin, China, in bottles of 40 capsules.

Pinyin Name	Pharmaceutical Name	Percent	TCM Function
Su He Xiang	Styrax Liquidis	8	Open Orifices
Bing Pian	Borneol	15	Aromatically Open Orifices
Tan Xiang	Lignum Santali Albi	31	Move Qi; Stop pain
Ru Xiang	Gummi Oliganum	15	Promote Blood circulation; Stop pain; Move Blood Stagnation
Mu Hu Die	Semen Oroxyli Indici	31	Move Qi

Note: 1. This formula is a modification of the formula, Su He Xiang Wan, developed during the Song Dynasty (960-1279) to treat Bi syndrome. Su He Xiang Wan was also used to Open Heart Orifices and waken the patient from unconsciousness associated with Zhong Feng (apoplexy).

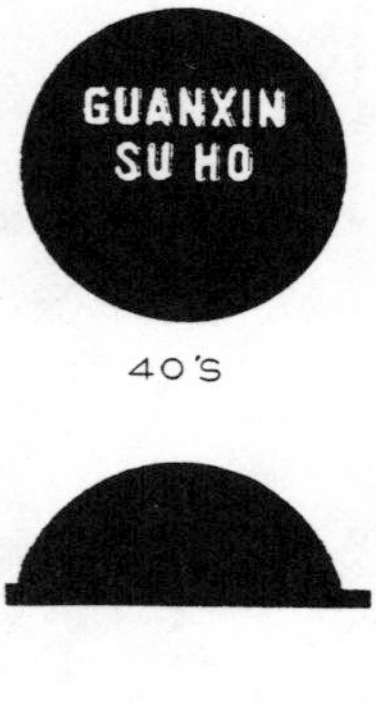

Chapter 6. Treat Tremors and Spasms due to Wind

(Includes Patent Medicines used with stroke cases; also some used to reduce itching)

Section A. **Dispel External Wind**

Section B. **Extinguish Internal Wind**

6.1 天 麻 丸

Tian Ma Wan

-------Gastrodiae-------- pills

Source: Jing Yue Quan Shu, (Jing Yue's Complete Works), Ming Dynasty, 1368-1644.

Function: 1. Dispel Wind; Promote Blood circulation
2. Relax the tendons; Stop pain

Application: 1. Use to treat headaches due to OPI Wind-Cold

2. Use to treat migraine headaches.

3. Use to treat numbness of the limbs due to poor Blood circulation or stroke (Zhong Feng)

4. Use to treat rheumatic pain caused by Wind-Cold or Dampness (Bi syndrome)

5. Use to treat post-stroke paralysis for face, arm or leg.

6. Use to treat Bell's Palsy (this formula is especially effective for this). See also 6.3, Da Huo Luo Dan.

Dose: 4-6 tablets, 2 or 3 times a day.

Tian Ma Wan is produced by the Min-Kang Drug Manufactory, I-Chang, China, in bottles of 100 pills.

Pinyin Name	Pharmaceutical Name	Percent	TCM Function
Tian Ma	Rhizoma Gastrodia Elata	8.2	Expel Wind; Stop pain
Du Zhong	Eucommia Ulmoides	9.6	Supplement Liver, Kidney; Strengthen tendons and bones
Niu Xi	Radix Achyranthis Bidentatae	8.2	Supplement Liver, Kidney. Strengthen tendons and bones
Du Huo	Radix Duhuo	6.9	Expel Wind-Cold; Stop lower body pain
Qiang Huo	Rhizoma et Radix Notopterygii	13.7	Expel Wind-Cold; Stop upper body pain
Dang Gui	Angelica Sinensis	13.7	Tonify Blood; Promote Blood circulation
Bi Xie	Rhizoma Dioscoreae	8.2	Eliminate Dampness
Di Huang	Radix Rehmanniae Glutinosae Conquitae	21.9	Nourish Yin; Tonify Blood
Xuan Shen	Radix Scrophulariae Ningpoensis	8.2	Nourish Yin
	Medium to 100%		

Notes: 1. In the original source, Tian Ma Wan was labelled Yi LaoTian Ma Wan and included Fu Zi, which is not always included today. Currently, when a manufacturer makes this Patent Medicine, a slight change is made in the original formula, and a new name is added. Five examples with new names are given below:

1) The Patent Medicine, Tian Ma Wan, made by the Min-Kang Drug Manufactory, I Chang, China, is made with the original formula, however, Fu Zi has been omitted.

2) The Patent Medicine, Tian Ma Tou Feng Pian, made in Tientsin, China, is made with the same formula as Yi Lao Tian Ma Wan and includes Fu Zi.

3) The Patent Medicine, Qu Feng Tian Ma Wan, is made by other manufactories outside of Tientsin using the same formula as Yi Lao Tian Ma Wan.

4) The Patent Medicine, Tian Ma Qu Feng Bu Pian, (Kunming Native Drugs Factory, Yunnan, China) is made with the Yi Lao Tian Ma Wan formula, however, 3 herbs are omitted, Yuan Shen, Du Huo and Bi Xie; and one is added, Rou Gui. This formula omitted two herbs which Expel Wind and Wind Cold Dampness, and omitted Yuan Shen which has a Cold property. One very Hot property medicine was added, Rou Gui. Thus, this formula is more Warming and Tonifying than the original formula. The Patent Medicine, Tian Ma Qu Feng Bu Pian, is used to treat patients who have more Cold syndrome with Def. Yang; it will have a better effect in warming the Meridian circulation. It is especially useful for treating elderly patients or chronic cases.

5) The Patent Medicine, Tian Ma Hu Gu Wan, has omitted several ingredients from the original formula for Tian Ma Wan. The omitted ingredients are strong medicines to eliminate Wind, Cold and Dampness, including Du Huo, Qiang Huo, and Fu Zi. These herbs are very Warm and very Dry; they may damage the Blood or body fluid (Yin). Tian Ma Hu Gu Wan uses a gentle herb, Gao Ben, to eliminate Wind and Dampness. Tian Ma Hu Gu Wan also contains several Tonic herbs which were not included in the original formula for Tian Ma Wan, including Ginseng and Os Tigris. Thus, this formula is especially well-suited for use with elderly patients who have rheumatism or arthritis, which is mostly related to Def. Liver and Kidney causing weakness of the tendons and bones. This formula is similar in function to #13.18, Jian Bu Hu Qian Wan.

2. Case History: MN was treating a 35 year old woman in Boston for chronic migraine headaches using Tian Ma Wan. The patient also had a one year history of TMJ pain on the same side as the migraine headaches. After using the Tian Ma Wan for a few weeks, the migraine headaches were reduced as well as the TMJ pain. The patient continued to use Tian Ma Wan for a few months to help prevent the return of the headaches and the TMJ pain.

3. Case History: MN was treating a 39 year old woman in Boston with hypersomnia, Raynaud's and amenorrhea using combination of Patent Medicines, including Tian Ma Wan, 6.1; Ren Shen Lu Rong Wan, 13.24 (because there were signs of Cold, and Def. Kidney Yang); and Wu Ji Bai Feng Wan, 12.12 (because the period was originally an 8 week cycle). After two months, the sleep episodes were less severe; after several months, the period was regulated to 6 weeks, then 4 weeks; the Raynaud's was also less severe.

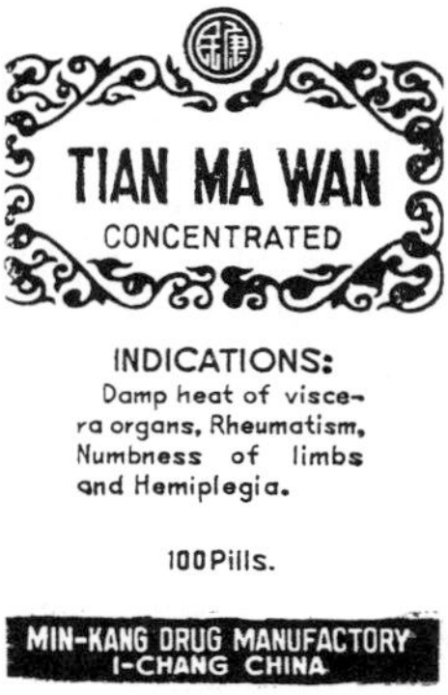
TIAN MA WAN
CONCENTRATED
INDICATIONS:
Damp heat of viscera organs, Rheumatism, Numbness of limbs and Hemiplegia.
100Pills.
MIN-KANG DRUG MANUFACTORY
I-CHANG CHINA

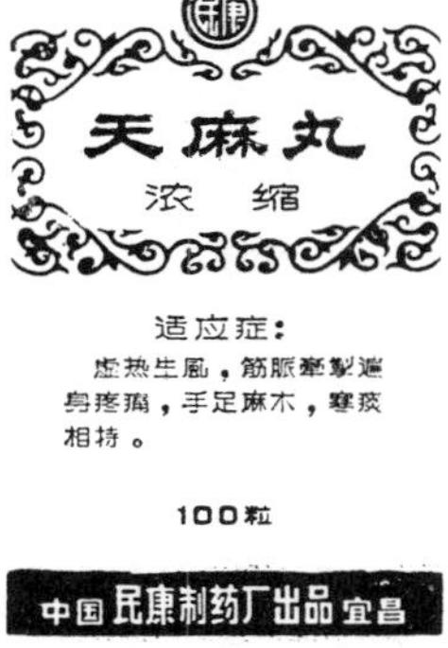
天麻丸
浓缩
适应症：
100粒
中国民康制药厂出品宜昌

6.2 花 蛇 解 瘙 丸

Hua	She	Jie	Yang	Wan
-------colorful snake-------		eliminate	itching	pills

Function: 1. Strengthen Qi; Nourish Blood

2. Eliminate Wind; Stop itching

Application: 1. Use to treat itching on the skin due to Wind Factor. This medicine is especially useful in treating chronic itching seen in cases with Deficiency. In TCM theory, itching on the skin is due to Wind Factor. The Wind Factor accumulates on the surface of the skin. Two types of herbal medicines are used to Eliminate the Wind and stop the itching: 1) Herbs which Expel Wind and 2) Herbs which Extinguish Wind by Nourishing the Blood. This Patent Medicine contains herbs which Eliminate Wind both by Expelling the Wind and by Nourishing the Blood.

2. Some Western medicine disease applications include the following: Erythematous eczema; and itching caused by drug allergy.

Contraindication: Do not eat seafood, bamboo shoots, or goose while taking this medicine.

Dose: Adults: 5 pills, 3 times per day Children: Use half-dose

Hua She Jie Yang Wan is produced as "Kai Yeung Pill" by the Hanyang Pharmaceutical Works, Hong Kong, in bottles of 50 pills.

The herbs are listed below in 3 separate groups according to function.

Pinyin Name	Pharmaceutical Name	Percent	TCM Function
Group 1			
Huang Qi	Radix Astragali	10	Strengthen Qi; Strengthen Yang
Ren Shen	Radix Ginseng	10	Energy on the surface of the body
Group 2			
Dang Gui	Radix Angelicae Sinensis	10	Nourish Blood;
Chuan Xiong	Radix Ligustici Wallichii	10	Extinguish Internal Wind
Sheng Di	Radix Rehmanniae Glutinosae	5	
Group 3			
Bai Zhi	Radix Angelicae	10	Expel Wind; Dry Dampness;
Fang Feng	Radix Ledebouriellae Sesloidis	5	Stop itching
Cang Er Zi	Fructus Xanthii	5	
Bai Hua She	Agkistrodon seu Bungarus	10	
Wu Shao She	Zaocys Dhumnades	5	
She Chuang Zi	Semen Cnidii Monnieri	10	
Cang Zhu	Rhizoma Atractylodis	10	

Note: 1. The Patent Medicine, San She Jie Yang Wan is similar to Hua She Jie Yang Wan. The formula in Hua She Jie Yang Wan contains more herbs to Expel Wind and Nourish Blood; this is most effective for use when the weather is windy and cold, or when the weather is suddenly changing to increased wind and cold. The formula in San She Jie Yang Wan contains several Cold property medicines, such as Niu Huang and Dan Pi, to Clear Heat. Hence, this formula is also good to use to treat a Damp Heat syndrome. For example, San She Jie Yang Wan is used when itching is accompanied by a rash which has a darker color than that observed when Hua She Jie Yang Wan is used. (The patient may not even have a rash where the Hua She Jie Yang Wan is used.) When San She Jie Yang Wan is used, the patient may have a dark red rash or even blistering (due to Dampness). San She Jie Yang Wan is also useful in treating other disorders where Dampness is present, such as leukorrhea with itching.

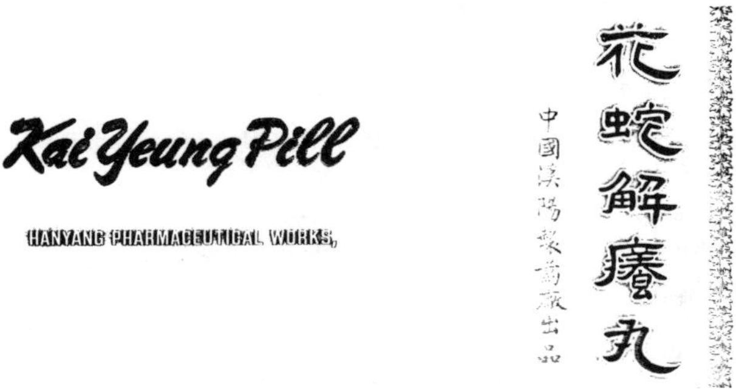

Another Patent Medicine used to reduce itching, Chuan Shan Jia Chu Shi Ching Du Wan, produced as "Armadillo Counter Poison Pill" by the United Pharmaceutical Works, Guangdong, is shown below. The dose is 4 pills, 3 times a day.

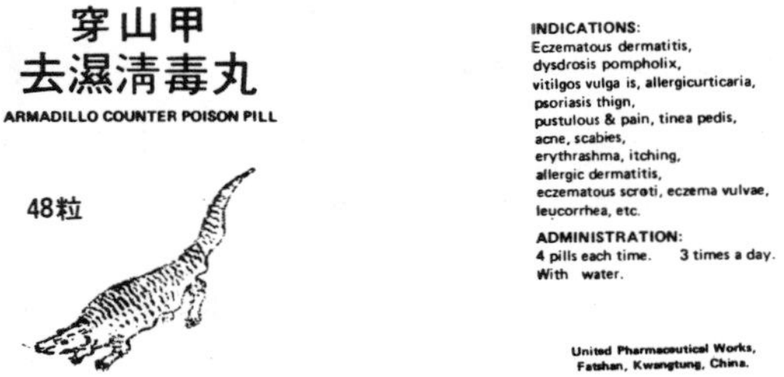

Case History: MN was treating a 36 year old woman in Boston for problems with hives which occurred especially during the last 2 weeks of the menstrual cycle. She had had this problem for over 3 years, and had been treated with antihistamines, with only minimal results. After using the "Chuan Shan Jia Chu Shi Ching Du Wan," shown above, (for Wind, and the External Heat signs), plus #13.20, Zhi Bai Di Huang Wan (for Deficient Yin, and signs of Empty Fire, Internal Heat), for one month, her hives were greatly reduced with the next menstrual cycle, and she was able to reduce the amount of the antihistamines by more than half.

63 大 活 络 丹

Da	Huo	Luo	Dan
great	activate	Meridians	pill

Source: Lan Tai Gui Fan, (Regulations from Lan Tai), Qing Dynasty, 1644-1911.

Function: 1. Promote (stimulate) smooth circulation of Blood and Qi to relax muscles and tendons.

2. Expel Wind and Cold.

3. Stop spasm; Stop pain.

Applications: 1. Use to treat limb numbness due to Wind Evil, Zhong Feng (Apoplexy); rheumatism or poor circulation.

2. Use to treat back pain, leg pain or stiff limbs (rheumatism) when Exogenous Wind Evil has affected the patient who usually has Def. Qi.

3. Use to treat sequelae of stroke (Zhong Feng, apoplexy) as soon as possible after the patient's medical and neurological conditions are stable. (Do not use while bleeding is still occurring in hemorrhage cases.) Can also be used for sequelae from head injury cases after the medical and neurological conditions are stable. Symptoms: Facial paralysis, limb paralysis (paralysis may be spastic or flaccid), impaired speech and articulation. The patient should also be receiving Physical Therapy and Speech Therapy while taking this herbal medicine, if possible.

4. Use to treat facial paralysis due to Bell's Palsy. This is more effective if it is used as soon as possible following onset. Acupuncture with needles and/or low-energy laser are also helpful (Kitamura A, Inokuchi T: The use of electroacupuncture in the treatment of ideopathic facial paralysis. Am. J. Acupuncture, 1989, 17: 125-129.)

Contraindication: Do not use with pregnant women.

Dose: One 3-gram honey pill, 2 times a day, taken with warm water. It can also be taken with 60 proof Chinese Yellow Wine; the wine will help to move the Blood circulation. In paralysis or rheumatism cases, it is common to use this for several months.

Da Huo Luo Dan is produced by the Tientsin Drug Manufactory, Tientsin, China in tubes of 40 coated pills. Da Huo Luo Dan is also produced by the Beijing Tung Jen Tang pharmacy in boxes of 10 honey pills.

This herbal formula contains 52 different ingredients; the major 22 ingredients are listed below.

Pinyin Name	Pharmaceutical Name	Percent	TCM Function
Xi Jiao	Cornu Rhinoceri Asiatici	1	Clear Heat
Hu Gu	Os Tigris	3	Expel Wind; Stop pain, Strengthen bones and tendons
He Shou Wu	Radix Polygoni Multiflori	2.84	Tonify Liver and Kidney
Chen Xiang	Lignum Aquilariae	2.84	Move Stuck Qi; Clear Meridians
Tian Ma	Rhizoma Gastrodiae	2.84	Stop Wind; Stop spasm
Qiang Huo	Rhizoma et Radix Notopterygii	2.84	Expel Wind Cold; Stop pain
Gui Ban	Plastrum Testudinis	2.84	Nourish Liver, Kidney Yin; Strengthen tendons and bones
Dang Gui	Radix Angelicae Sinensis	2.13	Strengthen Blood; Promote circulation
Xi Xin	Herba Asari Cum Radice	1.42	Expel Wind Cold; Stop pain
Ding Xiang	Flos Caryophylli	1.42	Move Qi; Stop pain; Clear Meridians
Niu Huang	Calculus Bovis	1	Clear Heat
She Xiang	Secretio Moschus moschiferi	0.72	Open Orifices; Move Stuck Qi
Ren Shen	Radix Ginseng	4.26	Strengthen Qi and Blood
Huang Lian	Rhizoma Coptidis	2.84	Clear Heat
Mu Xiang	Radix Saussureae seu Vladimiriae	2.84	Move Stuck Qi
Rou Gui	Cortex Cinnamomi Cassiae	2.84	Warm the Meridians
Shu Di Huang	Radix Rehmanniae Glutinosae Conquitae	2.84	Nourish Yin; Tonify Blood
Wu Yao	Radix Linderae Strychnifoliae	2.84	Move Stuck Qi
Wei Ling Xian	Radix Clematidis Chinensis	2.84	Expel Wind Damp
Ru Xiang	Gummi Olibanum	1.42	Promote Blood circulation; Stop pain
Fang Feng	Radix Ledebouriellae Sesloidis	3.55	Expel Wind
Qing Pi	Pericarpium Citri Reticulatae Viride	1.42	Move Stuck Qi; Clear Meridians

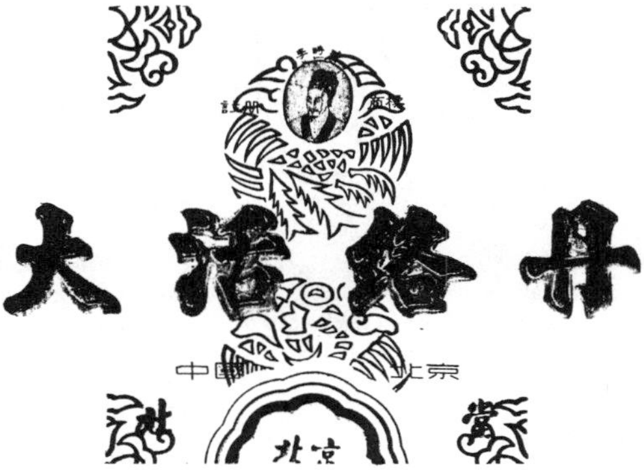

6.4 人 參 再 造 丸

Ren	Shen	Zai	Zao	Wan
----------Ginseng----------		----------reform---------		pill

Source: From Experience, developed for the Imperial Palace, Qing Dynasty, 1644-1911. It is also in the current Pharmacopoeia of the People's Republic of China.

Function:
1. Calm Internal Wind; Dispel External Wind; Eliminate Phlegm
2. Promote Blood circulation; Clear the Stuck Qi and Stuck Blood in the Meridians caused by Wind and Mucous.

Application:
1. Use to treat sequelae of stroke (Zhong Feng, apoplexy) as soon as possible after the patient's medical and neurological conditions are stable. (Do not use while bleeding is still occurring in hemorrhage cases.) Can also be used for sequelae from head injury cases after the medical and neurological conditions are stable. Symptoms: Facial paralysis, limb paralysis (paralysis may be spastic or flaccid), impaired speech and articulation. The patient should also be receiving Physical Therapy and Speech Therapy while taking this herbal medicine, if possible.

2. Use to prevent stroke in patients who have already had transient ischemic attacks (TIA's) or other neurological problems sometimes associated with a pre-stroke condition - i.e. motor, sensory or visual abnormalities from which there has been rapid recovery.

Contraindication: Do not use with pregnant women.

Dose: Honey Pills (9 grams, each pill): 1 pill, 2 times a day, taken with warm water.
Small Coated Pills: 10 pills, once a day.

Note: This medicine should be taken at least 6 months, by a stroke patient with paralysis.

Ren Shen Zai Zao Wan is produced by the Shanghai Chinese Medicine Works, Shanghai, China, in boxes of 10 honey pills. It is also produced as "Tsaitsaowan" by the Tientsin Drug Manufactory, Tientsin, China in bottles of 50 coated pills.

This formula contains 58 herbs. The majority of herbs (41) are listed below in 7 groups by TCM function.

Pinyin Name	Pharmaceutical Name	Grams	TCM Function
Group 1			
Ren Shen	Radix Ginseng	20	Strengthen Qi and Blood; NourishYin;
Huang Qi	Radix Astragali	20	Strengthen Kidney and Strengthen
Shou Di	Radix Rehmanniae Glutinosae Conquitae	20	bones and tendons
He Shou Wu	Radix Polygoni Multiflori	20	
Gui Ban	Plastrum Testudinis	10	
Hu Gu	Os Tigris	10	
Gu Sui Bu	Rhizoma Gusuibu	10	
Group 2			
Quan Xie	Buthus Martensi	15	Calm Internal Wind;
Di Long	Lumbricus	5	Release contractures;
Tian Ma	Rhizoma Gastrodiae Elatae	20	Stop Spasm
Jiang Can	Bombyx Batryticatus	10	

Group 3			
Qi She Rou	Agkistrodon acutus	20	Expel Wind;
Sang Ji Sheng	Ramus Loranthi seu Visci	20	Clear Meridians
Bi Xie	Rhizoma Dioscoreae	20	
Song Jie	Lignum Pini Nodi	10	
Wei Ling Xian	Radix Clemetidis Chinensis	15	
Ma Huang	Herba Ephedrae	20	
Xi Xin	Herba Siegesbeckiae Orientalis	10	
Fang Feng	Radix Ledebouriellae Sesloidis	20	
Qiang Huo	Rhizoma et Radix Notopterygii	20	
Bai Zhi	Radix Angelicae	20	
Ge Gen	Radix Puerariae	15	
Chuan Xiong	Radix Ligustici Wallichii	20	
Group 4			
Chen Xiang	Lignum Aquilariae	10	Move Stuck Qi;
Wu Yao	Radix Linderae Strychnifoliae	10	Promote Blood circulation;
Xiang Fu	Rhizoma Cyperi Rotundi	10	Move Stuck Blood
Xue Jie	Sanguis Draconis	7.5	
Ru Xiang	Gummi Olibanum	10	
Mo Yao	Myrrha	10	
San Qi	Radix Pseudoginseng	5	
Dang Gui	Radix Angelicae Sinensis	10	
Group 5			
Ju Hong	Pericarpium Citri Erythrocarpae	40	Regulate Qi;
Bai Zhu	Rhizoma Atractylodis Macrocephalae	18	Strengthen Spleen;
Fu Ling	Sclerotium Poriae Cocos	10	Increase or Strengthen Source of
Gan Cao	Radix Glycyrrhizae Uralensis	20	Acquired Jing
Dou Kou	Semen Alpiniae Katsumadai	10	
Shen Qi	Massa Fermentata	40	
Group 6			
Niu Huang	Calculus Bovis	2.5	Clear Heart Heat;
Shui Niu Jiao	Cornu Bubali	15	Eliminate Phlegm
Zhu Huang	Concretio Silicea Bambusae	10	
Group 7			
Bing Pian	Borneol	2.5	Open Heart Orifices;
She Xiang	Secretio Moschus moschiferi	5	Waken consciousness

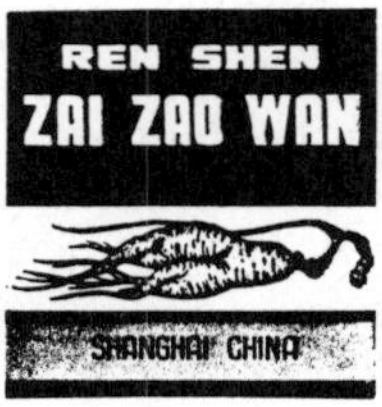

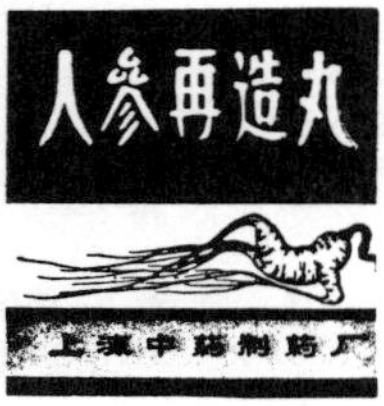

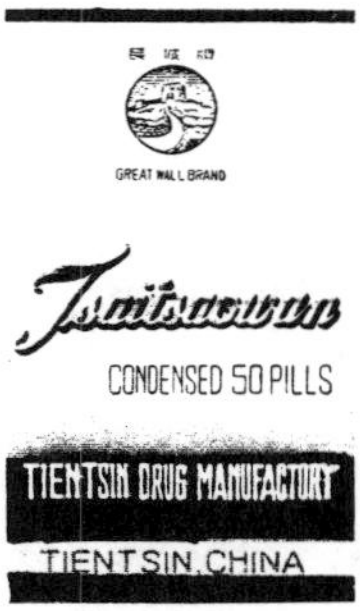

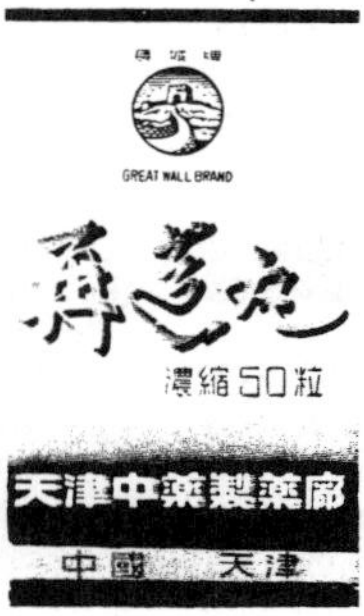

6.5 琥 珀 抱 龍 丸

Hu	Po	Bao	Long	Wan
---------Succinum--------		hold	dragon	pills

Source: This formula is a modification of the formula Bao Long Wan, which originally appeared in the book, Shou Shi Bao Yuan, (Protection of Vital Energy for Longevity), Ming Dynasty, 1368-1644.

Function:
1. Clear Heart Heat; Eliminate Phlegm in children
2. Stop Convulsions; Calm the Spirit in children

Application:

1. Use to treat Phlegm Heat in the Lung syndrome in children. Symptoms: Fever, cough, phlegm congestion in the lung with problems breathing, wheezing may be present. In serious cases, the patient may have agitation or loss of consciousness due to the fever; convulsions may be present.

2. Some Western medicine disease applications include the following: (Note, in order to use this formula for these diseases, the patient must have fever.) Acute Bronchitis, pneumonia; epidemic encephalitis B, epidemic cerebrospinal meningitis; tetanus, spasms caused by high grade fever including opisthotonos, lockjaw; high-grade fever associated with measles; unconsciousness due to high grade fever.

Dose: Child is less than 1 month of age: One-third pill, 2 times a day; for serious cases, use 3 times a day.
Child is 1 to 3 months of age: One-half pill, 2 times a day; for serious cases, use 3 times a day.
Child is 1 year or older: 1 pill, 2 or 3 times a day

Hu Po Bao Long Wan is produced as "Po Lung Yuen Medical Pills" in Hong Kong, with 10 honey pills per box.

The contents are listed below in 7 groups according to the function.

Pinyin Name	Pharmaceutical Name	Percent	TCM Function
Group 1			
Niu Huang	Calculus Bovis	7.8	Clear Heart Heat; Detoxify Fire Poison; Calm the Spirit
Group 2			
Tian Zhu Huang	Concretio Silicea Bambusae	7.8	Clear Heat; Eliminate Phlegm
Dan Nan Xing	Pulvis Arisaemae cum Felle Bovis	3.1	
Group 3			
She Xiang	Secretio Moschus moschiferi	0.6	Open Heart Orifices; Waken consciousness
Group 4			
Quan Xie	Buthus Martensi	4.7	Calm the Excess Liver Wind;
Jiang Can	Bombyx Batryticatus	15.5	Stop convulsions
Group 5			
Zhu Sha	Cinnabaris	4.7	Calm the Spirit; Tranquilize;
Hu Po	Succinum	7.8	Help Niu Huang Clear Heart Heat

Group 6			
Xiong Huang	Realgar	1.6	Detoxify Fire Poison
Group 7			
Chi Fu Ling	Sclerotium Poriae Cocos Rubrae	15.5	Clear Damp Heat; Promote urination

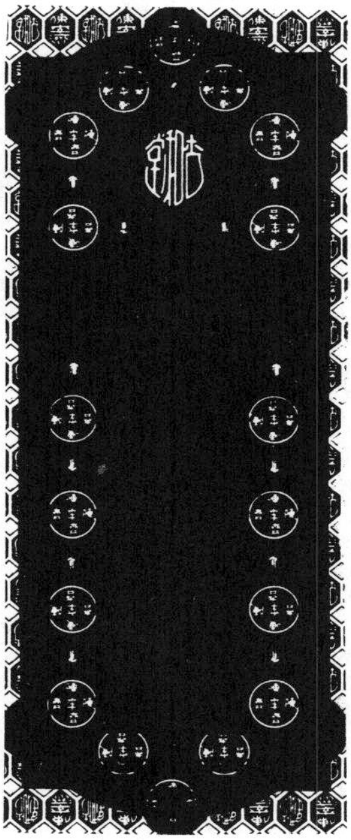

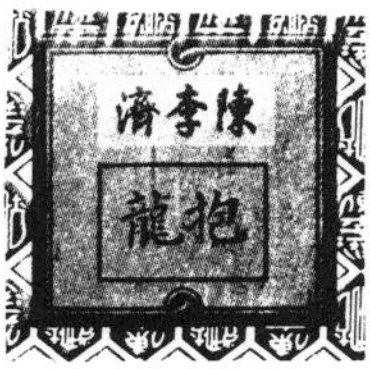

6.6 牛黄清心丸

Niu	Huang	Qing	Xin	Wan
cow	gallstone	Clear Heat	Heart syndrome	pills

Function: 1. Clear Excess Heat, Calm the patient

Application: 1. Use to treat sequelae of stroke (arm, leg or facial paralysis, speech impairment, dizziness). This is also especially useful to help calm a stroke patient who is agitated, with Heat signs, such as red face, easily angered, rapid Pulse, etc.

Dose: Adults: One 3-gram honey pill, 2 times a day
Children less than 1 year: One-half honey pill, 2 times a day

Niu Huang Qing Xin Wan is produced as "Niu Huang Ching Hsin Wan" by the Beijing Tung Jen Tang Pharmacy in boxes of 10 honey pills.

Pinyin Name	Pharmaceutical Name	Percent	TCM Function
Niu Huang	Calculus Bovis	8	Clear Heat, Open Heart Orifices
Ling Yang Jiao	Cornu Antelopis	9	Clear Heat in Liver
Dang Gui	Radix Angelicae Sinensis	6	Tonify Blood, Promote Blood circulation
Chuan Xiong	Rhizoma Ligustici Wallichii	6	Promote Blood circulation
Gan Cao	Radix Glycyrrhizae	5	Catalyst for other herbs
Bai Shao	Radix Paeoniae Lactiflorae	5	Relax muscles, Smooth Liver Wind
Xi Jiao	Cornu Rhinoceri	5	Clear Heat in Heart
Ren Shen	Radix Ginseng	10	Tonify Qi
Rou Gui	Cortex Cinnamomi Cassiae	8	Warming
Fang Feng	Radix Ledebouriellae Sesloidis	6	Stop Wind
A Jiao	Asini Gelatinum	7	Strengthen Yin and Blood
She Xiang	Secretio Moschus moschiferi	5	Open Orifices
	Honey	20	

Notes: 1. There are a variety of formulas similar to Niu Huang Qing Xin Wan, depending on the manufacturer. Wan Shi Niu Huang Qing Xin Wan, #5.3, is a formula directed mainly at Clearing Heat and Unblocking Obstruced Orifices. Niu Huang Qing Xin Wan, #6.6, can Clear some Excess Heat, but is more directed at treating the sequelae of stroke (arm, leg or facial paralysis, speech debility, dizziness). Both are produced by the Beijing Tung Jen Tang Pharmacy.

2. This is a well-known medicine in China and it is considered to be a good medicine. It is frequently used in China; therefore, frequently sold out and difficult to get. While MN was observing stroke cases in hospitals in Shanghai and Beijing in 1985, she asked about the use of this and was told several times, "We would have used this, but it was not available."

MN's observation on the use of this with a few stroke cases in Boston indicated good results in calming the agitated stroke patient (Excess Liver Yang type). The family members were very grateful for having this available for the patient, after having returned home from the hospital. One case had good results with taking only one-half honey pill, only in the morning (the formula is relatively expensive). He took this starting at 3 months after stroke onset for a month, and then again at 11 months after stroke onset. There were no negative side effects from this herbal formula, no drowsiness, etc.; the patient and family members were especially pleased about this.

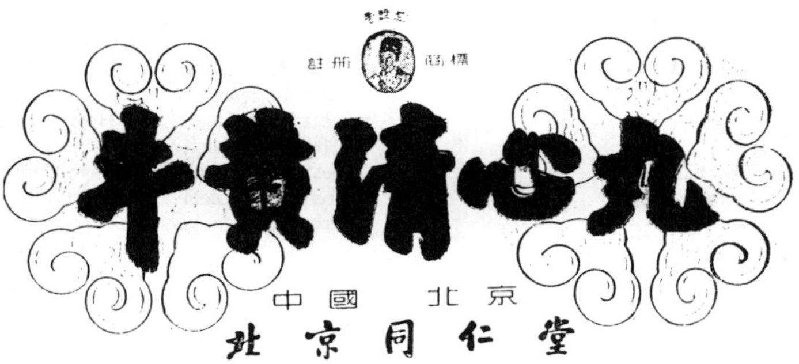

6.7 牛 黄 解 压 丸

Niu	Huang	Jiang	Ya	Wan
cow	gallstone	decrease	(blood) pressure	pills

Function: 1. Clear Heat in Heart
2. Remove Phlegm Heat Accumulation
3. Calm the Spirit; Reduce high blood pressure

Application: 1. Use to treat Excess Liver Yang syndrome which has promoted Liver Wind which has affected the head. Symptoms: Headache, dizziness, vertigo, impatience and irritabiliy, high blood pressure, insomnia, red face, bitter taste in the mouth. The Tongue is red; the Pulse is wiry.

2. Use to remove Phlegm Heat Accumulation which has blocked the flow of Qi in the Meridians producing paralysis, limb numbness, aphasia or coma. The Pulse is Slippery and Wiry.

Dose: 1 or 2 honey pills, 2 times a day. Each pill weighs 1.6 grams.

Niu Huang Jiang Ya Wan is produced by Tientsin Da Ren Tang, Tientsin, China, in boxes of 10 honey pills.

The percents for each ingredient are not available.

Pinyin Name	Pharmaceutical Name	TCM Function
Ling Yang Jiao	Cornu Antelopis	Clear Heat; Reduce Excess Liver Yang
Niu Huang	Calculus Bovis	Clear Heart Heat; Detoxify Fire Poison
Zhen Zhu	Magarita	Calm the Spirit
Bing Pian	Borneol	Clear Heart Heat; Open Heart Orifices; Refresh the Spirit
Yu Jin	Tuber Curcumae	Move Stuck Liver Qi; Relieve Depression
Huang Qi	Radix Astragali	Strengthen Spleen Qi; Prevent other herbs from weakening the patient

6.8 保 嬰 丹

保	嬰	丹
Bao	**Ying**	**Dan**
protect	infant	powder

Source: Yao Dian, (Chinese Pharmacopoeia).

Function: 1. Clear Heat; Eliminate Phlegm in children
2. Extinguish Liver Wind due to Excess Heat in children

Application: 1. Use to treat high-grade fever; semi-unconsciousness or unconsciousness in children. A lot of phlegm may be present in the chest; breathing may be difficult.

2. Some Western medicine disease applications include the following: Acute pneumonia; acute bronchitis.

Dose: Powder Form: Each vial of powder contains 0.3 grams of the medicine.
Child is less than 1 month: Use 0.1 gram, 2 or 3 times per day.
Child is 1 month to 1 year: Use 0.3 grams, 2 or 3 times per day.
Child is more than 1 year: Increase the dose accordingly, but no greater than 0.9 grams, 2 or 3 times per day.

Pill Form: Each pill contains 0.5 grams of the medicine
Child is more than 1 year: 1 pill, 3 times per day
Child is less than 1 year: Decrease the dose proportionately

Bao Ying Dan is produced by the Guangzhou United Pharmaceutical Manufactory, Guangzhou, China, in powder form.

The herbs are listed below in 5 groups, according to their function.

Pinyin Name	Pharmaceutical Name	Percent	TCM Function
Group 1			
Niu Huang	Calculus Bovis	1.33	Clear Heat; Detoxify Fire Poison; Stop Convulsions
Group 2			
Dan Nan Xing	Pulvis Arisaemae cum Felle Bovis	33.22	Clear Phlegm Heat
Zhu Huang	Concretio Silicea Bambusae	11.63	
Xiong Huang	Realgar	8.3	
Group 3			
Jiang Can	Bombyx Batryticatus	9.97	Extinguish Liver Wind;
Quan Xie	Buthus Martensi	4.98	Stop Convulsions
Group 4			
Hu Po	Succinum	8.3	Calm the Spirit;
Zhu Sha	Cinnabaris	4.98	Stop Convulsions
Fu Ling	Sclerotium Poriae Cocos	16.6	

Group 5			
She Xiang	Secretio Moschus moschiferi	0.66%	Open Orifices; Waken the patient from coma

Notes: 1. The Patent Medicine, Hou Zao San, is similar to Bao Ying Dan. The major ingredient, Hou Zao (Calculus Macacae Mulattae), Clears Excess Phlegm Heat in the Lung which may block the Heart Orifice, causing high grade fever or even unconsciousness in cases of pneumonia or bronchitis in children.

2. The Patent Medicine, Xiao Er Qi Li San, is similar to Bao Ying Dan; the effect is also similar. Xiao Er Qi Li San is used to Clear Excess Lung Heat and Eliminate Excess Liver Wind which has caused spasms in children. Thus, it is used to treat the following symptoms due to OPI Wind-Heat: High-grade fever, cough, excess phlegm and difficult breathing. If the symptoms progress to convulsions, this formula may also be used to help stop the convulsions.

Contraindication for Xiao Er Qi Li San: Do not use with a child who has been diagnosed as having measles. In the early stage of measles, herbs which Expel Wind and Clear Heat (such as Yin Qiao Jie Du Pian, or Sang Ju Gan Mao Pian) are used to induce the measles to come out. Xiao Er Qi Li San contains too many very Cold property herbs to use in treating the early stage of measles; it would prevent the eruption of the measles.

The medicine is in powder form and available in vials. Each vial contains 0.26 grams of the powder. It should be taken 3 times per day. Children under 1 year of age should take 0.13 grams each time (one-half vial); children over 1 year of age should take 0.26 grams each time (whole vial). Because the taste is bitter, the powder can be given with some other liquid which has been sweetened, for example, with honey.

Another Patent Medicine, Zhu Bo Qi Li San, made in Hong Kong, has a formula similar to Xiao Er Qi Li San and it has a similar effect.

Another Patent Medicine, 12.3, Qi Li San, is a completely different medicine, which is used to treat bruises and contusions associated with sports injuries; it should not be confused with Xiao Er Qi Li San or Zhu Bo Qi Li San.

Chapter 7. Clear Heat

(Includes Patent Medicines used to reduce infections, sore throat, treat wounds, etc.)

Section A. **Clear Heat, Dry Dampness**

Section B. **Clear Heat, Reduce Excess Fire**

Section C. **Detoxify Fire Poison**

7.1 黃 連 上 清 片

Huang	Lian	Shang	Qing	Pian
----Rhizoma Coptidis----		upper	clear	tablets

Source: Wan Bing Hui Chun, (Recovery of Ten Thousand Patients), Ming Dynasty, 1368-1644.

Function: 1. Relieve Fire; Dispel Wind-Heat

2. Clear Wind-Heat in Upper Warmer and Middle Wamer

3. Promote bowel movement

Application: 1. Use to treat Wind-Heat syndrome associated with common cold or flu. Symptoms: Fever, headache, dizziness, tinnitus, mouth ulcer, swollen gums, sore throat, conjunctivitis, toothache, or constipation.

2. Use to treat hypertension with dizziness, headache, red eyes, flushed face associated with Wind-Heat syndrome.

3. Some Western medicine disease applications include the following: (Note, the patient must have Heat signs to use this formula.) Tonsillitis, parotitis, otitis media, acute bronchitis, acute pneumonia, pulmonary abscess, and skin infections including sores, carbuncles, boils.

Contraindication: Do not use with pregnant women.

Dose: 4 tablets, 1 or 2 times a day.

Huang Lian Shang Qing Pian is produced as "Huang Lien Shang Ching Pien" by the Tientsin Drug Manufactory, Tientsin, China, in vials of 8 tablets.

Pinyin Name	Pharmaceutical Name	Percent	TCM Function
Huang Lian	Rhizoma Coptidis	7.86	Clear Heat; Disperse Fire
Chuan Xiong	Rhizoma Ligustici Wallichii	3.15	Expel Wind; Stop headache
Jing Jie	Herba seu Flos Schizonepetae Tenuifoliae	6.29	Expel Wind
Fang Feng	Radix Ledebouriellae Sesloidis	3.15	Expel Wind
Huang Qin	Radix Scutellariae Baicalensis	6.29	Clear Heat
Jie Geng	Radix Platycodi Grandiflori	6.29	Open Lung Energy; Soothe throat; Discharge pus
Shi Gao	Gypsum	3.15	Clear Lung Heat
Ju Hua	Flos Chrysanthemi Morifolii	12.58	Expel Wind Heat; Clear Liver Heat
Bai Zhi	Radix Angelicae	6.29	Expel Wind
Gan Cao	Radix Glycyrrhizae Uralensis	3.15	Harmonize other herbs
Da Huang	Rhizoma Rhei	25.16	Disperse Heat through bowel movement
Man Jing Zi	Fructus Viticis	16.64	Expel Wind; Stop headache

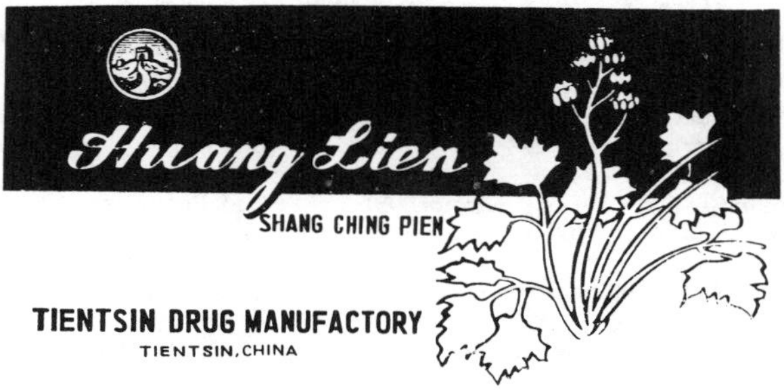
Huang Lien
SHANG CHING PIEN
TIENTSIN DRUG MANUFACTORY
TIENTSIN, CHINA

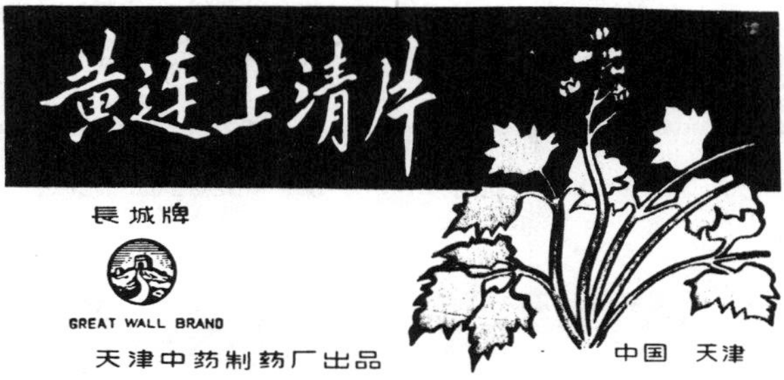
黄连上清片
長城牌
GREAT WALL BRAND
天津中药制药厂出品
中国 天津

7.2 牛 黄 上 清 丸

Niu	**Huang**	**Shang**	**Qing**	**Wan**
cow	gallstone	upper	clear	pills

Source: Yi Xue Ru Men, (Elements of Medicine), Ming Dynasty, 1368-1644.

Function: 1. Clear Heat; Disperse Fire; Reduce inflammation

Application: 1. Use to treat sore or ulcer on the tongue.

2. Use to treat stomatitis (inflammation or infection in the mouth, may be viral, with or without fever); oral Herpes.

3. Use to treat Wind-Heat syndrome with any of the following symptoms: Fever, sore throat, toothache, conjunctivitis, constipation, uneasiness (due to Heat in the Heart).

Contraindication: Do not use with pregnant women.

Dose: Honey pill: 1 honey pill, 2 times a day   Coated Pills: 10 coated pills, once a day.

Niu Huang Shang Qing Wan is produced as "Niuhuang Shang Ching Wan" by the Tientsin Drug Manufactory, Tientsin, China, in bottles of 50 coated pills.

Pinyin Name	Pharmaceutical Name	Percent	TCM Function
Niu Huang	Calculus Bovis	10	Clear Heat; Disperse Fire
Huang Lian	Rhizoma Coptidis	15	Clear Heat; Disperse Fire
Dang Gui	Radix Angelicae Sinensis	15	Move Blood
Bing Pian	Borneol	5	Clear Heat; Open Orifices; Awaken the Spirit
Da Huang	Rhizoma Rhei	20	Disperse Heat through bowel movement
Ju Hua	Flos Chrysanthemi Morifolii	15	Expel Wind Heat; Clear Liver Heat
Jie Geng	Radix Platycodi Grandiflori	5	Open Lung Energy; Soothe throat; Discharge pus
Lian Xin	Plumula Nelumbinis Nuciferae	5	Clear Heat in Heart
Gan Cao	Radix Glycyrrhizae Uralensis	2	Harmonize other herbs

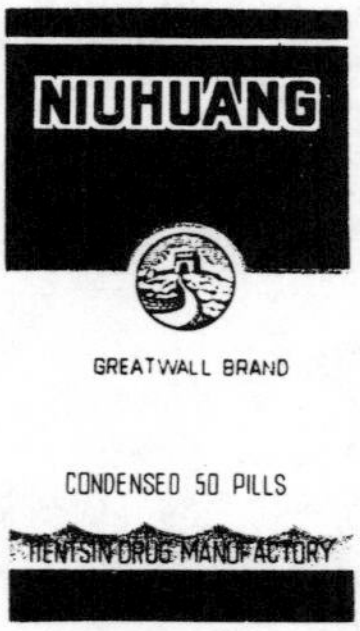

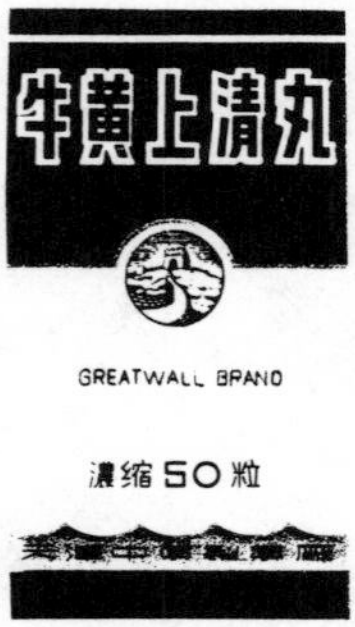

7.3 雙 料 喉 風 散

Shuang	**Liao**	**Hou**	**Feng**	**San**
double	ingredient	----sore throat disease----		powder

Function: 1. Clear Heat; Eliminate inflammation
2. Soothe throat; Stop pain

Application: 1. Use to treat oral infections or disorders - e.g. stomatitis, tonsillitis, pharyngitis, mouth ulcer, canker sore, toothache, scarlet fever or other throat disorders caused by Heat.

2. Use to treat nasal infections or disorders - e.g. runny nose, sinus headache, nasal secretions which are yellow, pus-like, caused by sinusitis.

3. Use to treat ear infections or disorders - e.g. ear pain with pus-like discharge and diminished hearing caused by otitis media.

4. Use to treat skin infections such as carbuncles or boils with an open wound; skin blisters.

Contraindication: For external use only.

Dose: For mouth infections, blow powder onto the infected area. For tonsillitis, use 1/6 vial, 3 times a day.
For nasal infections, sniff it up the nostril. Use 1/10 vial, 5 times a day.
For ear infections, use hydrogen peroxide solution to wash the ear, then blow powder into the ear. Use 1/10 vial, once a day.
For skin infections, first wash the area with strong black tea, then apply the powder to the open wound in an appropriate amount, once a day. The black tea will act as an astringent.

Shuang Liao Hou Feng San is produced as "Superior Sore Throat Powder" by the Meizhou City Pharmaceutical Manufactory, Guangdong, China, in small vials containing the powder.

Pinyin Name	Pharmaceutical Name	Percent	TCM Function
Niu Huang	Calculus Bovis	5	Clear Heat; Detoxify Fire Poison
Bing Pian	Borneol	25	Clear Heat; Stop Pain
Gan Cao	Radix Glycyrrhizae Uralensis	15	Clear Heat
Qing Dai	Indigo Pulverata Levis	5	Clear Blood Heat; Detoxify Fire Poison
Zhen Zhu	Magarita	5	Tranquilize Heart Spirit; Stop pain; Promote Healing
Huang Lian	Rhizoma Coptidis	30	Clear Heat; Detoxify Fire Poison
Shan Dou Gen	Radix Sophorae Subprostratae	15	Clear Heat; Detoxify Fire Poison Benefit throat

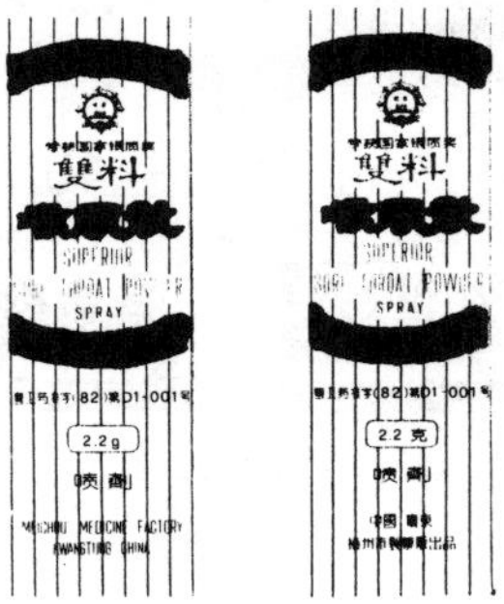

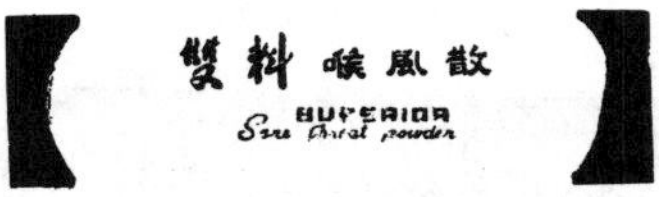

7.4 黃連素片

Huang	Lian	Su	Pian
-----------Coptidis---------		extract	tablets

Function: 1. Subside inflammation; Detoxify Fire Poison

Application: 1. Use to treat intestinal infection and inflammation including dysentery, primarily due to bacilli (rod-shaped bacteria). Symptoms: Frequent bloody or watery stools, abdominal pain, vomiting, fever.

2. Use to treat chronic amebic dysentery.

3. Use to treat carbuncles and sores on the skin with pus; conjunctivitis.

Dose: Adults: 2 or 3 tablets, 3 times a day, taken with warm water.
Children: 1/2 to 1 tablet, 3 times a day, taken with warm water.

Huang Lian Su Pian is produced as "Huang Lien Su Tablets" by the Min-Kang Drug Manufactory, I-Chang, China, in vials containing 12 tablets and as "Superior Tabellae Berberini" by the Min-Kang Drug Manufactory, I-Chang, China.

Pinyin Name	Pharmaceutical Name	Percent	TCM Function
Huang Lian	Rhizoma Coptidis	100	Clear Heat; Detoxify Fire Poison

Notes: 1. Laboratory researach in China has shown the function of this herb to be similar to that of a broad spectrum antibiotic. It is effective in reducing the bacterial counts for the following bacteria: Bacillus dysenteriae; Staphylococcus; Pneumococcus; Meningococcus; Corynebacterium diphteriae; Streptococcus; Mycobacterium tuberculosis var. hominis; Leptospira.

2. In China, the active ingredient is extracted chemically and sold in drug stores, as well as in herb shops. This medicine is very effective, and it is used frequently.

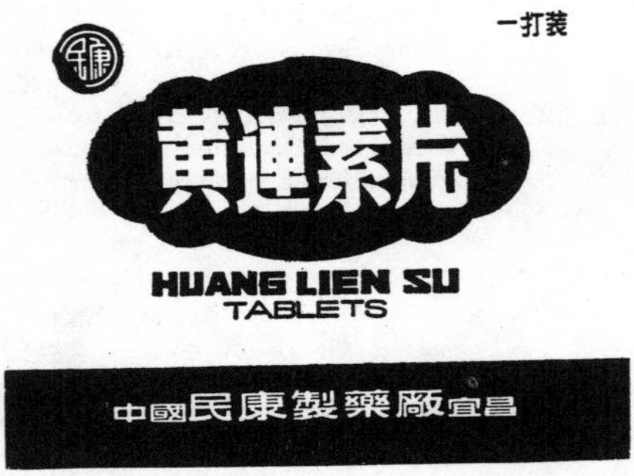

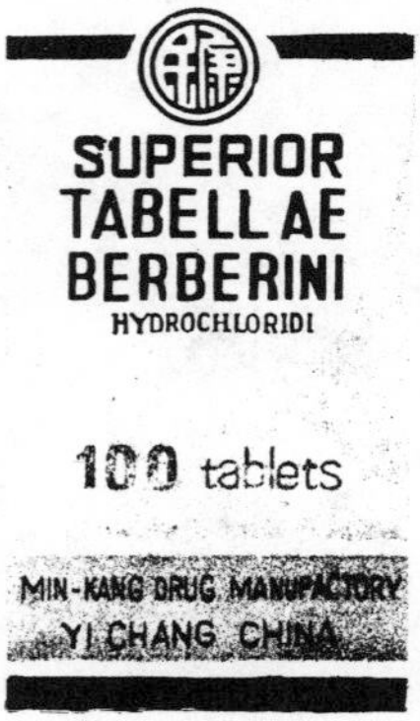

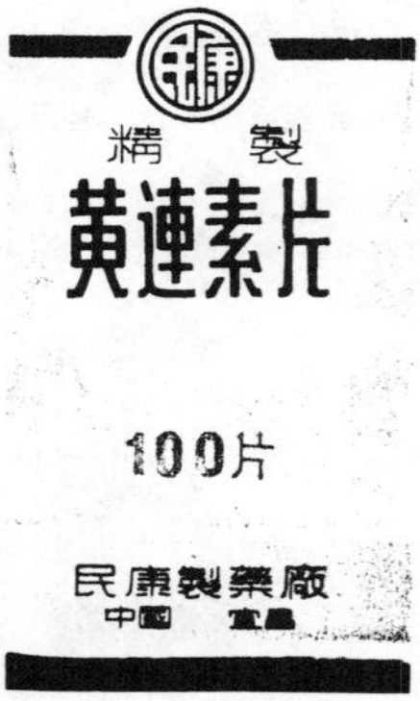

7.5 加味香連片

加	味	香	連	片
Jia	**Wei**	**Xiang**	**Lian**	**Pian**
extra	ingredients	---herbal formula name---		tablets

Source: Experience in the Chinese military. The formula is in the text, Hui Min He Ji Jiu Fang, (Formulas of the People's Welfare Pharmacy), Song Dynasty, 960 - 1279.

Function: 1. Clear Heat; Dry Dampness
2. Promote circulation of Qi; Remove Stagnation of Qi

Application: 1. Use to treat dysentery (acute bacillary) due to Damp Heat. Symptoms: Possible fever (in very serious cases with shock, fever may be absent); abdominal pain; urgent sensation to have a bowel movement several times a day; diarrhea with blood and pus may be present.

Dose: 2 tablets, 2 to 4 times a day. Take with warm water.

Jia Wei Xiang Lian Pian is produced as "Chiawei Hsianglienpian" by the Peking Pharmaceutical Manufactory, Beijing, China, in vials of 8 tablets.

The ingredients are listed in 3 groups which are arranged according to function.

Pinyin Name	Pharmaceutical Name	Percent	TCM Function
Group 1			
Mu Xiang	Radix Saussureae seu Vladimiriae	10.81	Promote Intestinal Qi circulation;
Bing Lang	Semen Arecae Catechu	5.4	Remove Intestinal Qi Stagnation;
Zhi Qiao	Fructus Citri seu Ponciri	10.81	Dry Dampness; Stop pain
Hou Po	Cortex Magnoliae Officinalis	10.81	
Wu Zhu Yu	Fructus Evodiae Rutaecarpae	5.4	
Group 2			
Huang Lian	Rhizoma Coptidis	16.22	Clear Heat; Detoxify Fire Poison;
Huang Bai	Cortex Phellodendri	5.4	Eliminate Dampness
Huang Qin	Radix Scutellariae Baicalensis	10.81	
Group 3			
Yuan Hu	Rhizoma Corydalis Yanhusuo	5.4	Regulate Blood circulation;
Bai Shao	Radix Paeoniae Lactiflorae	10.81	Stop pain
Dang Gui	Radix Angelicae Sinensis	5.4	
Gan Cao	Radix Glycyrrhizae Uralensis	2.7	Regulate the Middle Warmer; Stop pain; Harmonize other herbs

Notes: 1. The original name for this Patent Medicine was Jia Wei Xiang Lian Wan (pills), with the same ingredients. The present formula is available in tablet form. The tablet form is more convenient, because with the pill form, a large number of pills had to be taken each time.

2. This formula is a modification of the Xiang Lian Wan formula. In a 1955 study, Xiang Lian Wan was used to treat acute bacillary dysentery in 38 patients. It controlled the fever in an average of 32.5 hours and the diarrhea, in 4 days; the culture was negative on the third day. (Journal of Traditional Chinese Medicine, 1955, Issue Number 8.) The modified formula, Jia Wei Xiang Lian Pian, 7.5, is more effective than Xiang Lian Wan, because it has more ingredients.

7.6 华 佗 膏

Hua	**Tuo**	**Gao**
Hua Tuo (Chinese Physician)		ointment

Function: 1. Expel Wind; Eliminate Dampness; Stop itching

Application: 1. Use to treat athlete's foot (tinea pedis) or fungus infection of the hand. The skin may be rough, thick and peeling off; itching may be present.

2. Use to treat dermatitis (eczema). Symptoms: Superficial inflammation of the skin characterized by vesicles (when acute), redness, edema, oozing, crusting, scaling, itching.

How to use: 1. Wash the affected area with warm water.
2. Apply the ointment to the skin twice a day, morning and evening. If the ointment is applied between the toes, use a cotton ball between the toes during the day and at night.

When treating skin infection on the palm of the hand where the surface is thick and rough, first soak the hand in warm water to soften the skin surface, before applying ointment.

Caution: While using this ointment on the skin, do not use soap, Lysol or H_2O_2 on the skin. Also, do not use alcohol, tincture of iodine or sulphur on the skin. These may cause irritation.

Hua Tuo Gao is produced by the Shanghai Chinese Drug Pharmaceutical Works, Shanghai, China.

Contents	Percent
Salicylic acid	5
Benzoic Acid	10
Cera Chinensis	2
Camphora	2
Vaseline	80
Chimonanthus Praecox-Link Oil	1

Notes: 1. If after using this ointment for a few day there is no effect, it is recommended that the patient soak the affected area in the following herbal solution. (Soak the area with this solution before applying the ointment, twice a day.) This solution has three ingredients (Fang Feng, Jing Jie, Ming Fan) in equal parts. Use 15 grams of each. Place into a pot with 2 to 4 cups of water. Bring to a boil and simmer for 30 minutes, cooking down the liquid by one cup. Cool the solution to a comfortable temperature (it should still be a little hot). Leave the herbs in the liquid and soak the area with the solution. The unused solution may be used three days. Store in the refrigerator. Before using each time, re-heat the solution (and herbs). After soaking the affected area, do not rinse it off. Apply the ointment after soaking the area.

2. If the patient desires to remove the ointment from the skin, use a solution of baking soda; do not use soap and water. A black tea (or other tea) solution may also be used to remove the ointment.

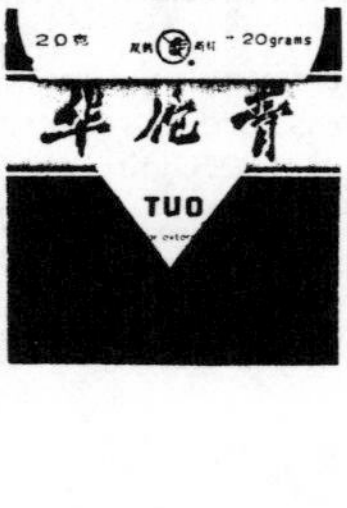

7.7 愈 带 丸

愈	带	丸
Yu	**Dai**	**Wan**
heal	leukorrhea	pills

Source: Zheng Zhi Zhun Sheng, (Standards for Diagnosis and Treatment), Ming Dynasty, 1368-1644.

Function: 1. Clear Damp Heat in the Lower Warmer.
2. Stop leukorrhea

Application: 1. Use to treat Damp Heat that has settled in the Lower Warmer, causing leukorrhea. Here the Dampness has already combined with Heat, and the leukorrhea has a yellow color; it may be accompanied by itching and pain, as well as odor. In some cases, the leukorrhea may also be bloody. Additional symptoms of Damp Heat in the Lower Warmer may include burning urination, abdominal pain, a bitter taste in the mouth, and dry throat.

2. Use to treat other disorders associated with Damp Heat in the Lower Warmer, including dysentery.

Contraindication: Do not use this medicine if the leukorrhea is due to Def. Spleen, where Dampness has developed in the Lower Warmer, but has not combined with Heat. In this case, the leukorrhea is clear or white in color. In treating leukorrhea due to Def. Spleen use Qian Jin Zhi Dai Wan, #12.11.

Dose: 8 to 10 pills, 3 times a day.

Yu Dai Wan is produced as "Yudai Wan (Leucorrhea Pills)" by the Lanzhou Fo Ci Pharmaceutical Factory, Lanzhou, China.

The 7 herbs are listed below in 4 groups according to function.

Pinyin Name	Pharmaceutical Name	Percent	TCM Function
Group 1 (Consists of the formula, Si Wu Tang, the essential and most common formula used to treat gynecological disorders)			
Shou Di Huang	Radix Rehmanniae Glutinosae Conquitae	12.5	Regulate and Strengthen the Blood; Astringent property to stop the leukorrhea
Bai Shao	Radix Paeoniae Lactiflorae	15.62	
Dang Gui	Radix Angelicae Sinensis	9.37	
Chuan Xiong	Radix Ligustici Wallichii	3.13	
Group 2			
Huang Bai	Cortex Phellodendri	6.25	Clear Heat; Dry Dampness
Group 3			
Chun Gen Pi	Ailanthus altissima (Mill.) Swingle	46.88	Astringent property to stop leukorrhea; Cold property to Clear Heat; Bitter taste to Dry Dampness

Group 4

Gao Liang Jiang	Rhizoma Alpiniae Officinari (Carbonized)	6.25	The Warm property of this herb will prevent any damage to Stomach Qi from the Cold property medicines with Bitter Taste in this formula. The carbonized form of this will stop bleeding.

Notes: 1. The formula listed here is a modification of the formula in the original source which contained only 4 herbs including the last 3 herbs listed here plus Bai Shao. The original formula did not contain all four herbs listed in the Si Wu Tang, which are included in the present formula.

2. In the original source, the formula with 4 herbs was called Chun Pi Wan. Today, there is still a Patent Medicine available in China with the name, Chun Pi Wan, which contains only the 4 herbs, but has a function similar to this Patent Medicine,Yu Dai Wan, which contains the 7 herbs listed above.

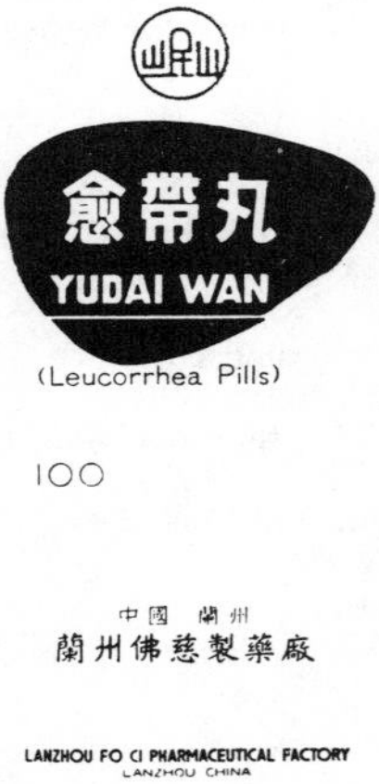

7.8 牛 黄 解 毒 片

Niu	Huang	Jie	Du	Pian
cow	gallstone	------detoxification-----		tablets

Source: Bian Zheng Zhun Sheng Fu Yu Ji, (Differentiation Standards from the Volume on Gynecology and Pediatrics), Ming Dynasty, 1368-1644.

Function:
1. Clear Heat; Reduce inflammation
2. Detoxify Fire Poisoon

Application:
1. Use to treat strong Fire Evil in the Upper Warmer. Symptoms: Throat pain, mouth dryness, throat dryness, tongue ulcer, mouth ulcer, toothache with or without swollen gums, headache.

2. Use to treat constipation caused by Excess Heat (not Def. Yin type of constipation).

3. Use to treat skin infections including sores, carbuncles, boils.

4. Some Western medicine disease applications include the following: (The patient must have the above-mentioned Heat signs.) Tonsillitis or pharyngitis with symptoms such as fever, throat pain, swollen tonsils (with or without pus); conjuncitivitis; parotitis; otitis media.

Contraindication: Do not use with pregnant women. This formula contains Da Huang, which is contraindicated during pregnancy because it could cause a miscarriage. Do not use with cases who have Deficiency, especially not in cases with Def. Spleen syndrome where loose stools or diarrhea may already be present. Use only in cases with Excess Fire.

Dose: Uncoated Tablets: 2 tablets, 2 times a day. In more severe cases, especially with toothache, use 2 tablets, 3 or 4 times a day. Honey Pills: 1 or 2 honey pills, 2 times a day.

Niu Huang Jie Du Pian is produced as "Niu Huang Chieh Tu Pien" by the Beijing Tung Jen Tang pharmacy in vials of 8 uncoated tablets; by the Tianjin Drug Manufactory in bottles of 20 coated tablets; and by the Shanghai Chinese Medicine Works in bottles of 20 coated tablets.

Pinyin Name	Pharmaceutical Name	Percent	TCM Function
Niu Huang	Calculus Bovis	2.5	Clear Heat; Detoxify Fire Poison
Huang Lian	Rhizoma Coptidis	14	Clear Heat; Disperse Excess Fire; Dry Dampness
Bing Pian	Borneol	7.5	Clear Heat; Open Orifices; Awaken patient from unconsciousness
Jing Yin Hua	Flos Lonicerae Japonicae	20	Clear Heat; Detoxify Fire Poison
Bo He	Herba Menthae	7	Expel Wind-Heat
Huang Qin	Radix Scutellariae Baicalensis	14	Clear Heat; Detoxify Fire Poison; Dry Dampness
Bai Zhi	Radix Angelicae	8	Expel Wind; Discharge pus; Decrease swelling; Stop pain
Zhi Zi	Fructus Gardeniae Jasminoidis	10	Clear Heat; Calm down patient
Da Huang	Rhizoma Rhei	10	Clear Intestinal Heat; Move stool
Chuan Xiong	Radix Ligustici Wallichii	7	Stop pain; Reduce Wind

Notes: 1. When taking this medicine, the patient may have increased bowel movements; some of the ingredients in the formula have a strong laxative effect.

2. The effect of this formula is similar to a broad spectrum antibiotic.

3. This is a popular and commonly-used formula for the early stages of a Seasonal Febrile Disease where fever and sore throat are present. It is common to combine it with #1.4, Yin Qiao Jie Du Pian.

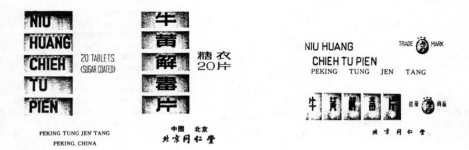

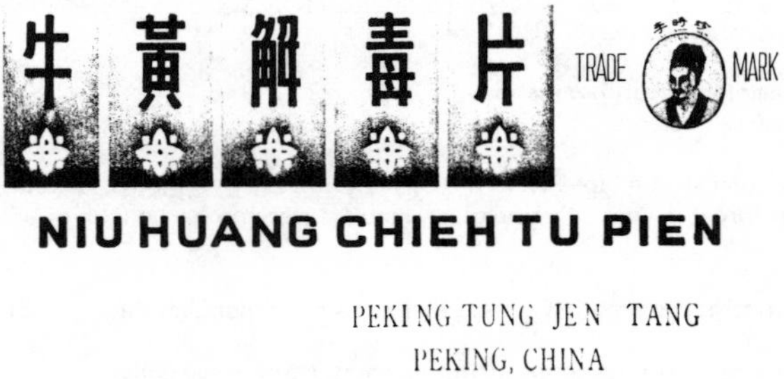

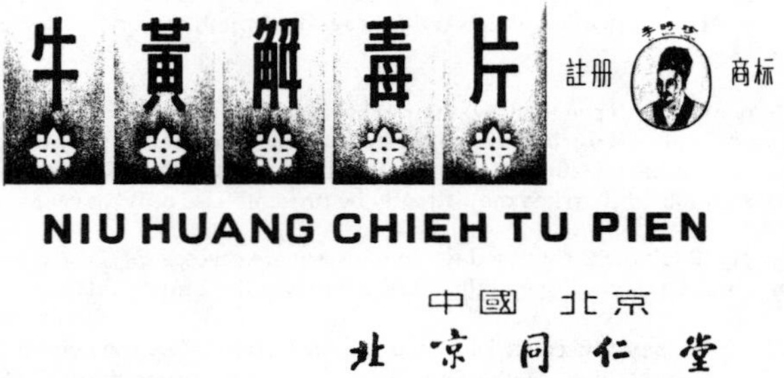

7.9 六 神 丸

六	神	丸
Liu	**Shen**	**Wan**
six	spirit	pills

Source: Formula by Lei Yuenshang, Dictionary of Chinese Medicine. Song Dynasty, 960-1279.

Function:
1. Detoxify Fire Poison
2. Decrease inflammation
3. Stop pain

Application:
1. Use to treat severe swollen sore throat as seen in Scarlet fever, Vincent's angina, diphtheria, strep throat, tonsillitis or parotitis.

2. Use to treat stomatitis.

3. Use to treat skin disorders including carbuncles, sores or boils. It is very effective in treating these.

Contraindication: Do not use with pregnant women. Avoid smoking, drinking and hot, spicy, pungent foods while taking this formula for sore throat. These would further irritate the throat.

Dose: These pills are very tiny (0.3 grams per pill). Adults: 10 pills, 1 to 3 times a day.
Children less than 3 years: 1 pill per year of age (Age 1, 1 pill; Age 2, 2 pills, etc.)
Children 4 to 8 years: 5 or 6 pills Children 9 to 15 years: 8 pills

The patient should try to keep the pills in the mouth and swallow them slowly. If this is not possible, take the pills with warm water.

External Use: Dissolve 10 pills in cold water or vinegar and make a paste. Spread the paste over the skin several times daily and keep the area damp.

Liu Shen Wan is produced as "Lu Shen Wan" by the Shanghai Chinese Medicine Works in small bottles containing 30 or 100 of these tiny pills.

Pinyin Name	Pharmaceutical Name	Percent	TCM Function
Niu Huang	Calculus Bovis	20	Clear Heat; Detoxify Fire Poison
She Xiang	Secretio Moschus moschiferi	20	Decrease inflammation; Detoxify Fire Poison
Zhen Zhu	Magarita	20	Detoxification; Promote tissue regeneration
Chan Su	Secretio Bufonis	13.3	Detoxification; Decrease swelling ; Stop pain
Bing Pian	Borneol	13.3	Clear Heat; Promote tissue regeneration
Xiong Huang	Realgar	13.3	Detoxify Fire Poison; Decrease swelling

Notes: 1. In China, this formula is commonly used; it is very effective in treating serious sore throat, etc. The formula is relatively expensive. It is not the "first choice" formula for treating the average sore throat, rather it is often used in more serious cases of sore throat when the "first choice" was not effective. The Patent Medicine #7.8, Niu Huang Jie Du Pian is often used as a "first choice."

2. The contents in this formula are all unusual medicines, hence the name, six "spirits." There are no herbal contents in the formula, they are all animal products such as musk, toad "cakes," etc.

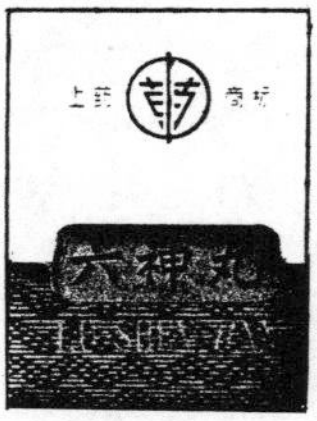

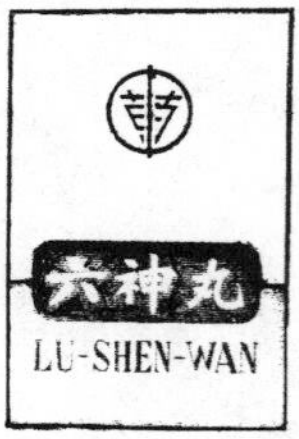

7.10 西 瓜 霜

西	瓜	霜
Xi	**Gua**	**Shuang**
--------water melon--------		frost

Source: The Complete Works for the Treatment of Sores, Qing Dynasty, 1644-1911.

Function:
1. Eliminate swelling
2. Stop pain

Application:
1. Use to treat diseases in the mouth including sores, stomatitis, ulcer.

2. Use to treat throat infections or toothache by placing the powder topically. (Put the powder in a short straw and blow it onto the inflammed area. A rubber atomizer, similar to that used to clean the ears, can also be used to spray the powder topically.)

3. Use to treat burns on the skin. (Mix 2 vials of the powder with some cooking oil. Use this mixture topically for a few days until the burn is healed.)

Contraindication: Do not eat greasy, oily food when taking this formula.

Dose: Internal Use: Each vial contains 2 grams of the powder. Mix 1 to 2 grams of the powder with water and take this amount 2 or 3 times a day.

External Use: Use it topically every 2 or 3 hours. May be used both internally and externally at the same time. The taste is salty and the patient will feel some local pungency.

Xi Gua Shuang is produced as "Water Melon Frost" by the Kweilin Drug Manufactory in Kwangsi, China, in vials containing 2 grams of the powder.

Pinyin Name	Pharmaceutical Name	Percent	TCM Function
Xi Gua Shuang	Watermelon frost	50	Stop pain; Decrease swelling
Chuan Bei Mu	Bulbus Fritillariae Cirrhosae	12	Clear Heat; Moisten Lung
Huang Bai	Cortex Phellodendri	8	Clear Heat; Detoxify Fire poison
Bo He Nao	Menthol	4	Clear Heat
Huang Lian	Rhizoma Coptidis	12	Clear Heat; Detoxify Fire poison
Huang Qin	Radix Scutellariae Baicalensis	8	Clear Heat; Detoxify Fire Poison
Bing Pian	Borneol	4	Stop pain
Zhu Sha	Cinnabaris	2	Clear Heat; Calm Spirit

Notes: 1. "Watermelon frost" is produced using the following process:

1) An entire watermelon is cut into small pieces.

2) These small pieces are mixed with Na_2SO_4 and $NaNO_3$.

3) This mixture is then placed into a clay jar.

4) The clay jar is sealed.

5) The sealed jar is placed in an area where air can circulate around it.

6) After awhile, the liquid from the mixture seeps through the clay jar and crystals form on the outside of the jar.

7) The crystals are continuously scraped off for several collections, until no more crystals are formed.

8) These crystals, called "Xi Gua Shuang" are then mixed with the other ingredients. Hence, the label, "Fu Fang Xi Gua Shuang" (Compound Watermelon Frost) is often used.

2. This formula is now available in lozenge form, as well as in liquid spray form. The lozenge form is a tablet which should be dissolved slowly in the mouth, not swallowed. The taste is a little sweet and very cooling. The spray form is designed to be sprayed directly onto the inflammed area in the throat or the pharynx. The lozenge form is called Xi Gua Shuang Run Ho Pian (Run means "moisten," Ho means "throat," and Pian means "tablet"). The spray form is called Xi Gua Shuang Pen Ji (Pen means "spray," Ji means "form").

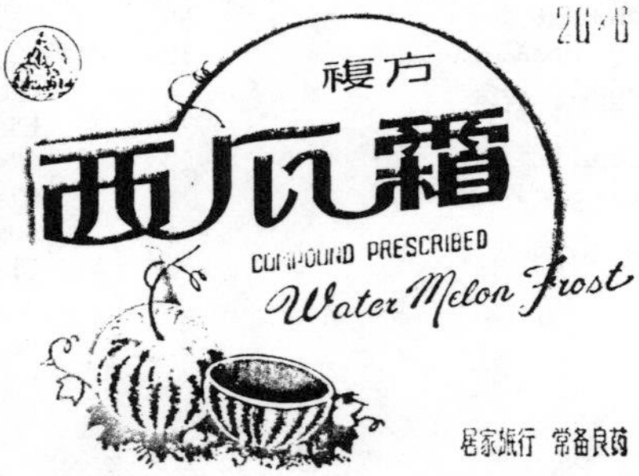

7.11 清 音 丸

Qing	**Yin**	**Wan**
clear	voice	pills

Source: Lan Tai Gui Fan, Qing Dynasty, 1644-1911.

Function:
1. NourishYin and Clear Heat in the Lung
2. Promote production of body liquid to strengthen body fluids and quench thirst
3. Promote salivation

Application:
1. Use to treat throat diseases due to Wind-Heat or Fire Evil which have accumulated in the Lung, so that the Lung Qi cannot Open. Thus, the patient has hoarseness, swollen and painful throat, and dry mouth.

2. Use to treat sore throat associated with tonsillitis, Scarlet fever or early febrile disease.

3. Use to treat throat narrowing and stop pain in Vincent's angina.

4. Use to treat voice hoarseness due to Lung problems. This formula will promote salivation and reduce mouth dryness.

Contraindication: Do not eat greasy, spicey food while taking this formula

Dose: 1 honey pill, 2 times a day. Slowly dissolve the pill in the mouth, or take with warm water.

Qing Yin Wan is produced by the Beijing Tung Jen Tang pharmacy in boxes of 10 honey pills.

Pinyin Name	Pharmaceutical Name	Percent	TCM Function
Ge Gen	Radix Puerariae	15	Promote increase in body fluid into the upper half of the body including the neck and throat; Clear Heat
He Zi Rou	Fructus Terminaliae Chebule	15	Soothe throat
Fong Mi	Honey	25	Moisten Lung
Tian Hua Fen	Radix Trichosanthis	20	Promote salivation; Stop thirst
Chuan Bei Mu	Bulbus Fritillariae Cirrhosae	25	Open Lung Qi; Moisten Lung

Note: 1. There are additional Patent Medicines with the same name, "Qing Yin Wan." The formula listed above is made by the Beijing Tung Jen Tang pharmacy. Another formula listed below, is made in Tianjin. The Tianjin formula contains more ingredients than the Beijing formula.

The Tianjin formula contains Yuan Shen, Jie Geng, Shan Dou Gen, Pang Da Hai, Bo He, Pang Sha, Jin Guo Lan, She Gan, Huang Lian, Jin Yin Hua, Mai Men Dong, He Zi Rou, Huang Qing, Zhi Zi, Jin Deng Long, Chuan Bei Mu and Gan Cao. The Tianjin formula is used to treat Stomach Heat which has damaged the Yin and body fluids, as well as Lung Heat.

There is a third formula made in Shanghai which is even more cooling because it contains some minerals.

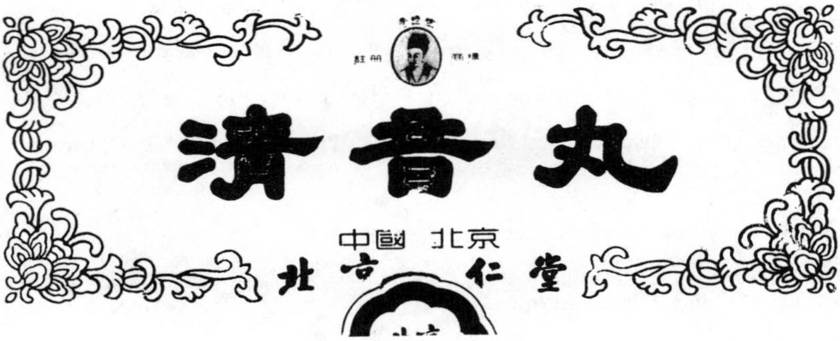

7.12 龍 膽 瀉 肝 丸

龍	胆	瀉	肝	丸
Long	**Dan**	**Xie**	**Gan**	**Wan**
dragon	Gall Bladder	discharge	Liver	pills

Source: Yi Zong Jin Jian, (The Golden Mirror of Medicine), Qing Dynasty, 1644 -1911.

Function: 1. Discharge Liver/Gall Bladder Damp Heat Accumulation
2. Discharge Excess Liver Fire

Application: 1. Use to treat Excess Liver Heat syndrome. This will drain the Excess Liver Fire in the upper portion of the body, including red, swollen eyes, headache, bitter taste in the mouth, earache, sudden deafness due to Excess Liver/Gall Bladder Heat. Pain in the hypochondriac region may also be present. Due to Excess Damp Heat Accumulation, the urine may be dark in color and scanty.

2. Some Western medicine disease applications include the following: (Note, in order to use this formula for the following disorders, the patient must have signs of Excess Liver Fire, Damp Heat Accumulation.) Acute conjunctivitis, acute otitis media, acute nasal furuncle, acute furuncle in the external auditory canal, hypertension due to excess Liver Fire, acute hepatitis with jaundice, acute cholecystitis, acute pyelonephritis, acute cystitis, acute urethritis, acute pelvic inflammatory disease, acute vulvitis, prostatitis.

Dose: 8 pills, 3 times a day

Long Dan Xie Gan Wan is produced as "Lung Tan Xie Gan Pill" by the Guangzhou Pharmaceutical Company, Guangzhou, China, in bottles of 100 pills.

The ingredients are listed below in 6 groups according to function.

Pinyin Name	Pharmaceutical Name	Percent	TCM Function
Group 1 (Primary ingredients)			
Long Dan Cao	Radix Gentianae Scabrae	15.38	Discharge Excess Damp Heat in the Liver/Gall Bladder
Zhi Zi	Fructus Gardeniae Jasminoidis	7.6	
Huang Qin	Radix Scutellariae Baicalensis	7.69	
Group 2 (Assistant ingredients)			
Ze Xie	Rhizoma Alismatis Plantago-aquaticae	15.38	Clear Heat; Promote Urination; Discharge Damp Heat Accumulation
Mu Tong	Caulis Mutong	7.69	
Che Qian Zi	Semen Plantaginis	7.69	
Group 3			
Chai Hu	Radix Bupleuri	15.38	Smooth Liver Qi; Regulate Liver Qi
Group 4			
Dang Gui	Radix Angelicae Sinensis	7.69	Strengthen Blood; Nourish Liver
Sheng Di Huang	Radix Rehmanniae Glutinosae	7.69	
Group 5			
Gan Cao	Radix Glycyrrhizae Uralensis	7.69	Harmonize other herbs

Notes: 1. This Patent Medicine is also available in tablet form. The formula used in this prepared formula is an especially well-organized formula. This means that there is a monarch medicine, Long Dan Cao; minister medicines, Zhi Zi, Huang Qin, Zi Xie, Mu Tong, and Che Qian Zi; assistant medicines, Chai Hu; Dang Gui, and Sheng Di Huang; and a guide medicine, Gan Cao. Formulas which contain four portions (monarch, minister, assistant and guide medicines) are considered to be well-organized formulas. Whenever herbs are used to Discharge Damp Heat, additional herbs are also used to Nourish Blood and Nourish Yin to prevent the possible side effects from the strong Cooling medicines.

2. Most medicines in this formula have a bitter taste (Cold property), thus, if used for a long period of time, it may damage the Spleen or Stomach. Therefore, this medicine should be stopped promptly, after the patient recovers.

3. A formula similar to this formula is also available in liquid, tincture form as "Quell Fire" in the Jade Pharmacy product line, available through Crane Enterprises, Plymouth, MA, etc. See bottom of page 343.

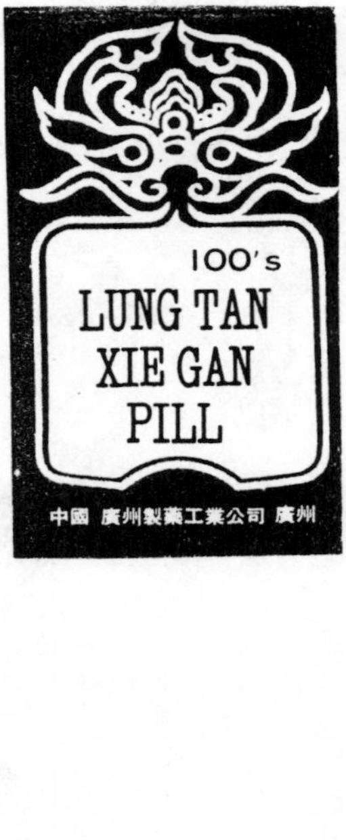

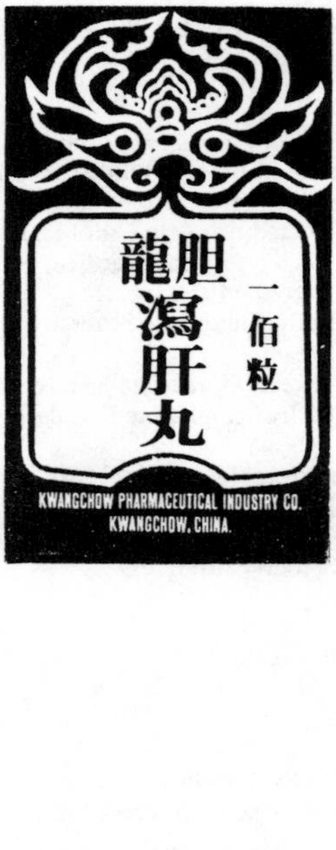

7.13 喉 炎 丸

喉	炎	丸
Hou	**Yan**	**Wan**
larynx	inflammation	pills

Function: 1. Clear Heat; Detoxify Fire Poison, Stop pain.

Application: 1. Use to treat throat diseases such as pharyngitis, tonsillitis, laryngitis.

2. Use to treat spasms or seizures in children due to high-grade fever or central nervous system infection.

3. Use to treat furuncles or carbuncles of the skin and subcutaneous tissue. Use externally and internally with furuncles and carbuncles. When used externally, this medicine is most effective when used with a red, swollen furuncle or carbuncle without pus on the inside. If the furuncle or carbuncle has turned to an open wound with pus, do not use this medicine externally.

Contraindication: Do not use with pregnant women.

Dose: Internal Use: 3 times a day, taken with warm water.
Adults: 10 pills, 3 times a day.
Children: Children 1 Year: 1 pill each time. Children 2 Years: 2 pills each time.
Children 3 Years: 3-4 pills each time. Children 4-8 Years: 5-6 pills each time.
Children 9-15 Years: 7-9 pills each time.

External Use: Stir at least 10 pills into a small amount of cold water or vinegar. Apply this mixture onto the periphery of the red and swollen skin area. Cover the affected area with gauze moistened with a saline solution; it is important to keep the affected area wet, otherwise the herbal medicine will not be absorbed. Store the unusued solution in the refrigerator and use this same mixture several times a day. Continue to apply this mixture until the swelling and infection have disappeared.

Hou Yan Wan is produced as "Laryngitis Pills" by the Szechuan Chengtu Chinese Medicine Works, Szechuan, China, in small vials, each containing 10 pills; there are 3 vials per box.

The percentage of each ingredient in this formula is not available. The herbs are grouped according to function when possible. There are a few herbs which must be listed separately.

Pinyin Name	Pharmaceutical Name	TCM Function
Group 1		
Xi Jiao	Cornu Rhinoceri	Clear Heat; Detoxify Fire Poison
Xiong Dan	Fel Ursi	
Niu Huang	Calculus Bovis	
Huang Lian	Rhizoma Coptidis	
Peng Sha	Borax	
Separate Herbs		
She Xiang	Secretio Moschus moschiferi	Decrease swelling; Remove Heat Accumulation
Chan Su	Secretio Bufonis	Decrease swelling; Detoxify Fire Poison; Stop pain
Zhen Zhu	Magarita	Detoxify Fire Poison; Promote tissue regeneration

Note: 1. There is another Patent Medicine, Hou Zheng Wan, which is similar in name and function to this Patent Medicine, Hou Yan Wan. In Hou Zheng Wan, there are several additional ingredients, and no She Xiang. The additional ingredients include Ban Lan Gen, Xuan Ming Fen, Qing Dai and Bai Cao Shuang. Hou Zheng Wan is often used at the beginning stage of tonsillitis, pharyngitis, laryngitis, etc. Hou Yan Wan and Liu Shen Wan are effective even if pus has developed in tonsillitis, whereas Hou Zheng Wan is not. In addition, Hou Yan Wan and Liu Shen Wan are more effective in treating carbuncles.

川江牌
TRADE MARK
CHUAN JIANG PAI

LARYNGITIS PILLS

喉炎丸

中國四川省製藥總廠成都分廠出品

PREPARED BY

CHINA SZECHUAN PROVINCIAL PHARMACEUTICAL FACTORY, CHENGTU BRANCH.

7.14 降 压 平 片

Jiang	Ya	Ping	Pian
decrease	pressure	normalize	tablets

Function: 1. Clear Liver Heat; Settle Excess Liver Yang; Reduce Internal Wind; Primary function is to decrease high blood pressure.

2. Soften blood vessels (i.e. soften the "hardened arteries"), yet also strengthen them so they will not be easily torn or broken.

3. Decrease high cholesterol levels in the blood.

Applications: 1. Use to treat hypertension, especially in the early stage. In this stage, the blood vessels are not yet seriously hardened and the atherosclerosis is not yet severe. Also, the high blood pressure has not yet affected the heart, brain or kidney function. The high blood pressure should start to be reduced within two weeks of treatment. After using this formula, additional symptoms including dizziness, headache, tinnitus and excess anger will also improve. This formula can be used for several years with no negative side effects.

Dose: 4 tablets, 3 times a day over at least 3, two-week Courses. After Course 1, the HBP should be decreased. After Courses 2 and 3, the HBP should be within normal limits. If the blood pressure is not WNL after 3 Courses, it can be continued for a few more Courses.

Jiang Ya Ping Pian is produced as "Hypertension Repressing Tablets" by the Liaoyuan Pharmaceutic Works, Liao Yang, China.

Pinyin Name	Pharmaceutical Name	Percent	TCM Function
Xia Ku Cao	Spica Prunellae Vulgaris	25	Clear Liver Heat; Disperse Liver Fire; Decrease blood pressure
Huang Qin	Radix Scutellariae Baicalensis	25	Clear Heat; Disperse Fire; Decrease blood pressure; Calm the patient
Di Long	Lumbricus	20	Clear Liver Heat; Calm the Wind; Decrease blood pressure
Ju Hua	Flos Chrysanthemi Morifolii	15	Clear Liver Heat; Extinguish Wind; Dilate coronary arteries;
Huai Hua	Flos Sophorae Japonicae Immaturus	15	Cool the blood; Decrease blood pressure; Treat atherosclerosis; Decrease fragility of small blood vessels

Note: 1. This Patent Medicine is most effective in treating hypertension in the early stage.

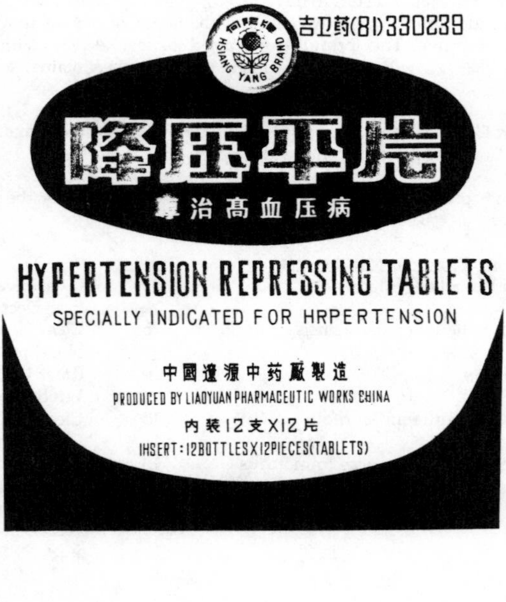

7.15 降 壓 丸

Jiang	Ya	Wan
decrease	pressure	pills

Source: This formula was developed by Dr. Shi Chin-Mo, in the 20th c.

Function: 1. Clear Heat from Excess Yang; Lower high blood pressure in cases with Excess Yang.
2. Calm the Internal Wind; Promote Blood circulation

Application: 1. Use to treat hypertension due to Excess Yang Heat or Internal Wind.
Symptoms: Hypertension with dizziness, uneasiness, stiff neck, distending type of headache and red face.

2. Use to treat Excess type of hypertension cases who are in a "pre-stroke condition" who have already had one or more Transient Ischemic Attacks (TIA's) resulting in temporary neurological symptoms such as facial or limb paralysis, diminished visual field, abnormal sensations in face or limbs, etc.

Contraindications: Do not use with pregnant women; this formula contains herbs which will promote Blood circulation, Remove Stagnation, bring down Qi, and could cause a miscarriage.

Use this formula with Excess Yang type cases only. It will get into the Liver and Heart Channels and Clear Excess Yang Heat. When an Excess Yang case who is taking this formula contracts a Wind-Cold OPI syndrome, this formula should temporarily be stopped; it contains several Cold Property herbs.

Dose: 20 pills, 2 times a day, taken with warm water.

Jiang Ya Wan is produced as "Chiang Ya Wan" by Beijing Tung Jen Tang pharmacy in bottles of 200 pills.

Pinyin Name	Pharmaceutical Name	Percent	TCM Function
Chong Yu Zi	Semen Leonuri Heterophylli	15	Clear Liver Heat; Promote Blood circulation
Huang Lian	Rhizoma Coptidis	3	Clear Heat
Ling Yang Jiao	Cornu Antelopis	3	Clear Liver Heat; Extinguish Liver Wind
Gou Teng	Ramulus Uncariae Cum Uncis	7	Clear Liver Heat; Extinguish Liver Wind; Clear Meridians; Decrease blood pressure
Hu Po	Succinum	3	Tranquilize the Spirit; Promote Blood circulation; Promote urination
Dang Gui	Radix Angelicae Sinensis	8	Tonify Blood; Remove Blood Stasis
Chen Xiang	Lignum Aquilariae	5	Move Stuck Qi
Chuan Xiong	Rhizoma Ligustici Wallichii	5	Promote Blood circulation; Stop headache
Tian Ma	Rhizoma Gastrodiae Elatae	4	Stop Liver Wind; Clear Meridians
Da Huang	Rhizoma Rhei	4	Clear Heat; Treat constipation
Sheng Di Huang	Radix Rehmanniae Glutinosae	10	Clear Heat; Cool Blood
A Jiao	Gelatinum Asini	10	Nourish Blood and Nourish Yin
Xia Ku Cao	Spica Prunellae Vulgaris	5	Clear Liver Heat; Decrease blood pressure
Mu Dan Pi	Cortex Moutan Radicis	5	Clear Heat; Promote Blood circulation; Decrease blood pressure
Niu Xi	Radix Achyranthis Bidentatae	13	Remove Blood Stasis; Promote blood circulation; Decrease blood pressure

Note: 1. This formula is commonly used with cases who are either in the early, or more developed stages of hypertension with headache and dizziness; as well as with cases who have developed temporary central nervous system symptoms such as facial or limb paralysis or numbness or speech problems.

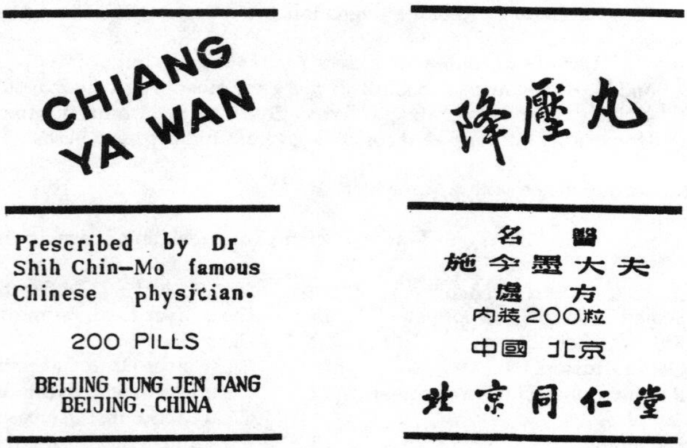
CHIANG
YA WAN
Prescribed by Dr
Shih Chin-Mo famous
Chinese physician.
200 PILLS
BEIJING TUNG JEN TANG
BEIJING. CHINA
降壓丸
名醫
施今墨大夫
處方
内装200粒
中國 北京
北京同仁堂

7.16 杜 仲 片

Du Zhong Pian

-----Cortex Eucommiae----- tablets

Function:
1. Nourish Kidney Yang; Lower high blood pressure in Def. Kidney Yang cases.
2. Decrease cholesterol.
3. Reduce hardening of the arteries and blood vessels.
4. Calm the Spirit and tranquilize

Application:

1. Use to treat earlier stages of high blood pressure in cases with Def. Kidney Yang. Symptoms: High blood pressure in patients with a pale face who feel cold and complain of lumbago; limb numbness and/or edema may also be present.

2. Use to treat earlier stages of high blood pressure in cases with Excess Liver Wind syndrome. Symptoms: High blood pressure with agitation, uneasiness, insomnia, excess anger.

3. Use to treat atherosclerosis.

Dose: 5 tablets, 3 times a day, taken with warm water. If the patient has problems above the acupuncture point CV 8 (umbilicus), take after a meal; if the patient has problems below CV 8, take before a meal

Du Zhong Pian is produced as "Compound Cortex Eucommiae Tablets" by the Kweichow United Pharmaceutical Manufactory, Kweichow, China, in bottles of 100 coated tablets.

Pinyin Name	Pharmaceutical Name	Percent	TCM Function
Du Zhong	Cortex Eucommiae	50	Strengthen Liver, Kidney; Decrease blood pressures; Tranquilize
Gou Teng	Ramulus Uncariae Cum Uncis	20	Calm Liver Wind; Decrease blood pressure; Tranquilize
Huang Qin	Radix Scutellariae Baicalensis	10	Clear Heat; Tranquilize; Decrease blood pressure
Xia Ku Cao	Spica Prunellae Vulgaris	20	Decrease blood pressure; Clear Liver Heat; Reduce Excess Liver Yang

Note: 1. It is common to take this formula in conjunction with anti-hypertensive Western medicines. It is important to monitor the blood pressure, and eventually, the amount of Western medicine may be reduced or eliminated. This herbal formula will have a gradual effect in reducing the high blood pressure. It has no side effects and may be taken for a long period of time.

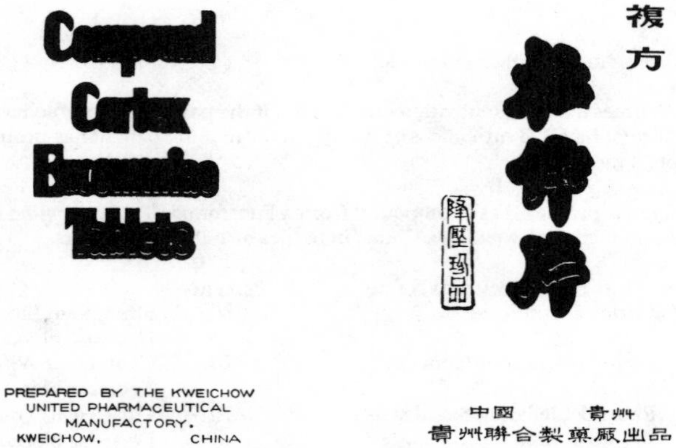

7.17 黃 連 羊 肝 丸

Huang	Lian	Yang	Gan	Wan
----Rhizoma Coptidis----		goat	liver	pills

Source: Tai Ping Hui Min He Ji Ju Fang, (Formulas of the People's Welfare Pharmacy), Song Dynasty, 960-1279.

Function: 1. Disperse Liver Fire; Brighten the eyes

Application: 1. Use to treat eye disorders due to Excess Liver Fire. Symptoms: Poor vision, especially at night, photophobia, pterygium of the eye extending over a part of the cornea; plus other Liver Fire symptoms such as headache, dizziness, bitter taste in the mouth, restlessness and eye redness

2. Some Western medicine disease applications include the following: (Note, these Western medicine eye disorders must be associated with Excess Liver Fire, to use this formula.) Glaucoma, cataracts, night blindness.

Dose: 1 honey pill, 2 times a day.

Pinyin Name	Pharmaceutical Name	Grams	TCM Function
Huang Lian	Rhizoma Coptidis	20	Clear Heat; Detoxify Fire Poison
Mi Meng Hua	Flos Buddleiae Officinalis	40	Clear Liver Heat; brighten eyes; Remove pterygium
Jue Ming Zi	Semen Cassiae Torae	40	Clear Heat in Liver and Large Intestine; Brighten eyes; Laxative
Shi Jue Ming	Concha Haliotidis	40	Clear Liver Heat; Decrease Excess Liver Yang; Brighten the eyes
Chong Wei Zi	Semen Leonuri Heterophylli	40	Cool the Liver; Brighten the eyes; Remove pterygium
Ye Ming Sha	Excrementum Vespertilii Murini	40	Clear Heat; Nourish eyes; Improve night vision (High level of Vitamin A)
Long Dan Cao	Radix Gentianae Scabrae	20	Clear Liver Heat
Huang Bai	Cortex Phellodendri	20	Clear Heat; Detoxity Fire Poison
Huang Qin	Radix Scutellariae Baicalensis	40	Clear Heat; Detoxify Fire Poison
Hu Huang Lian	Rhizoma Picrorrhizae	40	Clear Heat; Detoxify Fire Poison
Chai Hu	Radix Bupleuri	40	Smooth Liver; Move Stuck Liver Qi
Qing Pi	Pericarpium Citri Reticulatae Viride	40	Move Stuck Liver Qi; Reduce depression
Mu Zei	Herba Equiseti Hiemalis	40	Expel Wind Heat; Remove pterygium
Yang Gan	Fresh Lamb Liver	160	Nourish Liver Yin; Strengthen vision

7.18 利 肝 片

Li	**Gan**	**Pian**
benefit	Liver	tablets

Function: 1. Clear Heat
2. Soothe Liver; Clear bile ducts

Application: 1. Use to treat acute hepatitis with or without jaundice.

2. Use to treat chronic hepatitis and chronic cholecystitis. This formula will decrease pain in the liver area and help relieve the symptoms. This formula can also be used to help expel gallstones.

Dose: 2 to 4 pills, 3 times a day, after meals.

Li Gan Pian is produced as "Liver Strengthening Tablets, Ligan Pian" by the Zhengjiang Chinese Medicine Works, Kiangsu, China, in bottles of 100 coated tablets.

Pinyin Name	Pharmaceutical Name	Percent	TCM Function
Jin Qian Cao	Lysimachia christinae	70	Clear Heat; Decrease Jaundice; Promote urination; Expel urinary tract or biliary stones
Dan Zhi	Selenarctos thibetanus	30	Clear Heat; Decrease inflammation of liver or gallbladder; Assist in digestion of fat

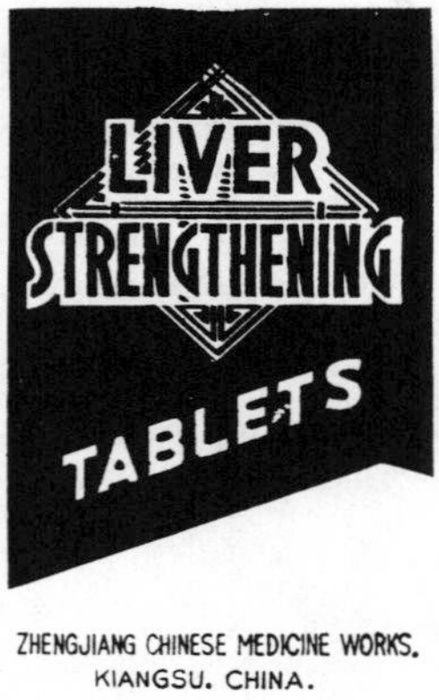

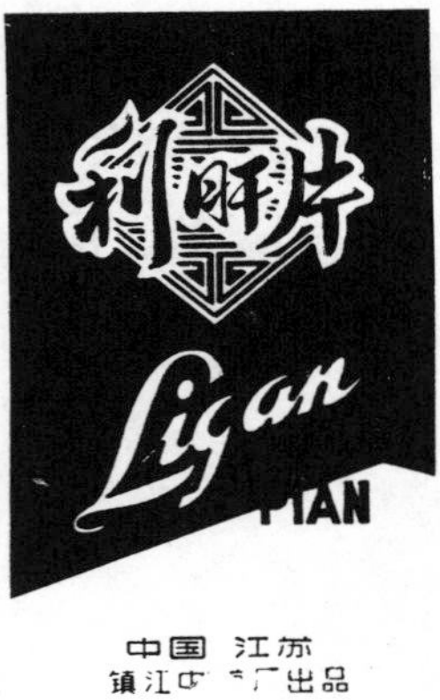

7.19 利 胆 片

Li	Dan	Pian
benefit	Gall Bladder	tablets

Function: 1. Clear bile ducts; eliminate inflammation

Application: 1. Use to treat acute jaundice due to Damp Heat (Yang Jaundice).

2. Use to treat acute or chronic inflammation in the bile ducts, or acute or chronic cholecyctitis.

3. Use to treat gallstones (cholecystolithiasis); this formula will help to expel the smaller stones, less than 1 cm in diameter (Nankai Hospital, Tianjin, China).

Dose: 4 to 6 tablets, 3 times a day.

Li Dan Pian is produced as "Lidan Tablets" by the Tsingtao Pharmaceutical Works, Tsingtao, China, in bottles of 120 tablets.

Pinyin Name	Pharmaceutical Name	Percent	TCM Function
Huang Qin	Radix Scutellariae Baicalensis	30	Clear Heat; Eliminate inflammation; Detoxify Fire Poison
Mu Xiang	Radix Saussureae seu Vladimiriae	16	Move Stuck Qi, Stop pain
Jin Qian Cao	Lysimachia christinae	10	Clear Heat; Decrease jaundice; Promote urination; Expel urinary tract or biliary stones
Jin Yin Hua	Flos Lonicerae Japonicae	10	Clear Heat; Decrease inflammation
Yin Chen	Herba Artemesiae Capillaris	10	Clear Damp Heat; Decrease jaundice
Chai Hu	Radix Bupleuri	10	Move Stuck Liver Qi; Clear bile ducts
Da Qing Ye	Isatis tinctoria L.	10	Clear Heat; Decrease inflammaton; Detoxify Fire Poison
Da Huang	Rhizoma Rhei	4	Clear intestinal heat; Promote bowel movement

Note: The Patent Medicine, Li Dan Pai Shi Pian, is similar to Li Dan Pian.

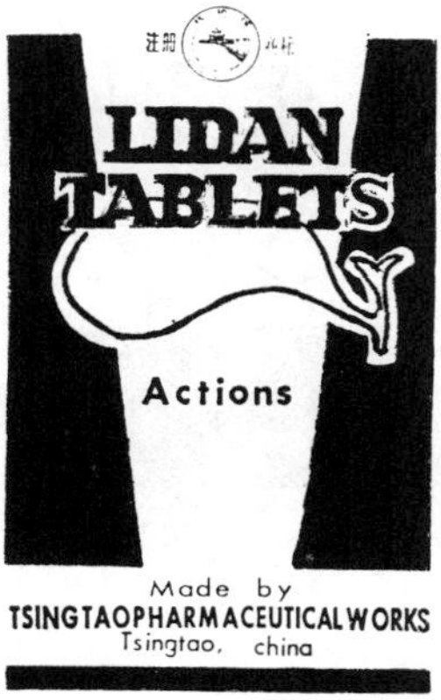

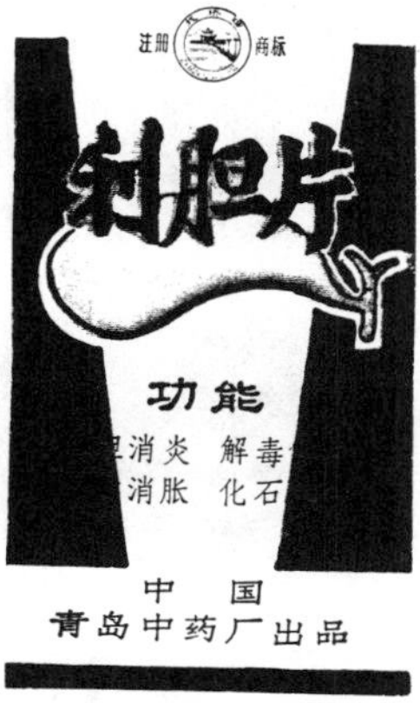

7.20 槐 角 丸

Huai	**Jiao**	**Wan**
Fructus Sophorae Japonicae		pills

Source: Dan Xi Xin Fa (Methods of Dr. Dan-Xi Zhu), Yuan Dynasty, 1279-1368.

Function:
1. Clear Heat in Large Intestine (LI)
2. Stop bleeding due to Wind in LI which produces stool with fresh blood

Application:
1. Use to stop intestinal bleeding where there is fresh blood with or without the stool.
2. Use to stop bleeding from hemorrhoids.
3. Use to treat intestinal bleeding associated with Excess Heat syndrome. Symptoms: Burning sensation around the anus, constipation or incomplete sensation following bowel movement (Damp Heat in LI), thirst; rapid Pulse

Dose: 9 pills, 3 times a day.

Huai Jiao Wan is produced as "Fructus Sophorae" by the Min-Kang Drug Manufactory, I-Chang, China, in bottles of 100 pills.

Pinyin Name	Pharmaceutical Name	Percent	TCM Function
Huai Jiao	Fructus Sophorae Japonicae	28.5	Clear Heat; Stop bleeding
Zhi Qiao	Fructus Citri seu Ponciri	14.3	Move Stuck Qi; Decrease distension
Dang Gui	Radix Angelicae Sinensis	14.3	Tonify Blood; Regulate Blood Function
Di Yu	Radix Sanguisorbae Officinalis	14.3	Cool Blood; Stop bleeding
Fang Feng	Radix Ledebouriellae Sesloidis	14.3	Eliminate Wind in Large Intestine; Stop bleeding
Huang Qin	Radix Scutellariae Baicalensis	14.3	Clear Heat; Reduce swelling

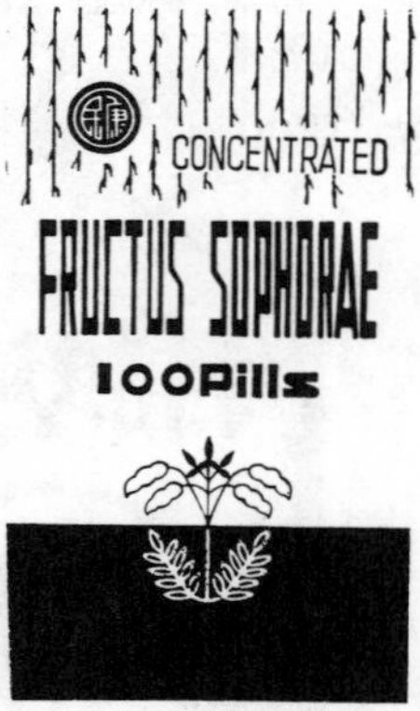

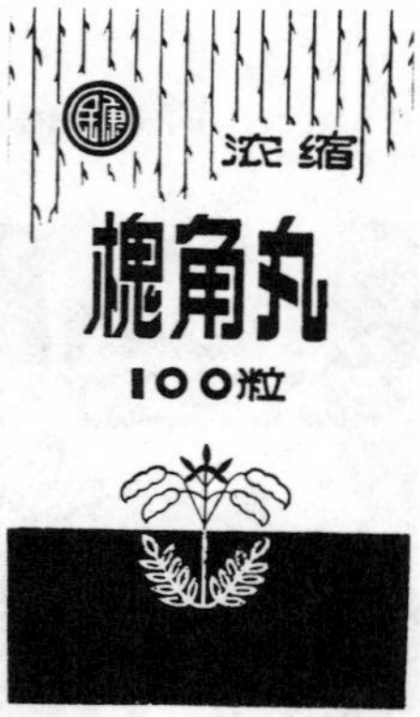

7.21 化 痔 灵 丸

化	痔	灵	丸
Hua	**Zhi**	**Ling**	**Wan**
eliminate	hemorrhoids	effective	pills

Function:
1. Clear Heat; Cool the Blood
2. Reduce swelling; Stop pain

Application:
1. Use to treat hemorrhoids due to Damp Heat collecting in the Lower Warmer.
   Symptoms: Swollen hemorrhoids with red color and severe pain.
2. Use to stop bleeding from hemorrhoids.
3. Use to treat prolapsed anus with bleeding, pain and swelling.

Dose: 4-6 pills, 3 times a day

Hua Zhi Ling Wan is produced as "Fargelin for Piles" by the United Pharmaceutical Manufactory, Guangzhou, China, in bottles of 60 coated pills.

Pinyin Name	Pharmaceutical Name	Percent	TCM Function
Wan Ge	Cyclian sinensis Gmelin	30	Stop bleeding; Stop prolapse; Astringent property
Shi Liu Pi	Pericarpium Punicae Granati	30	Stop bleeding; Stop prolapse; Astringent property
Huang Lian	Rhizoma Coptidis	10	Clear Heat; Detoxify Fire Poison
Tian Qi	Radix Pseudoginseng	17	Stop bleeding; Stop pain
Xiong Dan	Fel Ursi	3	Clear Heat; Cool Blood
Hu Po	Succinum	10	Disperse Stuck Blood; Aid in tissue regeneration

Other formulas may also contain the following ingredients:

Huai Hua	Flos Sophorae Japonicae Immaturus	Stop intestinal bleeding; Clear Heat
Wu Bei Zi	Galla Rhi Chinensis	Stop prolapse; Astringent property;
Xiong Huang	Realgar	Detoxify Fire Poison in the intestines

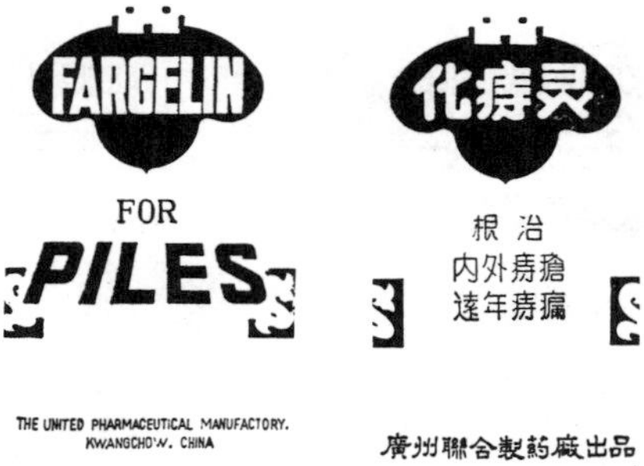

7.22

强	力	化	痔	灵
Qiang	**Li**	**Hua**	**Zhi**	**Ling**
-----extra strength-----		eliminate	hemorrhoid	effective

Function: 1. Clear Heat; Stop pain; Stop bleeding

Application: 1. Use to treat internal and/or external hemorrhoids; prolapsed anus. This formula will help to stop bleeding, stop pain and prevent infection.

Dose: 3 or 4 pills, 3 times a day. For serious cases, the dose can be doubled. Use at least 3 days.

Qiang Li Hua Zhi Ling is produced as "High Strength Fargelin for Piles" by the United Pharmaceutical Manufactory, Guangzhou, China, in bottles of 36 coated tablets.

Pinyin Name	Pharmaceutical Name	Percent	TCM Function
Hu Po	Succinum	15	Disperse Stuck Blood; Aid in tissue regeneration
Xiong Dan	Fel Ursi	5	Clear Heat; Cool Blood
Tian Qi	Radix Pseudoginseng	20	Stop bleeding; Stop pain
Huang Qin	Radix Scutellariae Baicalensis	15	Clear Heat; Detoxify Fire Poison
Yuan Hu	Rhizoma Corydalis Yanhusuo	5	Stop pain
Di Yu	Radix Sanguisorbae Officinalis	10	Stop bleeding
Huai Hua	Flos Sophorae Japonicae Immaturus	15	Stop bleeding; Cool the Blood
Zi Zhu Cao	Folium Callicarpae	15	Stop bleeding; Reduce inflammation

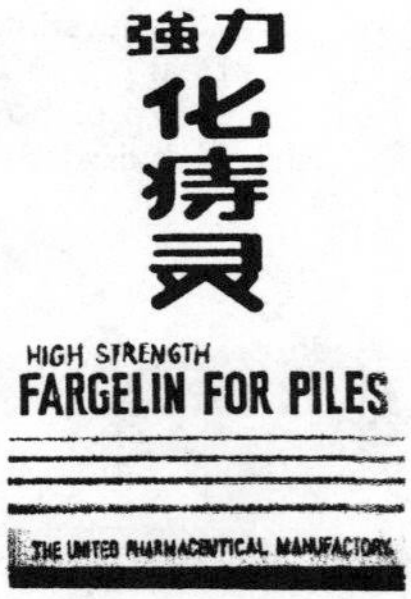

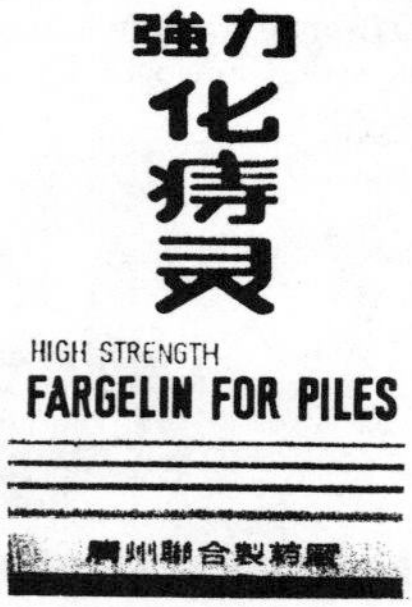

7.23 痔 丸

Zhi **Wan**

hemorrhoid pills

Source: Yang Yi Da Chuen, (Complete Book of Dermatology), Qing Dynasty, 1644-1911

Function:
1. Clear Heat; Decrease swelling
2. Promote Blood circulation; Remove Blood Stasis; Stop pain
3. Discharge pus

Application:
1. Use to treat infected hemorrhoids with swelling, pain and abscess with pus.

2. Use to stop bleeding from hemorrhoids.

3. Use to treat anal abscess with pus, bleeding and inflammation

4. Use to treat a thrombosed hemorrhoid that has hardened. A thrombosed hemorrhoid is one containing clotted blood. Pain is the primary problem associated with this condition. In addition to pain with a bowel movement, there is pain with sitting or coughing. When the hemorrhoid is examined, it is hard and there is a round-shaped node, purple in color. (This formula is especially effective for this condition.)

Dose: 6 pills, 2 or 3 times a day

Zhi Wan is produced as "Zhiwan" by the Min-Kang Drug Manufactory, I-Chang, China, in bottles of 100 pills.

Pinyin Name	Pharmaceutical Name	Percent	TCM Function
Ci Wei Po	Erinaceus europeous L.	18.8	Stop hemorrhoid bleeding
Chuan Shan Jia	Squama Manitis Pentadactylae	1.5	Move Stuck Blood; Decrease swelling
Jin Yin Hua	Flos Lonicerae Japonicae	18.8	Clear Heat; Detoxify Fire Poison
Hong Hua	Flos Carthami Tinctorii	3.7	Promote Blood circulation; Move Blood Stasis; Eliminate swelling
Huai Hua	Flos Sophorae Japonicae Immaturus	18.8	Stop bleeding; Cool the Blood
Bing Lang	Semen Arecae Catechu	4.7	Move Stuck Qi
Ru Xiang	Gummi Olibanum	2.8	Promote Blood circulation; Stop pain; Decrease swelling of the hemorrhoid
Mo Yao	Myrrha	1.5	Promote Blood circulation; Stop pain; Decrease swelling of the hemorrhoid
Bai Zhi	Radix Angelicae	2.8	Decrease swelling; Stop pain; Expel pus
	Subsidiary substances to 100%		

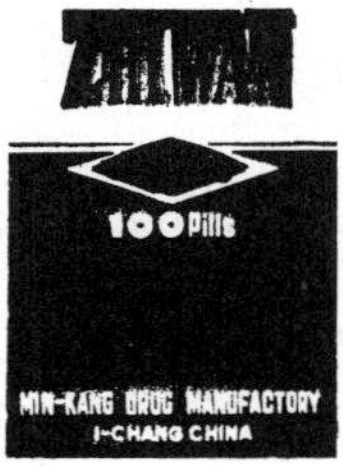

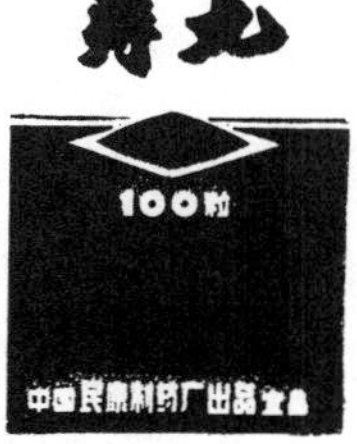

7.24 熊 胆 痔 瘡 膏

Xiong	Dan	Zhi	Ling	Gao
--------Fel Ursi-------		hemorrhoid effective		ointment

Function: 1. Clear Heat; Detoxify Fire Poison; reduce inflammation.
2. Stop pain; stop bleeding.

Application: 1. Use to treat hemorrhoids with inflammation and bleeding.
Symptoms: Swelling, burning sensation, itching, and constipation.

2. Use to treat anal fissure.

3. Pruritus ani

Dose: For External Use Only. Apply onto the anal region. The area should be clean before the ointment is applied. Apply the ointment, 1 to 3 times a day.

Xiong Dan Zhi Ling Gao is produced as "Hemorrhoid's Ointment" by the Chung-Lien Drug Works, Hangzhou, China in two sizes, 4 gram and 10 gram tubes.

Pinyin Name	Pharmaceutical Name	Percent	TCM Function
Group 1			
Xiong Dan	Fel Ursi	2.7	Clear Heat; Detoxify Fire Poison
Bing Pian	Borneol	1.6	
Zhen Zhu	Magarita	2.7	
Group 2			
Chi Shi Zhi	Halloysitum Rubrum	13.84	Stop bleeding; Astringent property; Eliminate mucous and inflammation
Extra ingredient not in a group			
She Xiang	Secretio Moschus moschiferi	0.16	Promote Blood circulation; Decrease swelling

Note: 1. This ointment is also useful to use to treat other skin sores such as carbuncles with or without open wound and pus.

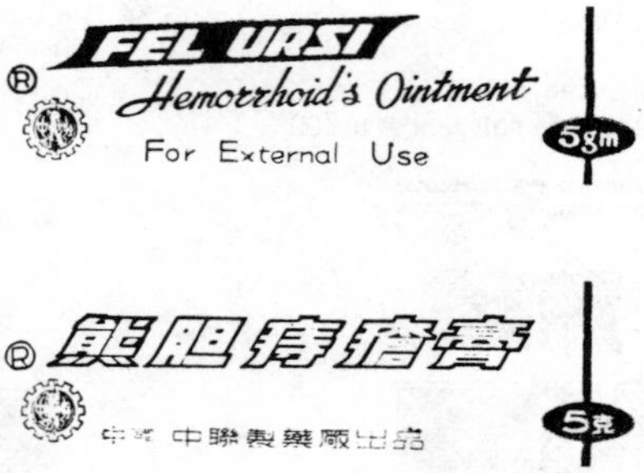

7.25 导 赤 片

Dao	Chi	Pian
lead, guide	heat (red)	tablets

Source: Xiao Er Yao Zheng Zhi Jue, (Pediatric Pharmaceutics), Song Dynasty, 960-1279.

Function: 1. Clear Heat, Reduce Excess Fire
2. Promote bowel movement and urination

Application: 1. Use to treat symptoms due to Excess Fire in the Heart Meridian. Symptoms: Swollen and sore throat; mouth or tongue sore (stomatitis), swollen gum with toothache; pink eye (conjunctivitis); difficult or burning, painful urination with dark yellow urine.

2. Use to treat Excess Heat in the Stomach or Large Intestine (LI) causing constipation.

3. Some Western medicine disease applications include the following: Bacterial infection in the urinary tract including cystitis, urethritis or pyelitis; stomatitis. (Note, for stomatitis, the patient may also apply some herbal medicine locally, e.g. Xi Gua Shuang, #7.10.)

Contraindication: Do not use with pregnant women; or someone who is weak, or someonw who has diarrhea.

Dose: 1 honey pill, 2 times a day. Each honey pill weighs 3 grams.

The 7 herbs are listed below in 4 groups, according to function.

Pinyin Name	Pharmaceutical Name	Percent	TCM Function
Group 1			
Sheng Di Huang	Radix Rehmanniae Glutinosae	15.69	Clear Heat; Nourish Yin; Reduce Heart Fire
Group 2			
Da Huang	Rhizoma Rhei	29.41	Clear Heat; Detoxify Fire Poison Promote bowel movement
Group 3			
Mu Tong	Caulis Mutong	7.84	Clear Heat in Heart;
Zhi Zi	Fructus Gardeniae Jasminoidis	23.53	Relieve painful urination;
Fu Ling	Sclerotium Poriae Cocos	7.84	Discharge Heat through urination
Hua Shi	Talcum	7.84	
Group 4			
Gan Cao	Radix Glycyrrhizae Uralensis	7.84	Harmonize other herbs; Clear Heat; Relieve painful urination

Note: 1. In the title, the word for red, Chi, refers to the color for the Heart (red) in TCM theory. The title refers to "leading away the red," or taking away the Heat in the Heart. In TCM theory, the Heart and Small Intestine are paired organs, and the Small Intestine relates to urination. A urinary tract infection can be referred to as "Heat pouring down from the Heart into the Small Intestine." Therefore, this herbal medicine is also appropriate for urinary tract infection.

If the patient has a urinary tract infection with bleeding, the best results will be obtained if this Patent Medicine is taken with a Yao Yin made of Bai Mao Gen (Rhizoma Imperatae Cylindricae). The Yao Yin should be made with 30 grams of Bai Mao Gen for one day.

7.26 黃 蓮 素 眼 膏

黃	蓮	素	眼	膏
Huang	**Lian**	**Su**	**Yan**	**Gao**
-----Rhizoma Coptidis---		extract	eyes	ointment

Source: Zheng Zhi Jue Sheng, (Regulations for Syndromes and Treatment), by Wang Ken-Tang, Ming Dynasty, 1368-1644.

Function: 1. Clear Heat; Detoxify Fire Poison

Application: 1. Use to treat red, swollen, inflammed eyes due to Excess Liver or Heart Heat.

2. Some Western medicine disease applications include the following: Conjunctivitis, keratitis, other eye infections

Dose: Apply underneath the eyelids, 3 times a day.

Huang Liang Su Yan Gao is produced as "Berberini Hydrochloridi" by the Guangzhou Pharmaceutical Industry Co., Guangzhou, China, in 2.5 gram tubes.

Pinyin Name	Pharmaceutical Name	Percent	TCM Function
Huang Lian	Rhizoma Coptidis	100	Clear Heat; Detoxify Fire Poison; Eliminate Dampness

Note: 1. Berberine, an active ingredient which comprises 5 - 8% of the entire herb, Huang Lian, is the only part used in Huang Lian Su Yan Gao. The original source used the entire herb, Huang Lian, to make a concentrate.

2.5gm BERBERINI HYDROCHLORIDI

2.5克 黃蓮素眼膏

7.27 穿 心 蓮 抗 炎 片

穿	心	蓮	抗	炎	片
Chuan	**Xin**	**Lian**	**Kang**	**Yan**	**Pian**
-------Andrographis Paniculatae-------			against	inflammation	tablets

Source: Chinese Pharmacopoeia

Function: 1. Clear Heat and reduce inflammation in the Upper, Middle and Lower Warmers

Application: 1. Use to treat Upper Warmer inflammation associated with Lung Heat - common cold, flu.

2. Use to treat cough or chronic asthma associated with Lung Heat. Sputum should be yellow

3. Use to treat pulmonary abscess, pneumonia, tuberculosis and other infections associated with Lung Heat.

4. Use to Clear Damp Heat in the Lower Warmer with symptoms such as urinary tract infection, diarrhea or dysentery. It is also useful as a preventative measure against urinary tract infection when travelling, etc.

Dose: 2 or 3 pills, 3 times a day. In severe cases, the dose may be increased to 6 pills, 3 times a day; it may also be combined with #7.8, Niu Huang Jie Du Pian.

Chuan Xin Lian Kang Yan Pian is produced as "Chuan Xin Lian Antiphlogistic Tablets" by the United Pharmaceutical Manufactory, Guangzhou, China, in bottles of 36 coated tablets.

Pinyin Name	Pharmaceutical Name	Percent	TCM Function
Chuan Xin Lian	Herba Andrographis Paniculatae	50	Clear Heat
Pu Gong Ying	Herba Taraxici Mongolici cum Radice	25	Clear Heat; Detoxify Fire Poison
Ban Lan Gen	Radix Isatidis seu Baphicacanthi	25	Clear Heat; Detoxify Fire Poison; Clear Blood Heat

Note: 1. Pharmacology research in China has observed this herbal formula to inhibit Bacillus dysentery and viruses. It has also been observed to inhibit growth of Streptococcus, Staphylococcus, and Diplococcus bactaeria (present in pneumonia).

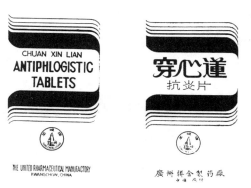

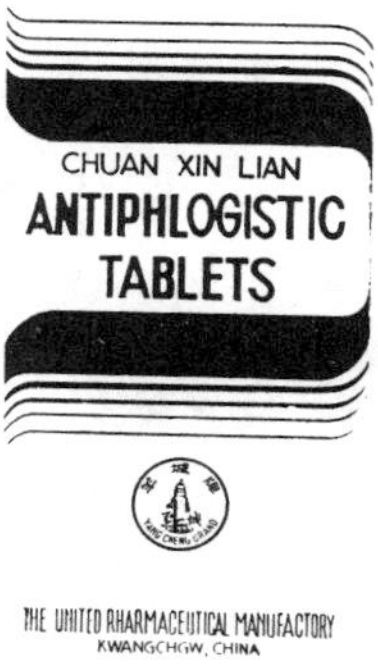

7.28 牛 黄 消 炎 丸

Niu	Huang	Xiao	Yan	Wan
cow	gallstone	eliminate	inflammation	pills

Source: Yao Dian, (Chinese Pharmacopoeia)

Function: 1. Clear Heat and relieve inflammation and fever due to Fire Poison

Application: 1. Use to treat serious tonsillitis and pharyngitis with throat swelling and pain associated with Fire Poison. Pus may be present.

2. Use to treat skin infections such as carbuncles and sores.

3. Use to treat mastitis.

Contraindication: Do not use with pregnant women. It may be used by a nursing mother, but it may cause some diarrhea in the baby.

Dose: Interal Use: Adults: 10 pills, 2 or 3 times a day. Children under 5 years: Use one-quarter the adult dose. Children over 5 years: Use one-half the adult dose, or less.

External Use: Use externally for carbuncles and sores. Crush the pills into powder form and use directly as a powder or mix with a small amount of vinegar, and place on the sore; cover with a sterile dressing. Apply once a day.

Niu Huang Xiao Yan Wan is produced as "Niuhuang Xiaoyanwan" by the Soochow Chinese Medicine Works, Kiangsu, China, in small vials containing 60 tiny pills.

Pinyin Name	Pharmaceutical Name	Percent	TCM Function
Niu Huang	Calculus Bovis	9.16	Clear Heat; Detoxify Fire Poison
Jen Zhu Mu	Concha Margaritifera Usta	19.23	Clear Liver Heat; Tranquilize Spirit
Tian Hua Fen	Radix Trichosanthis	19.23	Clear Heat; Decrease swelling; Discharge pus
Da Huang	Rhizoma Rhei	19.23	Disperse Heat through bowel movement
Qing Dai	Indigo Pulverata Levis	7.69	Clear Blood Heat; Detoxify Fire Poison; Reduce throat swelling
Chan Su	Secretio Bufonis	5.2	Reduce swelling; Detoxify Fire Poison; Stop pain
Xiong Huang	Realgar	19.81	Detoxify Fire Poison; Decrease inflammation

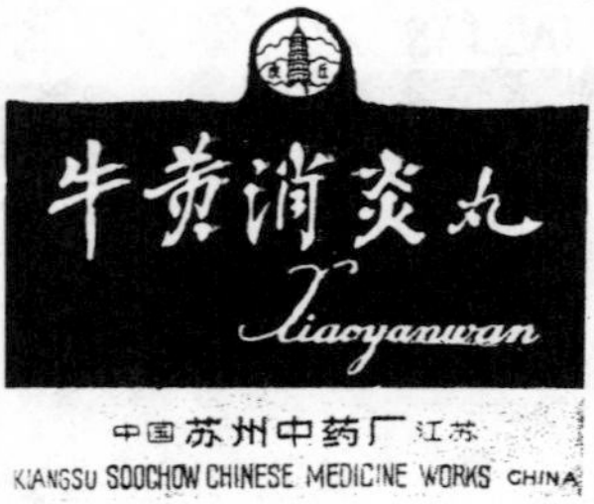

7.29 連翹敗毒片

Lian	Qiao	Bai	Du	Pian
---Forsythiae Suspensae---		------detoxification------		tablets

Source: Zheng Zhi Zhun Sheng, (Standards for Diagnosis and Treatment), Ming Dynasty, 1368-1644.

Function: 1. Clear Heat; Reduce inflammation

2. Eliminate swelling; Relieve pain

Application: 1. Use primarily to treat the early stage of carbuncles where the skin is red, but not yet erupted; pain is present. It is also appropriate to use this if pus is present. This will help to discharge the pus.

2. Use to treat skin infections or any kind of skin inflammation including carbuncles, boils, Poison Ivy, etc. This will Clear Wind Heat.

3. Use to treat eruption of skin, for example, itchy skin caused by allergies. This formula will help to expel Wind Heat in conditions such as psoriasis, etc.

Contraindication: Do not use with pregnant women. While taking this formula, do not eat greasy, spicy food.

Dose: 4-6 tablets, 3 times a day.

Lian Qiao Bai Du Pian is produced as "Lienchiaopaitu Pien" by the Tientsin Drug Manufactory, Tientsin, China in vials containing 8 tablets.

Pinyin Name	Pharmaceutical Name	Percent	TCM Function
Jin Yin Hua	Flos Lonicerae Japonicae	13.78	Clear Heat; Detoxify Fire Poison; Reduce swelling
Zhi Zi	Fructus Gardeniae Jasminoidis	10.34	Clear Heat; Detoxify Fire Poison
Huang Qin	Radix Scutellariae Baicalensis	10.34	Clear Heat; Detoxify Fire Poison
Chi Shao Yao	Radix Paeoniae Rubra	10.34	Clear Heat; Cool Blood; Disperse Blood Stagnation
Bai Xian Pi	Cortex Dictamni Dasycarpi Radicis	10.34	Expel Wind; Eliminate Damp Heat; Stop itching
Lian Qiao	Fructus Forsythiae Suspensae	13.78	Clear Heat; Detoxify Fire Poison; Reduce swelling
Chan Tui	Periostracum Cicadae	6.96	Expel Wind
Fang Feng	Radix Ledebouriellae Sesloidis	40.34	Expel Wind; Stop itching
Da Huang	Rhizoma Rhei	13.78	Detoxify Fire Poison; Promote bowel movement; Rid Fire through bowel movement

Notes: 1. This formula is also available in syrup form (for children) or pill form.

2. Other variations of this formula may contain an additional 9 herbs which have the effect to discharge pus and Clear Heat. These 9 herbs are the following: Huang Qing, Pu Gong Ying, Zhe Bei Mu, Jie Geng, Bai Zhi, Mu Tong, Di Ding, Xuan Shen, and Gan Cao.

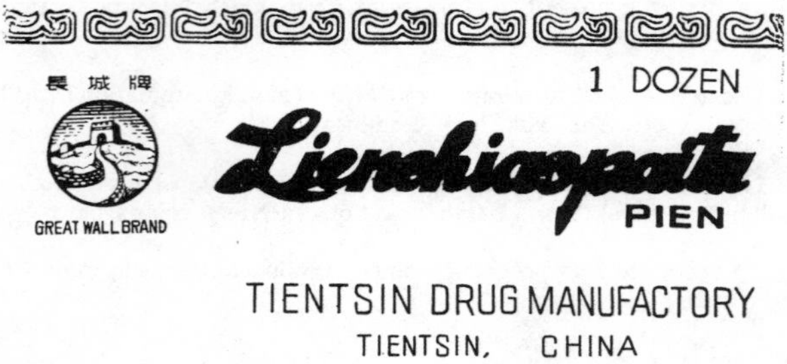

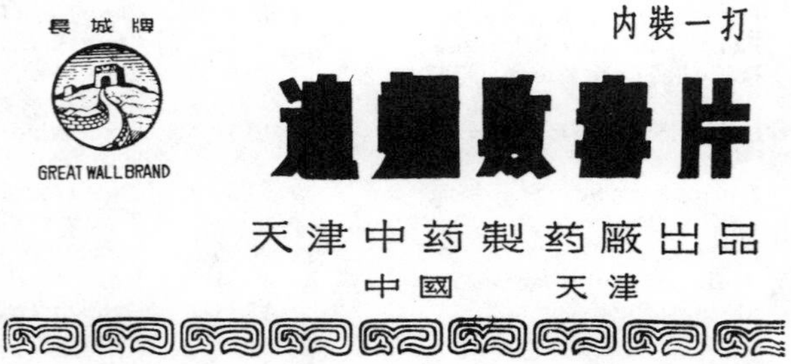

7.30 紫 金 定

Zi	**Jin**	**Ding**
purple	gold	Ding form of Patent Medicine

Source: Wai Ke Zheng Zong, (Orthodox Manual of Surgery), Ming Dynasty, 1368 - 1644. This prepared formula is also in the modern Chinese Pharmacopoeia.

Function:
1. Expel Summer Season Exogenous Evil; Detoxify Fire Poison
2. Decrease inflammation; Stop pain

Application:
1. Use to treat Summer Heat-Stroke with abdominal distension, abdominal pain, diarrhea, semi-unconsciousness.
2. Use to treat children's pneumonia, bronchitis.
3. Use to treat early stage of skin infection such as carbuncles.

Contraindication: Do not use internally with pregnant women.

Dose: The medicine is used either internally or externally.

Internal Use: 0.6 to 1.5 grams, 1 or 2 times a day. Dissolve the medicine in warm water before swallowing; or break the medicine up into pieces, before swallowing with warm water.

External Use: Use vinegar or cold water to soften the medicine and apply the paste onto the affected area. The area may then be covered.

Each Ding vial contains either 0.3 grams or 3 grams.

Pinyin Name	Pharmaceutical Name	Percent	TCM Function
She Xiang	Secretio Moschus moschiferi	4.68	Open Heart Orifice; Detoxify Fire Poison due to Summer Season Exogenous Evil; Promote Blood circulation; Remove Heat Accumulation (Carbuncles)
Shan Ci Gu	Bulbus Shancigu Tulipa edulis Bak.	31.25	Discharge Heat; Remove Accumulation; Decrease swelling
Xiong Huang	Realgar	3.13	Detoxify Fire Poison; Treat Carbuncles
Da Ji	Radix Euphorbiae seu Knoxiae	23.44	Remove Intestinal Accumulation
Qian Jin Zi Shuang	Euphorbia lathyris L.	15.63	Remove Intestinal Accumulation; Decrease swelling
Wu Bei Zi	Galla Rhi Chinensis	15.63	Stop diarrhea; astringent property
Zhu Sha	Cinnabaris	6.25	Calm the Spirit; Tranquilize

Notes: 1. This Patent Medicine also has another name, Yu Zhu Dan, which appeared in the original source.

2. This Patent Medicine contains two strong purgatives, Da Ji and Qian Jin Zi Shuang, which are not common medicines. In this formula, however, only a small dose of each of these two medicines is used. Also, the Qian Jin Zi Shuang form is a form without the oil in the seeds, therefore the purgative effect has been reduced, and no serious diarrhea will be produced. Also, in this formula, Wu Bei Zi, an astringent, is present, which will help to reduce the diarrhea effect.

7.31 鷄 骨 草 丸

Ji	Gu	Cao	Wan
------------------Herba Abri-----------------			pilla

Function: 1. Clear Liver Heat; Clear bile ducts, Detoxify Fire Poison
2. Decrease inflammation, Stop pain

Application: 1. Use to treat acute hepatitis, with or without jaundice.

2. Use to treat chronic hepatitis or chronic cholecystitis associated with Damp Heat

3. Use to treat Liver Heat syndrome and Eliminate Liver Fire.
Symptoms: Dizziness, vertigo, tinnitus, ear pain, burning urination.

Dose: 4 tablets, 3 times a day, after meals.

Ji Gu Cao Wan is produced as "Jigucao Wan" by the Yulin Drug Manufactory, Kwangsi, China, in bottles of 50 pills.

Pinyin Name	Pharmaceutical Name	Percent	TCM Function
Ji Gu Cao	Herba Abri	40	Clear Heat; Detoxify Fire Poison
She Dan	Snake Bile	15	Clear Heat; Clear bile ducts
Zhen Zhu	Magarita	3	Calm spirit; Nourish Heart
Niu Huang	Calcalus Bovis	10	Clear Heat; Detoxify Fire Poison
Dang Gui	Radix Angelicae Sinensis	10	Nourish Blood; Promote Blood circulation
Gou Qi Zi	Fructus Lycii Chinensis	7	Nourish Liver; Nourish Blood
Dan Shen	Radix Salviae Miltiorrhizae	15	Promote Blood circulation; Nourish Blood

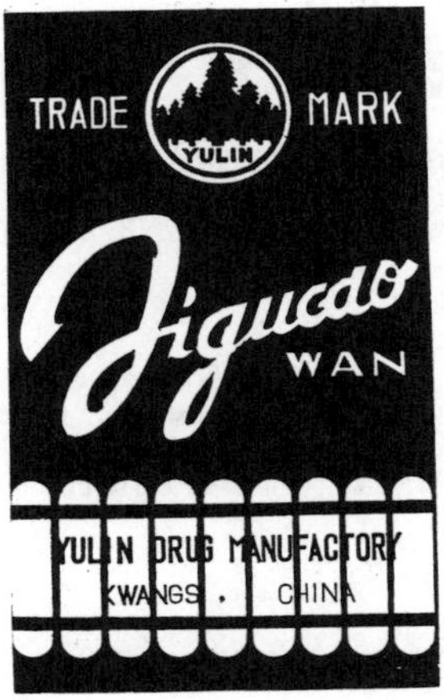

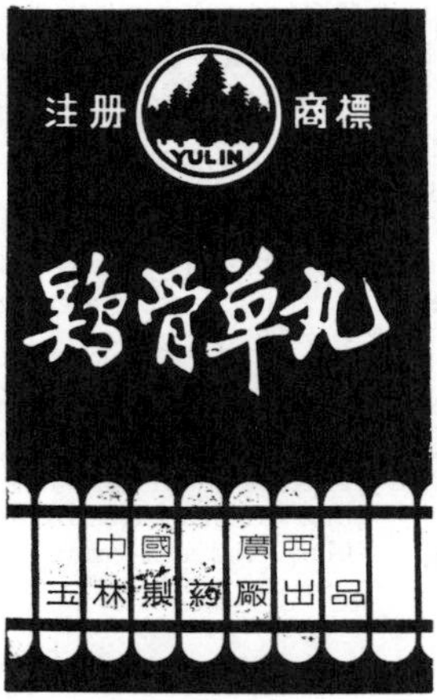

7.32 三 粒 回 春 丹

San	Li	Hui	Chun	Dan
three	unit of measure	-------return to spring------		pills
		--------recover health-------		

Source: Qian Shu-Tian, an herbal medicine physician from the Qing Dynasty, 1644-1911.

Function:
1. Clear Heat; Detoxify Fire Poison; Eliminate Phlegm
2. Open Heart Orifices; Reduce agitation; Waken consciousness

Application:

1. Use to treat the syndrome Phlegm Heat in the Lung, in children. Symptoms: Fever, cough, Phlegm congestion in the Lung with problems breathing, wheezing may be present. In serious cases, the patient may have agitation or loss of consciousness due to the fever; convulsions may be present.

2. Use to Regulate Spleen/Stomach Function in children where dysfunction has caused Stagnation of Qi with Phlegm Heat. Symptoms: Regurgitation and vomiting of milk; night-time crying; abdominal pain or diarrhea.

3. Some Western medicine disease applications in Pediatrics include the following: (Note, the child must have the above-listed Phlegm-Heat in the Lung symptoms or Spleen/Stomach symptoms where Stagnation of Qi has combined with Phlegm Heat, in order to use this formula.) Acute bronchitis, pneumonia, acute encephalitis, acute cerebro-spinal Meningitis, acute or chronic gastroenteritis.

Dose: The pills are packaged in various ways, for example in some packages, 3 pills are sealed into one wax ball; in some packages, 5 pills are sealed into one wax ball. The dose is measured by each pill, not by each wax ball.

Children less than 1 Year: 1 pill, 2 or 3 times a day
Children 1 - 2 Years: 2 pills, 2 or 3 times a day
Children 4 - 5 Years: 3 pills, 2 or 3 times a day
Children 8 - 12 Years: 5 pills, 2 or 3 times a day

San Li Hui Chun Dan is produced in Hong Kong, with 3 small pills per wax ball, 1 wax ball per envelope, and 10 envelopes per box.

The contents are listed below in 9 groups which are arranged according to function.

Pinyin Name	Pharmaceutical Name	Percent	TCM Function
Group 1			
Niu Huang	Calculus Bovis	1.4	Clear Heart Heat; Detoxify Fire Poison
Group 2			
Tian Zhu Huang	Concretio Silicea Bambusae	4.4	Clear Heat; Eliminate Phlegm
Chuan Bei Mu	Bulbus Fritillariae Cirrhosae	4.4	
Dan Nan Xing	Pulvis Arisaemae cum Felle Bovis	6.9	

Group 3			
She Xiang	Secretio Moschus moschiferi	1.4	Open Heart Orifices; Waken consciousness
Group 4			
Gou Teng	Ramulus Uncariae cum Uncis	27.7	Calm the Excess Liver Wind; Stop consulvions
Tian Ma	Rhizoma Gastrodiae Elatae	4.4	
Quan Xie	Buthus Martensi	4.4	
Jiang Can	Bombyx Batryticatus	4.4	
Group 5			
Da Huang	Rhizoma Rhei	6.9	Clear Heat; Extinguish Excess Fire; Disperse Intestinal Accumulation of Fire
Group 6			
Chen Pi	Pericarpium Citri Reticulatae	4.4	Regulate Stomach Qi; Eliminate Phlegm
Fa Ban Xia	Rhizoma Pinelliae Ternatae	4.4	
Group 7			
Bai Dou Kou	Fructus Amomi Cardomomi	4.4	Move Stuck Qi in Stomach and Intestines; Eliminate Phlegm; Prevent Accumulation of Phlegm Heat
Zhi Qiao	Fructus Citri seu Ponciri	4.4	
Mu Xiang	Radix Saussureae seu Vladimiriae	4.4	
Chen Xiang	Lignum Aquilariae	4.4	
Tan Xiang	Lignum Santali Albi	4.4	
Group 8			
Gan Cao	Radix Glycyrrhizae Uralensis	3.0	Clear Heat; Harmonize other herbs
Group 9			
Zhu Sha	Cinnabaris (Used to coat the pill)		Calm the Spirit; Tranquilize; Help Niu Huang Clear Heart Heat

Notes: 1. In TCM theory, pediatric diseases are usually caused by Exogenous Evil plus poor digestion of milk. This combination produces Internal Phlegm Heat. The development of this Phlegm Heat may cause gastric disorders such as vomiting and diarrhea which may later develop into acute convulsions. Sometimes the regurgitation and vomiting and diarrhea are the primary signs which show the presence of Phlegm Heat; this may later develop into high grade fever and convulsions. The purpose of this herbal formula is to treat four basic pathological changes including Heat, Phlegm, Wind and Convulsions. Therefore, this formula contains ingredients to Clear Heat, Eliminate Phlegm, Calm the Liver Wind and Stop convulsions.

2. In addition to this original formula, several similar formulas have been produced by different manufactories using the same name. The formula made in Shanghai has more ingredients to Stop Wind and Stop convulsions. Another formula made in Suzhou has more ingredients to Clear Heat and Open Orifices.

3. In China this is a commonly used medicine because it can successfully treat many digestive disorders and upper respiratory infections often seen in children.

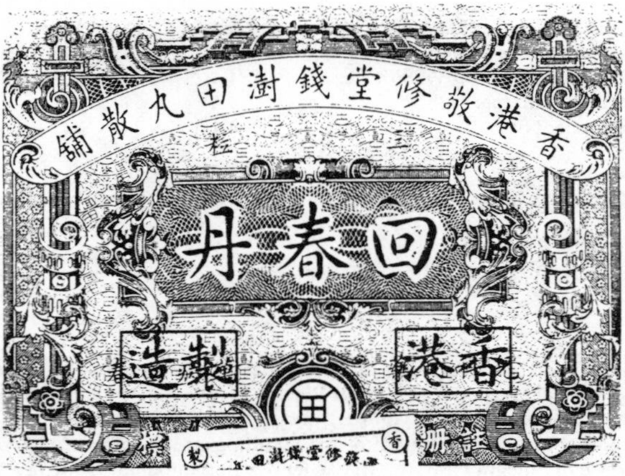
香港敬修堂錢澍田丸散舖
回春丹
香港
製造

7.33 京 万 红

Jing	Wan	Hong
capital city	many	red color

Function: 1. Stop pain; Decrease inflammation
2. Detoxification; Promote regeneration of damaged tissues due to burns

Application: 1. Use to treat any kind of burn on the body surface, including burns caused by steam, hot water, flame, hot oil, chemical burns, nuclear radiation burns (including burns from radiation therapy), sunburn, electrical burns.

2. Use to treat other disorders such as hemorrhoids and bedsores.

How to use the ointment: For above Application #1: For first or second degree burns, first clean the area, then rub the ointment directly on the surface area of the burn. Cover the area with gauze. Apply the ointment and change the gauze, daily. For third degree burns without infection, treat the same as first or second degree burns. For third degree burns with infection, the wound should be cleaned every day and larger amounts of the ointment should be used. Keep the wound covered.
For Application #2: Apply the ointment locally.

Jing Wan Hong ointment is produced as "Ching Wan Hung" by the Tientsin Drug Manufactory, Tientsin, China, in tubes of two sizes, 30 grams and 500 grams.

The ingredients are not published, however, the ingredients in this formula have the effect to Clear Heat and Detoxify Fire Poison (prevent infection and fight infection, if present); Clear Blood Heat, Dry Dampness (eliminate effusion); Decrease swelling; Stop pain and speed healing and regeneration of damaged tissues due to burns. After applying this ointment, the pain is usually stopped immediately.

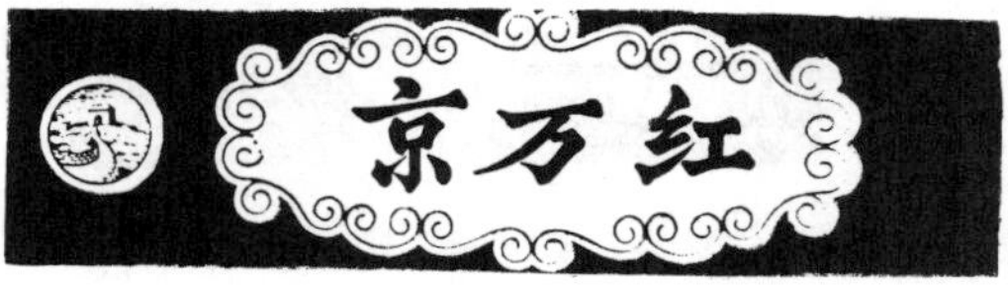

7.34 複 方 土 槿 皮 酊

Fu	Fang	Tu	Jin	Pi	Ding
---------complex---------		------herb name------		bark	tincture

Function: 1. Detoxify Fire Poison; Stop itching

Application: 1. Use to treat skin infections caused by fungi, tinea, or Sarcoptes scabiei (scabies).
Symptoms: Itching on the skin where irritation is present.

Caution: For external use only.

How to use this liquid: Each day, rub the liquid onto the skin once or twice until skin is healed. It is not necessary to cover the skin; the liquid will dry quickly.

Fu Fang Tu Jin Pi Ding is produced as "Composita Tujin Liniment" by the United Pharmaceutical Factory, Guangzhou, China, in 15 cc bottles.

Pinyin Name	Pharmaceutical Name		TCM Function
Mu Jin Hua	Tincture of Cortex Hibisci	6.00 cc	Clear Heat; Eliminate
Ben Jia Suan	Benzoic Acid	1.8 grams	Dampness; Treat fungus
Xue Yang Suan	Salicylic acid	0.90 grams	infection
	Ethyl alcohol	9.0 cc	

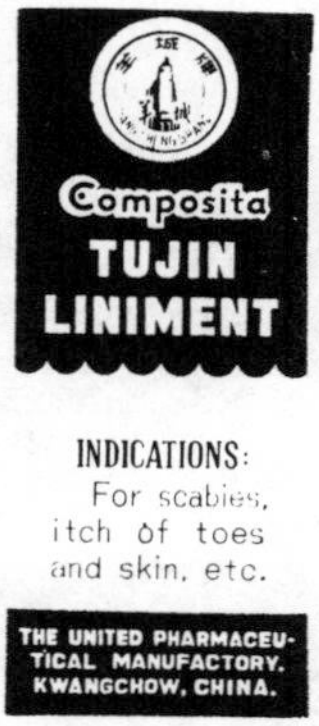

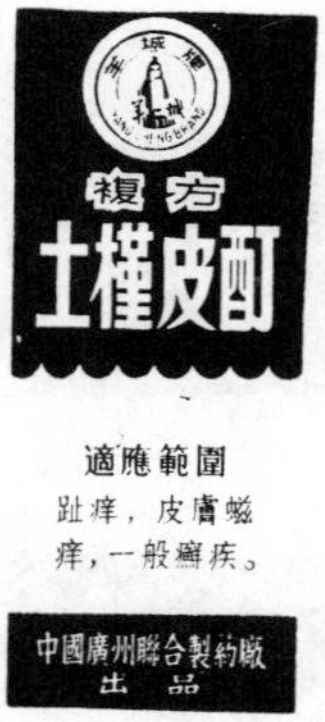

7.35 西 黄 丸

Xi	**Huang**	**Wan**
West	gallstone	pills

(Niu Huang produced in Northwestern China)

Source: Wai Ke Chuen Sheng Ji, (Volume on Surgery for Entire Life-span [Children and Adults]), Qing Dynasty, 1644-1911.

Function: 1. Reduce swelling; Detoxify Fire Poison
2. Move Stuck Blood and Phlegm Accumulation; Stop pain

Application: 1. Use to treat carbuncles.

2. Use to treat abscess due to Heat or Fire Poison including pulmonary abscess; breast abscess; intestinal abscess such as acute or chronic appendicitis, suppurative peritonitis, suppurative colitis, etc.

3. Use to treat abscess due to Phlegm Accumulation including abscess associated with scrofula, lymphadenitis, breast cancer, osteomyleitis.

Contraindication: Do not use with pregnant women.

Dose: 1 vial, 2 times a day.

The 4 herbs are listed below in 3 groups, according to function.

Pinyin Name	Pharmaceutical Name	Percent	TCM Function
Group 1			
Niu Huang	Calculus Bovis	1.38	Clear Heat; Detoxify Fire Poison
Group 2			
She Xiang	Secretio Moschus moschiferi	6.88	Promote Circulation of Qi in the Meridians using a strong aroma; Reduce Accumulation of Stuck Blood; Reduce Accumulation of
Group 3			
Ru Xiang	Gummi Olibanum	45.87	Promote Qi and Blood circulation;
Mo Yao	Myrrha	45.87	Remove Stagnation; Stop pain; Reduce swelling; Promote tissue regeneration

Notes: 1. In China, this medicine has been used to successfully treat infection due to Staphylococcus which was otherwise resistent to penicillin. (Journal of Traditional Chinese Medicine, December, 1964)

2. There is another Patent Medicine called Xing Xiao Wan which has the same ingredients except it has Xiong Huang (Realgar) instead of Niu Huang. The functions and applications are similar. Xing Xiao Wan is used primarily for carbuncles without pus; Xi Huang Wan is used for carbuncles with or without pus. Xing means "to wake up;" Xiao means "to disappear;" hence, it may "work overnight."

Chapter 8. Warm the Interior

Section A. **Warm the Middle-Warmer, Dispel Cold**

8.1 附 子 理 中 丸

Fu	**Zi**	**Li**	**Zhong**	**Wan**
---------Aconite---------		regulate	Middle Warmer	pills

Source: Tai Ping Hui Min He Ji Ju Fang, (Formulas of The People's Welfare Pharmacy), 1151 A.D., Song Dynasty, 960-1279. This formula is a modification of the original formula, Li Zhong Wan, which appeared in the Shang Han Lun, 219, A.D.

Function: 1. Warm the Middle Warmer; Dispel Internal Cold
2. Nourish Spleen/Stomach Qi

Application: 1. Use to Nourish Middle Warmer Yang which has been damaged by Cold.
Symptoms: Vomiting, loose stools, diarrhea, abdominal pain, clear urine, cold limbs; deep, thin Pulse and pale Tongue without much coating. (The stomach ache and Middle Warmer distension may be relieved by warmth.)

2. Some Western medicine disease applications include the following: (Note, the patient must have the Cold signs listed above, to use this formula.) Acute gastroenteritis, gastric ulcer, duodenal ulcer, colitis, gastroptosis, cholera.

Dose: Smaller Pills: 5 pills, 2 times a day   Honey Pills: 1 pill, 2 times a day.

Fu Zi Li Zhong Wan is produced as "Fu-Tzu Li-Chung Wan" by the United Pharmaceutical Manufactory, Guangzhou, China, in boxes with 10 honey pills; and by the Lanzhou Chinese Medicine Works, Lanzhou, China, in bottles with 100 smaller pills.

Pinyin Name	Pharmaceutical Name	Percent	TCM Function
Gan Jiang	Rhizoma Zingiberis Officinalis	21.74	Warm the Middle Warmer; Strengthen Yang
Bai Zhu	Rhizoma Atractylodis Macrocephalae	21.74	Strengthen Spleen; Dry Dampness
Dang Shen	Radix Codonopsis Pilosulae	21.74	Strengthen Middle Warmer Qi
Gan Cao	Radix Glycyrrhizae Uralensis	21.74	Warm the Middle Warmer; Harmonize other herbs
Fu Zi	Radix Aconiti Carmichaeli Praeparata	13.04	Strengthen Yang; Stop pain

Note: 1. This Patent Medicine has more warming properties than other Patent Medicines such as 9.1, Ren Shen Jian Pi Wan; 11.2, Mu Xiang Shun Qi Wan; 11.3, Chen Xiang Hua Qi Wan; and 11.4, Xiang Sha Liu Jun Wan.

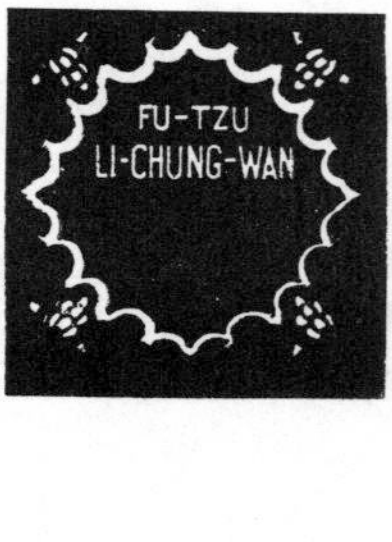

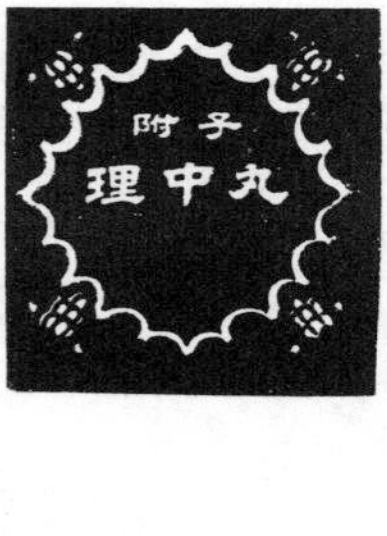

Chapter 9. Relieve Food Stagnation

Section A. **Transform Food Mass and Remove Food Stagnation**

Section B. **Remove Food Accumulation with Laxative Effect**

9.1 人 參 健 脾 丸

Ren	Shen	Jian	Pi	Wan
------------Ginseng----------		strengthen	Spleen	pills

Source: Zheng Zhi Zhun Sheng, (Standards for Diagnosis and Treatment), 1602.

Function:
1. Strengthen Spleen; Eliminate Dampness
2. Regulate Stomach and Spleen Energy; Move Food Mass

Application: 1. Use to treat Def. Spleen. Spleen/Stomach Symptoms: The patient frequently has Stuck Food Mass; poor appetite; Stomach distension; low energy; a pale face; and a weaker Pulse. Intestinal Symptoms: The patient frequently has diarrhea or loose stools due to Dampness associated with Def. Spleen Qi.

Contraindication: Do not use this formula with a woman who is nursing. The formula contains the herb Mai Ya, which has the additional function of restraining lactation.

Dose: 8 pills, 3 times a day. Take 30 minutes to one hour after meals.

Ren Shen Jian Pi Wan is produced as "Ginseng Stomachic Pills" by the Lanzhou Chinese Medicine Works, Lanzhou, China, in bottles of 200 pills.

Pinyin Name	Pharmaceutical Name	Percent	TCM Function
Dang Shen	Radix Codonopsis Pilosulae	16	Strengthen Spleen; Tonify Qi
Shan Zha	Fructus Crataegi	12	Move Food Mass; Strengthen Stomach
Bai Zhu	Rhizoma Atractylodis Macrocephalae	16	Supplement Spleen; Strengthen Stomach; Dry Dampness
Zhi Shi	Fructus Citri seu Ponciri Immaturus	24	Move Stuck Qi; Move Food Mass
Chen Pi	Pericarpium Citri Reticulatae	16	Regulate Stomach Qi; Strengthen Spleen; Dry Dampness; Stop vomiting or nausea
Mai Ya	Fructus Hordei Vulgaris Germinantus	16	Dissolve Food Mass; Strengthen Stomach

Note: 1. There are similar formulas which also use the name, Jian Pi Wan; their functions are similar.

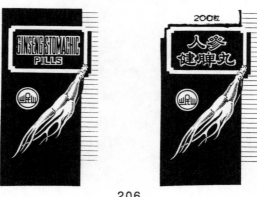

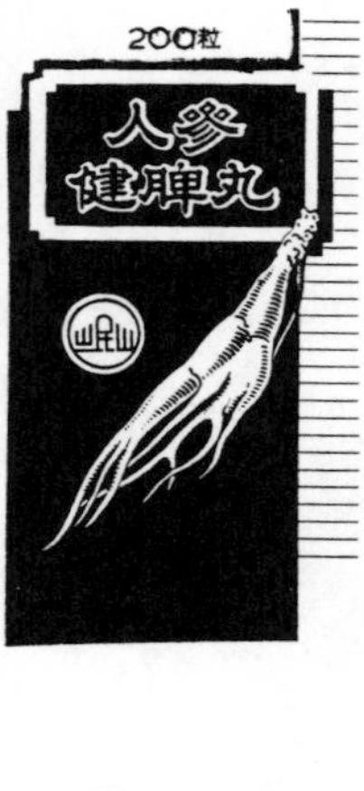

9.2 七 星 茶

七	星	茶
Qi	**Xing**	**Cha**
seven	star	tea

Function:
1. Strengthen Spleen; Improve digestion
2. Clear Heat
3. Calm uneasiness

Application:

1. Use to treat indigestion in babies and children. Symptoms: Poor appetite, regurgitation and vomiting of milk, breath odor associated with poor digestion, weight loss due to poor digestion, loose stools.

2. Use to Calm uneasiness. Symptoms: Poor sleep, awakening several times during the night; crying a lot, including at night (crying may be associated with poor digestion.)

3. Use to treat inflammation in the mouth, including oral ulcer. This may be due to Yeast or other infection. In this condition, the urine may be a darker or reddish color.

Dose: This herbal formula is available in liquid form in 100cc bottles. Use the dosages below and dilute in warm water.

Age 1 to 2 Years: 5 cc, 2 times a day   Age 2 to 12 Years: 10-20 cc, 2 times a day

Qi Xing Cha is produced as "Chi-Sing-Char" by the Sing-Kyn Drug House, Canton, China, in bottles containing 100 cc.

Pinyin Name	Pharmaceutical Name	Grams	TCM Function
Dan Zhu Ye	Herba Lophatheri Gracilis	9.4	Clear Heat; Promote urination
Yi Yi Ren	Semen Coicis Lachryma-jobi	12.5	Clear Heat; Promote urination; Strengthen Spleen; Stop diarrhea
Gu Ya	Fructus Oryzae Sativae Germinantus	12.5	Strengthen Spleen; Remove Food Mass
Gou Teng	Ramulus Uncariae cum Uncis	4.7	Clear Heat; Stop crying at night
Chan Tui	Periostracum Cicadae	8 pieces	Clear Heat; Expel Wind; Calm uneasiness; Stop crying
Shan Zha	Fructus Crataegi	6.25	Remove Food Mass; Improve digestion
Gan Cao	Radix Glycyrrhizae Uralensis	1.56	Clear Heat; Harmonize other herbs

Note: 1. This formula is commonly used with children in China, and families often keep it in the house. It is a safe and gentle formula, with a wide variety of uses for treating disorders in the early stage. It is especially useful in treating digestive disorders including those in the early stage (without Heat signs) or even in the later stage (with Heat signs.)

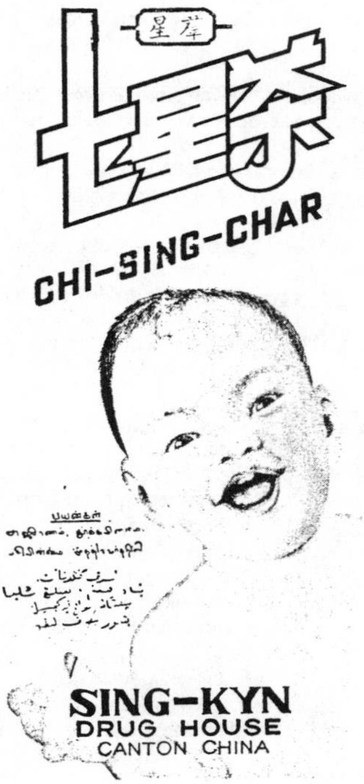
星羣
七星茶
CHI-SING-CHAR
SING-KYN
DRUG HOUSE
CANTON CHINA

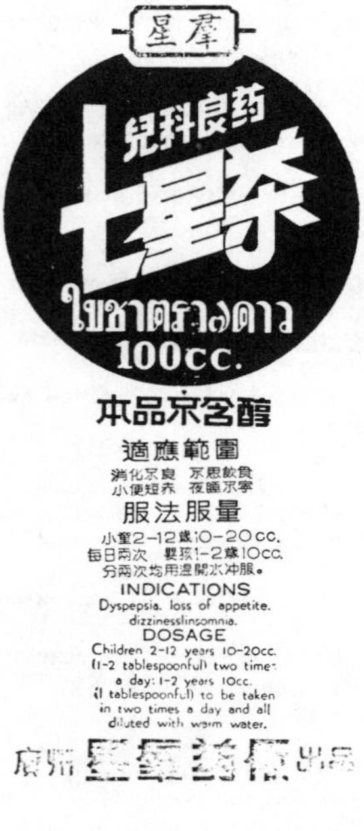
星羣
兒科良药
七星茶
ใบชาตราเจ็ดดาว
100cc.
本品不含醇
適應範圍
消化不良 不思飲食
小便短赤 夜睡不寧
服法服量
小童2-12歲10-20cc.
每日兩次 嬰孩1-2歲10cc.
分兩次均用溫開水沖服。
INDICATIONS
Dyspepsia. loss of appetite.
dizzinesslinsomnia.
DOSAGE
Children 2-12 years 10-20cc.
(1-2 tablespoonful) two time:
a day: 1-2 years 10cc.
(1 tablespoonful) to be taken
in two times a day and all
diluted with warm water.

9.3 潤 腸 丸

Run	**Chang**	**Wan**
moisten	intestines	pills

Function: 1. Clear Intestinal Heat
2. Moisten the stool; Promote bowel movement

Application: 1. Use to treat constipation due to Excess Internal Heat or Def. body fluid caused by Empty Heat/Def. Yin

Dose: 4 pills, 3 times a day. The dose may be increased up to 8 pills, 3 times a day if the regular dose produces no effect.

Run Chang Wan is produced as "Fructus Persica Compound Pills" by the Lanzhou Chinese Medicine Works, Lanzhou, China, in bottles of 200 pills.

Pinyin Name	Pharmaceutical Name	Percent	TCM Function
Huo Ma Ren	Semen Cannabis Sativae	28.6	Moisten the intestines. These seeds contain 31% oil.
Tao Ren	Semen Persicae	28.6	Moisten Dryness; Lubricate the intestines
Rou Cong Rong	Herba Cistanches	14.3	Moisten the intestines and strengthen Kidney
Dang Gui	Radix Angelica Sinensis	14.3	Moisten the intestines; Move the stool; Strengthen Yin; Strengthen Blood
Da Huang	Rhizoma Rhei	14.3	Clear Heat from large intestine; Promote bowel movement

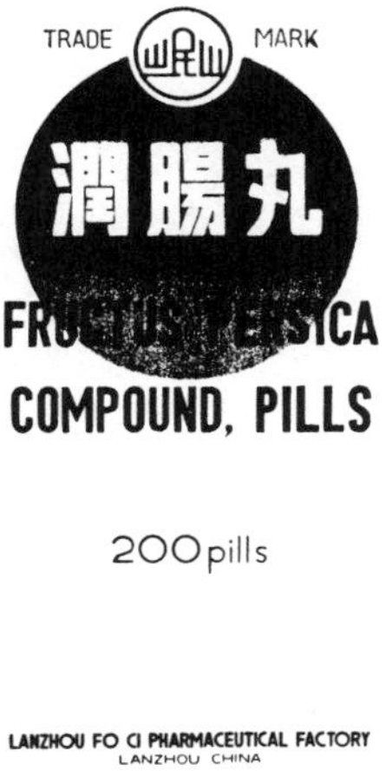

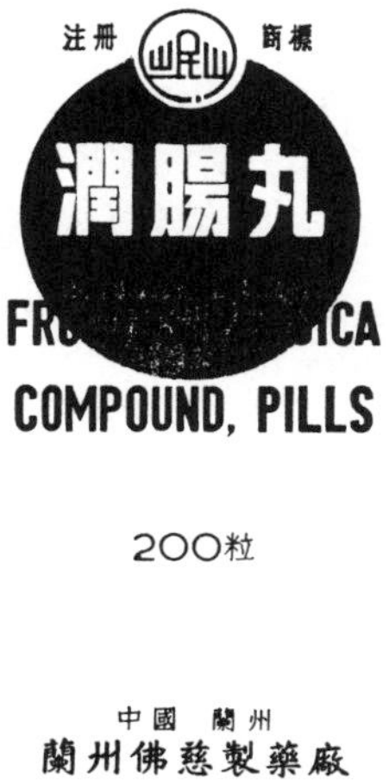

Chapter 10. Drain Dampness by Promoting Urination
(Includes a Patent Medicine used with Urinary Tract Infection, Kidney Stones, etc.)

Section A. **Treat Dysuria**

10.1 石 淋 通 片

Shi	Lin	Tong	Pian
stone	dysuria	open	tablets

Source: Zhong Guo Yao Dian, (Pharmacopoeia of the People's Republic of China), 1977. This medicine has been used for the problems listed below for at least 25 years.

Function:
1. Promote diuresis (especially for cases with difficult urination)
2. Clear Damp Heat in the Lower Warmer

Application:
1. Use to treat various disorders caused by Heat or Damp Heat in the urinary system. Symptoms: Frequent urination in small amounts (with or without blood in the urine); painful urination.

2. Some Western medicine disease applications include the following: Urinary tract stones (including kidney stones); urinary tract infection or inflammation; pyelonephritis; gallstones; hepatitis with jaundice; cirrhosis of the liver with ascites; edema associated with nephritis.

Dose: 6 tablets, 3 times a day. For serious cases, 8 or 9 tablets per dose is recommended.

Shi Lin Tong Pian is produced as "Shi Lin Tong" by the Swatow United Medicinal Factory, Swatow, China, in bottles of 100 tablets.

Pinyin Name	Pharmaceutical Name	Percent	TCM Function
Jin Qian Cao	Desmodium styracifolium	100	Eliminate Dampness; Promote urination; Clear Damp Heat; Reduce Jaundice

Note: 1. The Patent Medicine, Te Xiao Pai Shi Wan, is similar in function to Shi Lin Tong. They are both used to treat kidney stones, gallstones and reduce inflammation and treat infection.

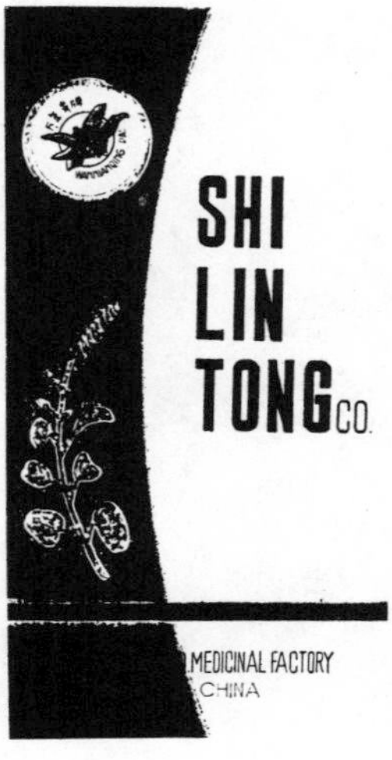

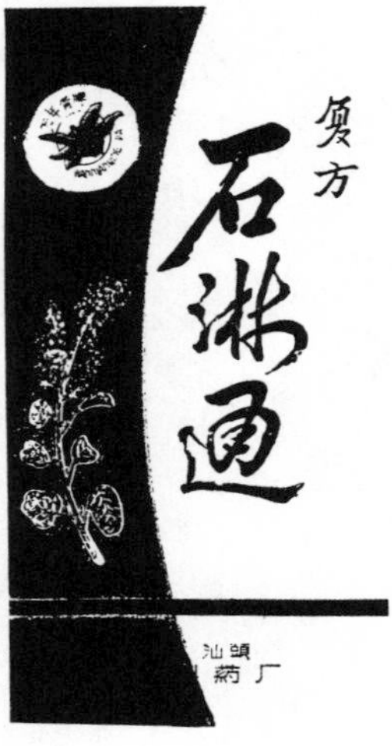

Chapter 11. Regulate Qi

(Includes Patent Medicines used with some Digestive Disorders; Liver/Gall Bladder Dysfunction, etc.)

11.1 舒 肝 丸

舒	肝	丸
Shu	**Gan**	**Wan**
comfort	Liver	pills

Source: Zhu Tian-Bi's formula, Ming Dynasty, 1368-1644.

Function:
1. Soothe Liver; Smooth Depressed Liver Qi
2. Aid digestion, Remove Food Mass
3. Stop pain in the Middle Warmer

Application:

1. Use to treat Stuck Liver Qi syndrome. Symptoms: Distension and pain in hypochondrium, or abdominal pain in liver or gall bladder areas (pain may travel to other parts as well, e.g. shoulder or lower abdomen).

2. Use to treat breast distension and pain associated with Premenstrual Syndrome. It is used the last week or more before the period begins.

3. Use to treat Spleen and Stomach syndrome associated with Stuck Liver Qi. Symptoms: Poor digestion, sensation of fullness in the stomach, especially after eating; nausea, burping, vomiting and regurgitation associated with hyperacidity.

4. Some Western medicine disease applications include the following: (Patients should have symptoms associated with Stuck Liver Qi or Spleen/Stomach syndrome in order to use this formula.) Chronic hepatitis, chronic cholecystitis and/or gallstones; acute or chronic gastritis; gastric or duodenal ulcer; idiopathic, functional, or hysteria-related digestive disorders; flatulence due to Stuck Liver Qi, or associated with drinking Chinese herbal decoctions (Flaws, B., Am. J. of Acupuncture, July-September, 1989, 17: 225-228).

Contraindication: Do not use with pregnant women.

Dose: 8 pills, 3 times a day.

Shu Gan Wan is produced as "Shu Kan Wan (Hepatico-Tonic Pills)" by the Lanzhou Chinese Medicine Works, Lanzhou, China, in bottles of 100 pills; and as "Shukan Wan Condensed" by the Tientsin Drug Manufactory, Tientsin, China, in bottles of 120 pills.

Pinyin Name	Pharmaceutical Name	Percent	TCM Function
Chuan Lian Zi	Fructus Meliae Toosendan	14.02	Move Stuck Qi; Stop pain
Jiang Huang	Rhizoma Curcumae	9.35	Smooth Depressed Liver Qi; Treat mental depression
Chen Xiang	Lignum Aquilariae	8.41	Lower Adverse Rising Qi; Stop pain
Yan Hu Suo	Rhizoma Corydalis Yanhusuo	8.41	Promote Blood circulation; Stop pain
Mu Xiang	Radix Saussureae	6.54	Move Stuck Qi; Stop pain
Dou Kou	Semen Alpiniae Katsumadae	4.67	Move Stuck Qi in Stomach; Remove Food Mass
Bai Shao	Radix Paeoniae Lactiflorae	13.08	Smooth Liver; Tonify Liver Yin
Fu Ling	Sclerotium Poriae Cocos	9.35	Strengthen Spleen; Discharge Dampness; Promote urination

Zhi Qiao	Fructus Citri seu Ponciri	8.41	Move Qi; Disperse stagnation
Chen Pi	Pericarpium Citri Reticulatae	6.54	Regulate Stomach Qi; Remove Food Mass
Sha Ren	Fructus seu Semen Amomi	6.54	Regulate Stomach Qi; Stop vomiting
Hou Po	Cortex Magnoliae	4.67	Move Stuck Qi; Lower Adverse Rising Qi

Notes: 1. This formula is effective when used alone. It is sometimes also used, however, as an adjunctive, supportive medicine with other formulas used for digestive disorders or liver/gallbladder problems.

2. The formula listed here is the original formula. There is another formula with the same name, in which two of the herbs listed here are omitted (Chuan Lian Zi and Fu Ling) and eight additional herbs are used (Xiang Fu, Gan Cao, Dan Pi, Chai Hu, Fo Shou, Qing Pi, Xiang Yuan, Tan Xiang). The major function is the same for the two formulas; the second formula is stronger to Move Stuck Liver Qi. The second formula is produced by the Lanzhou Chinese Medicine Works, Lanzhou, China.

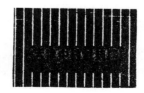

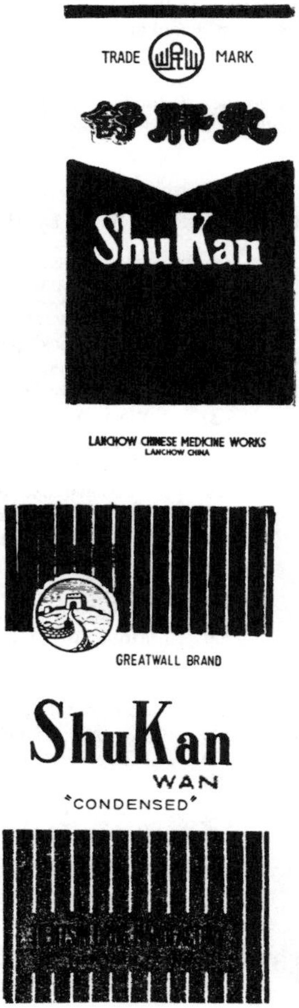

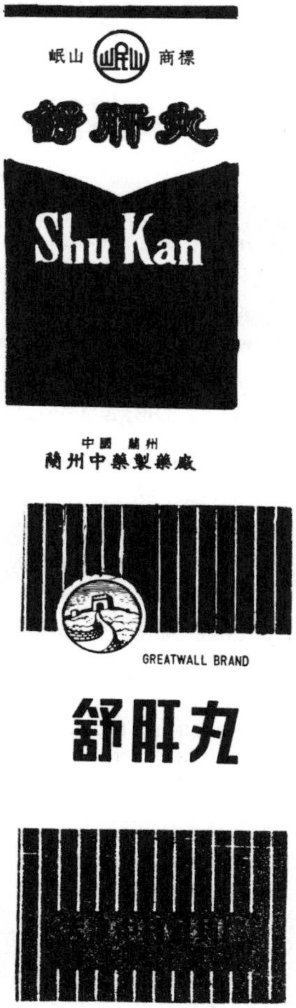

11.2 木香順氣丸

Mu	Xiang	Shun	Qi	Wan
----------Saussureae---------		regulate	Qi	pills

Source: Shen Shi Zun Sheng Shu, (Respect of Life Book), by Dr. Shen from the Qing Dynasty, 1644-1911.

Function:
1. Move Stuck Qi in the Middle Warmer; Stop pain
2. Strengthen Stomach; Disperse Food Mass

Application:
1. Use to treat feeling of fullness in the chest, diaphragm and hypochondrium due to Stuck Liver Qi or Food Mass.

2. Use to increase peristalsis in the stomach and remove Food Mass in the stomach due to improper eating. The patient may have a foul smell in the mouth and foul belching. (This is sometimes associated with hypoacidity and insufficient acid to digest food in Western medicine.)

3. Some Western medicine disease applications include the following: Chronic hepatitis, cirrhosis of the liver (early stage), chronic gastritis, intestinal spasms (abdominal pain).

Dose: 8 pills, 2 times a day.

Mu Xiang Shun Qi Wan is produced as "Aplotaxis Carminative Pills" by the Lanzhou Chinese Medicine Works, Lanzhou, China, in bottles of 200 pills.

Pinyin Name	Pharmaceutical Name	Grams	TCM Function
Mu Xiang	Radix Saussureae	200	Move Stuck Qi; Stop pain
Dou Kou	Semen Alpiniae Katsumadai	200	Move Stuck Qi in Stomach; Remove Food Mass
Cang Zhu	Rhizoma Atractylodis	150	Strengthen Spleen; Dry Dampness
Sheng Jiang	Rhizoma Zingiberis Officinalis Recens	200	Warm Middle Warmer; Stop nausea; Stop vomiting
Qing Pi	Pericarpium Citri Reticulatae Viride	200	Move Stuck Liver Qi; Decrease distension
Chen Pi	Pericarpium Citri Reticulatae	200	Regulate Stomach Qi; Strengthen Spleen
Fu Ling	Sclerotium Poriae Cocos	200	Strengthen Spleen; Discharge Dampness; Promote urination
Chai Hu	Radix Bupleuri	150	Move Stuck Liver Qi
Hou Po	Cortex Magnoliae Officinalis	200	Move Stuck Qi; Lower Adverse Rising Qi
Bing Lang	Semen Arecae Catechu	200	Decrease Middle Warmer and abdominal distension
Zhi Qiao	Fructus Citri seu Ponciri	200	Move Qi; Disperse Stagnation
Wu Yao	Radix Linderae Strychnifoliae	200	Move Stuck Qi; Stop pain
Lai Fu Zi	Semen Raphani Sativi	200	Move Stuck Qi in the Stomach; Remove Food Mass
Shan Zha	Fructus Crataegi	200	Remove Food Mass; Increase acid in the Stomach

Shen Qu	Massa Fermentata	200	Strengthen the Stomach; Remove Food Mass
Mai Ya	Fructus Hordei Vulgaris Germinantus	200	Strengthen the Stomach; Remove Food Mass
Gan Cao	Radix Glycyrrhizae Uralensis	150	Warm the Middle Warmer; Harmonize other herbs

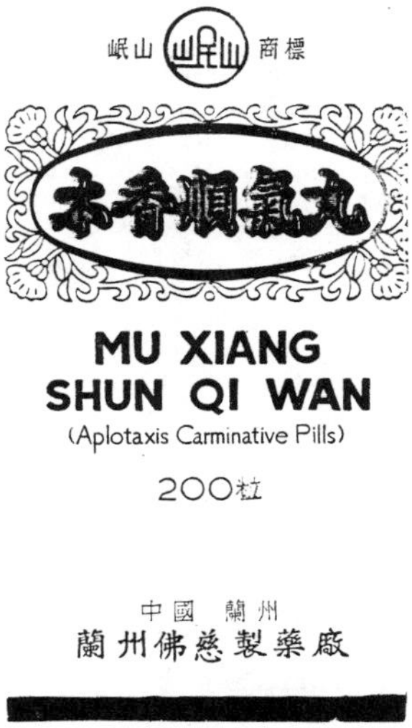

11.3 沉 香 化 氣 丸

Chen	Xiang	Hua	Qi	Wan
----------Aquilariae----------		move	Qi	pills

Source: Yu Yao Yuan Fang, Volume III, (Imperial Pharmacy Formulas), by Xu Guo-Zhen, Yuan Dynasty, 1279-1368.

Function:
1. Move Stuck Qi; Lower Adverse Rising Qi
2. Remove Food Stagnation in the Stomach

Application:
1. Use to treat abdominal distension and reduce feeling of fullness and pain in the hypochondrium and chest areas.

2. Use to treat gastric disorders including Food Mass in the stomach due to improper eating. Symptoms: Poor or no appetite, belching and sour regurgitation.

3. Some Western medicine disease applications include the following: Chronic hepatitis, gastritis, stomach ulcer, duodenal ulcer, intestinal obstruction, chronic cholecystitis, or other gastric disorders with the above-mentioned symptoms.

Contraindication: Do not use with Def. Yin cases, this formula contains some herbs with slightly warming properties.

Dose: 9 pills, 2 times a day, taken one-half hour before a meal or after a meal.

Chen Xiang Hua Qi Wan is produced by the Min-Kang Drug Manufactory, I-Chang, China, in bottles of 100 pills.

Pinyin Name	Pharmaceutical Name	Percent	TCM Function
Chen Xiang	Lignum Aguilariae	3.60	Lower Adverse Rising Qi; Move Stuck Qi; Stop pain
Bing Lang	Semen Arecae Catechu	4.86	Move Stuck Qi; Remove Food Mass
Cao Dou Kou	Semen Alpiniae Katsumadai	4.36	Strengthen Spleen; Dry Dampness; Aid Digestion
Sha Ren	Fructus seu Semen Amomi	2.43	Move Qi; Stop pain; Strengthen Stomach; Dry Dampness
Xiang Fu	Rhizoma Cyperi Rotundi	7.20	Smooth Liver; Regulate Liver and Stomach Qi; Stop pain
Hou Po	Cortex Magnoliae Officinalis	7.20	Move Qi; Lower Adverse Rising Qi
Fu Ling	Sclerotium Poriae Cocos	7.20	Strengthen Spleen; Harmonize the Middle Warmer; Tranquilize; Promote urination
Chen Pi	Pericarpium Citri Reticulatae	7.20	Move Middle Warmer Qi; Strengthen Spleen; Stop vomiting Lower Adverse Rising Qi;
Lai Fu Zi	Semen Raphani Sativi	4.86	Remove Food Mass; Decrease distension
Gan Cao	Radix Glycyrrhizae Uralensis	2.43	Strengthen the Middle Warmer; Stop stomach ache

Notes: 1. The primary functions of this formula are to 1) Lower Adverse Rising Qi and 2) Disperse Stagnation of Qi, especially associated with Food Mass.

2. The formula used in Chen Xiang Hua Qi Wan produced by the Lanzhou Chinese Medicine Works, Lanzhou, China is very different from the formula used for Chen Xiang Hua Qi Wan produced by the Min-Kang Drug Manufactory, I-Chang, China (the above-listed formula). In the formula produced by the Lanzhou Chinese Medicine Works there are only 5 ingredients; these ingredients have the effect of Strengthening the Stomach and Spleen, and Clearing Stomach and Intestinal Heat; they also have the effect of Removing Stuck Food Mass. This formula is especially suitable for use with a patient who has Stuck Food Mass due to Stomach and Intestinal Heat with symptoms such as foul odor to the breath, history of over-eating, constipation, and thick yellow coat on the Tongue. If the patient does not have constipation, the Da Huang may cause some loose stools.

Overall, both formulas are effective to remove stagnation in the Stomach and Intestines. The Lanzhou formula is especially effective for the patient with Stuck Food Mass due to Stomach and Intestinal Heat. The I-Chang formula is especially effective for the patient with Stagnation of Qi in the Middle Warmer.

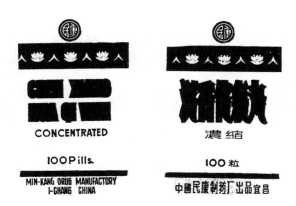

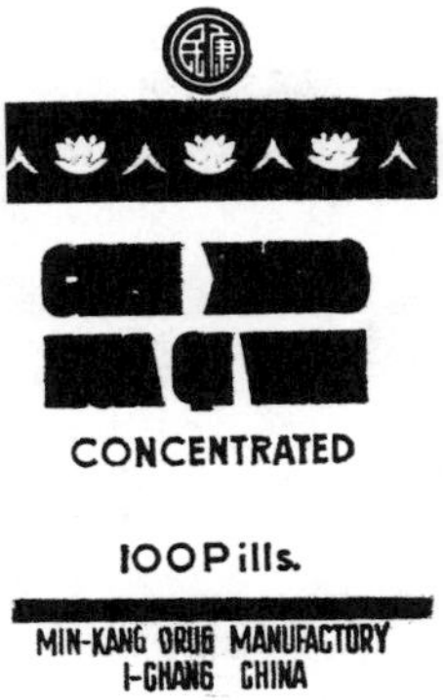

11.4 香砂六君丸

Xiang	Sha	Liu	Jun	Wan
Saussureae	Amomi	six	gentlemen	pills

Source: Shi Fang Ge Kuo, (Experienced Formulas Written in Rhyme), by Chen Xuo-Yuan, 1801, A.D.

Function: 1. Nourish Spleen/Stomach; Strengthen Qi
2. Stop pain; Eliminate Phlegm

Application: 1. Use to treat any symptoms caused by Def. Qi of Spleen or Stomach. This is a Tonic medicine for the Spleen/Stomach. Symptoms: Poor digestion with nausea, vomiting, burping, regurgitation, stomach gurgling, borborygmus, distension in the Middle Warmer, stomach ache, chronic diarrhea, a pale face, a pale Tongue, and a weaker or slow Pulse.

2. Some Western medicine disease applications include the following: (Note, the patient must have the above-mentioned Def. Spleen/Stomach symptoms to use this.) Gastric or duodenal ulcer, acute or chronic gastritis, chronic diarrhea, Crohn's disease.

Dose: 12 pills, 3 times a day, taken before meals. This medicine will be more effective if the patient avoids cold or raw food while taking it.

Xiang Sha Liu Jun Wan is produced as "Aplotaxis-Amomum Pills" by the Lanzhou Chinese Medicine Works, Lanzhou, China, in bottles of 100 pills.

Pinyin Name	Pharmaceutical Name	Percent	TCM Function
Dang Shen	Radix Codonopsis Pilosulae	17.2	Tonify the Middle Warmer and Strengthen Qi
Bai Zhu	Rhizoma Atractylodis Macrocephalae	17.2	Strengthen Spleen; Dry Dampness
Fu Ling	Sclerotium Poriae Cocos	17.2	Strengthen Spleen; Dry Dampness
Ban Xia	Rhizoma Pinelliae Ternatae	17.2	Dry Dampness; Eliminate Phlegm; Stop vomiting
Chen Pi	Pericarpium Citri Reticulatae	8.6	Regulate Middle Warmer Qi; Stop vomiting, nausea; Dry Dampness
Mu Xiang	Radix Saussureae seu Vladimiriae	6.9	Move Stuck Qi; Stop pain
Sha Ren	Fructus seu Semen Amomi	6.9	Move Middle Warmer Qi; Eliminate Dampness; Stop diarrhea
Gan Cao	Radix Glycyrrhizae	8.6	Strengthen Spleen; Harmonize other herbs

Notes: 1. This Patent Medicine is very effective and is commonly used.

2. The formula used in the Patent Medicine, Liu Jun Zi Pian, is similar to the formula used in Xiang Sha Liu Jun Wan; however, it contains two ingredients less than that used in Xiang Sha Liu Jun Wan. In Liu Jun Zi Pian, there is no Mu Xiang (Radix Saussureae seu Vladimiriae) or Sha Ren (Fructus seu Semen Amomi). Thus, Liu Jun Zi Pian is not as effective as Xiang Sha Liu Jun Wan in moving Stuck Qi in the Stomach. However, Liu Jun Zi Pian is more effective than Xiang Sha Liu Jun Wan in Strengthening the Spleen and Drying Dampness due to Def. Spleen. Liu Jun Zi Pian is also more effective in treating nausea and vomiting than is Xiang Sha Liu Jun Wan.

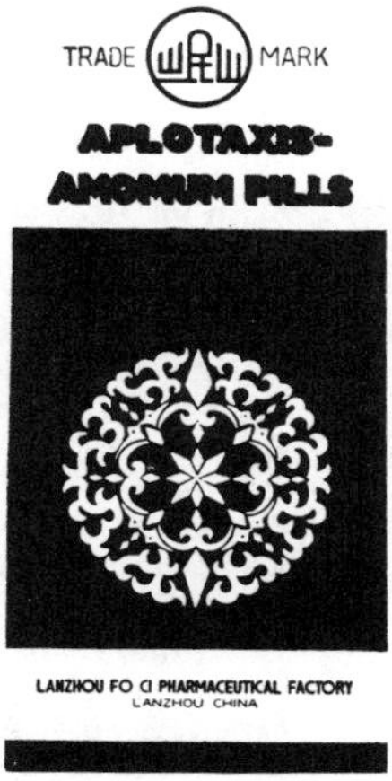

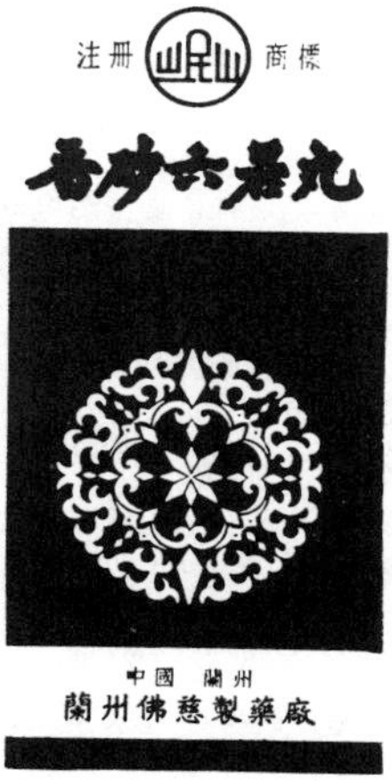

11.5 香 沙 养 胃 片

Xiang	Sha	Yang	Wei	Pian
Saussureae	Amomi	nourish	Stomach	pills

Source: Wan Bing Hui Chun, (Recovery of Ten Thousand Diseases), Ming Dynasty, 1368-1644.

Function: 1. Nourish Qi; Strengthen the Stomach
2. Remove Food Mass; Relieve stomach ache

Application: 1. Use to treat Def. Spleen/Stomach syndrome in weaker patients.
Symptoms: Low energy, poor appetite; gastric symptoms, especially following a meal, such as stomach distension, burping, heartburn, stomach ache, nausea; loose stools or diarrhea. This formula will Tonify the Spleen/Stomach Qi and thus reduce the above-mentioned symptoms.

2. Some Western medicine disease applications include acute or chronic gastritis (including ideopathic) and gastric or duodenal ulcer.

Dose: 4 tablets, 2 times a day.

Xiang Sha Yang Wei Pian is produced as "Hsiang Sha Yang Wei Pien" by the Tientsin Drug Manufactory, Tientsin, China, in bottles of 60 uncoated tablets.

Pinyin Name	Pharmaceutical Name	Percent	TCM Function
Bai Zhu	Rhizoma Atractylodis Macrocephalae	21.3	Strengthen Spleen/Stomach; Dry Spleen Dampness
Mu Xiang	Radix Saussureae seu Vladimiriae	5.7	Regulate Qi; Move Stagnation; Stop pain
Sha Ren	Fructus seu Semen Amomi	5.7	Regulate Stomach Qi
Bai Dou Kou	Fuctus Amomi Cardamomi	8.5	Regulate Stomach Qi; Warm the Middle Warmer
Dang Shen	Radix Codonopsis Pilosulae	24.2	Tonify the Middle Warmer; Strengthen Spleen Qi
Mai Ya	Fructus Hordei Vulgaris Germinantus	8.5	Remove Food Mass; Strengthen the Stomach
Chen Pi	Pericarpium Citri Reticulatae	14.2	Regulate Stomach Qi; Dry Spleen Dampness
Gan Cao	Radix Glycyrrhizae Uralensis	3.4	Warm the Middle Warmer; Harmonize other herbs
Shen Qu	Massa Fermentata	8.5	Remove Food Mass; Regulate Stomach Qi

Note: 1. The Patent Medicine listed above is usually found in tablet form. Some Patent Medicines in pill form may also contain 6 additional herbs - Cang Zhu, Huo Xiang, Fu Ling, Hou Po, Ban Xia Qu, and Xiang Fu. These additional herbs Dry Spleen Dampness and Move Stuck Qi.

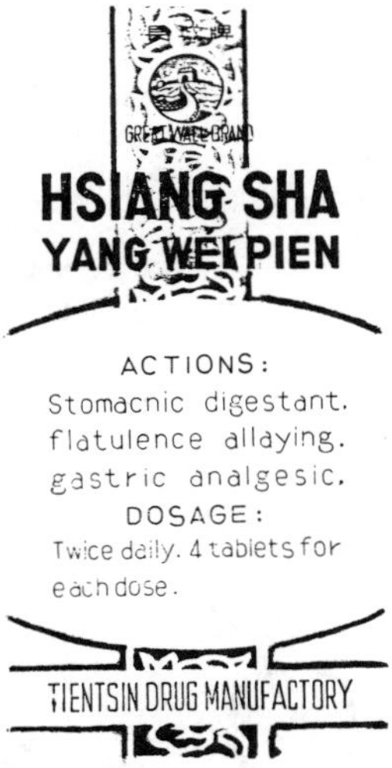
GREAT WALL BRAND
HSIANG SHA
YANG WEI PIEN
ACTIONS:
Stomacnic digestant.
flatulence allaying.
gastric analgesic.
DOSAGE:
Twice daily. 4 tablets for each dose.
TIENTSIN DRUG MANUFACTORY

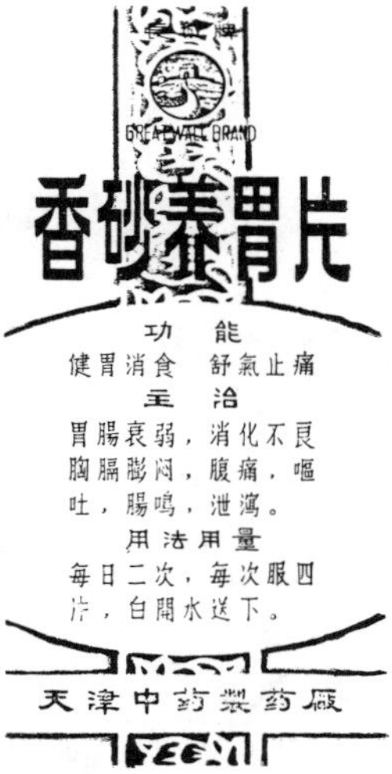
GREAT WALL BRAND
香砂養胃片
功　能
健胃消食　舒氣止痛
主　治
胃腸衰弱，消化不良
胸膈膨悶，腹痛，嘔
吐，腸鳴，泄瀉。
用法用量
每日二次，每次服四
片，白開水送下。
天津中药製药廠

11.6 胃 特 靈

Wei	Te	Ling
Stomach	special	effective

Function: 1. Strengthen Stomach
2. Relieve stomach ache
3. Neutralize excess acid in the stomach

Application: 1. Use to treat Stuck Qi in Spleen/Stomach which causes stomach ache, heartburn, burping.

2. Some Western medicine disease applications include gastric or duodenal ulcer, gastritis with hyperacidity in the stomach, stomach distension and gas.

Dose: 4-6 pills, 3 times a day, taken before a meal, or when necessary - i.e. when pain is present or there is heartburn.

Wei Te Ling is produced as "Wei Te Ling (Stomach Sedative)" by the Tsingtao Medicine Works, Tsingtao, China, in bottles containing 120 coated tablets.

Pinyin Name	Pharmaceutical Name	Percent	TCM Function
Wu Zei Gu	Os Sepiae seu Sepiellae	40	Neutralize excess stomach acid; Promote healing of ulcer; astringent property
Yuan Hu	Rhizoma Corydalis Yanhusuo	30	Stop pain
Fong Mi	Honey	30	Strengthen the Middle Warmer; Promote tissue regeneration

Note: 1. This Patent Medicine is a simple formula with only 2 main ingredients. It is most effective in relieving stomach pain and decreasing stomach acid. If the burping, distension and gas are also major problems, additional Patent Medicines may also be used in combination with this, including #11.5, Xiang Sha Yang Wei Pian; or #11.2, Mu Xiang Shun Qi Wan.

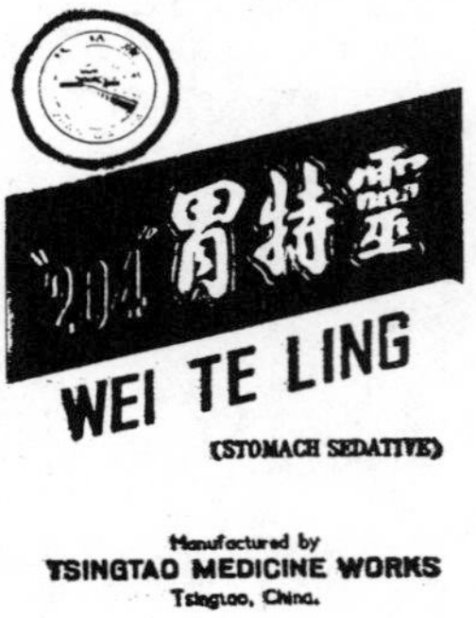

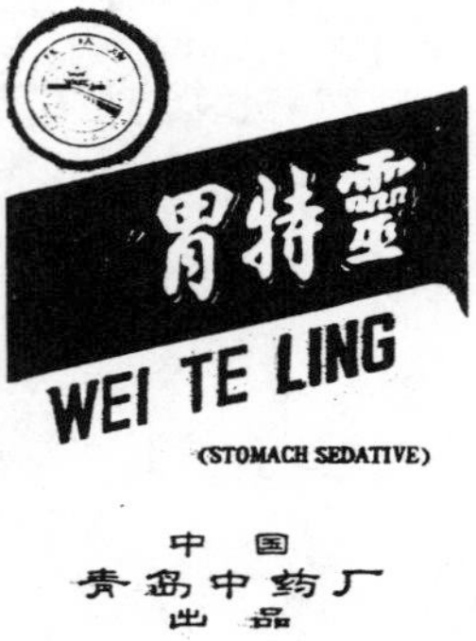

11.7 賽 霉 安

Sai Mei An

----------Name of the Manufacturer----------

Function: 1. Decrease excess stomach acid; Stop bleeding; Protect mucosa of the stomach
2. Stop stomach ache; Promote tissue regeneration

Application: 1. Use to treat gastric or duodenal ulcer due to hyperacidity in the stomach.

2. Use to treat acute or chronic gastritis with hyperacidity in the stomach.

3. Use to treat mouth ulcer or stomatitis. (Apply a small amount of the powder topically, 3 or 4 times a day.)

Contraindication: Do not take this in conjunction with any other alkaline substance, it would reduce the healing effect of the membrane.

Dose: 3 pills, 3 times a day, taken one-half hour before a meal. It must be taken on an empty stomach.

After being taken, this medicine will turn into a membrane in the stomach, which will cover the lining of the stomach, thus protecting the stomach ulcer. Food will not be able to touch the ulcer and irritation from the stomach contents will be reduced, thus relieving the stomach pain. The patient should continue to take this medicine at least 2 weeks after the symptoms are gone; this will aid tissue regeneration.

Sai Mei An is produced as "Sai Mei An Capsules" by the Sai Mei An Pharmaceutical Manufactory, Quanzhou, China, in bottles of 50 capsules.

Pinyin Name	Pharmaceutical Name	Percent	TCM Function
Zhong Ru Shi	Stalactitum	10	Neutralize hyperacidity in the stomach (high in Calcium)
Han Shui Shi	Calcitum	20	Neutralize hyperacidity in the stomach
Bing Pian	Borneol	10	Clear Heat; Stop pain
Zhen Zhu	Magarita	2	Neutralize hyperacidity in the stomach
Wa Leng Zi	Concha Arcae	20	Neutralize hyperacidity in the stomach
Bai Cao Shuang	Fuligo E Herbis	15	Stop bleeding
Hai Ge Ke	Concha Cyclinae Sinensis	23	Neutralize hyperacidity in the stomach

賽霉安

SAI MEI AN

CAPSULES

内服剂

中國泉州市
賽霉安製藥廠出品

11.8 胃 药

Wei — Stomach
Yao — medicine

Function: 1. Strengthen Spleen/Stomach
2. Neutralize excess acid in the stomach; reduce stomach pain

Application: 1. Use to treat Stuck Qi in the Stomach, which has produced Stomach pain. Use to Move Stuck Spleen Qi, decrease distension, reduce gas, stop pain, reduce burping and regurgitation of stomach acid.

2. Some Western medicine disease applications include acute or chronic gastritis due only to excess stomach acid. This formula will reduce and neutralize the stomach acid. This formula can also be used to treat gastric or duodenal ulcers. It will reduce acidity, stop the pain and promote tissue regeneration in the stomach mucosa and muscles.

Dose: 3 pills, 2 or 3 times a day, taken before meals or when necessary - i.e. when pain is present or there is heartburn.

Wei Yao is produced as "Gastropathy Capsules, Weiyao" by the Zhengjiang Chinese Medicine Works, Kiang Su, China, in bottles of 42 capsules.

Pinyin Name	Pharmaceutical Name	Percent	TCM Function
Yuan Hu	Rhizoma Corydalis Yanhusuo	21.1	Stop pain
Wu Zei Gu	Os Sepiae seu Sepiellae	10.5	Neutralize excess stomach acid; Promote healing of ulcer; astringent property
Qing Ma Xiang	Radix Aristolochiae	10.5	Clear Heat; Detoxify Fire Poison; Decrease swelling
Zhen Zhu Mu	Concha Margaritaferae	21.1	Neutralize excess stomach acid
Ming Fan	Alum	15.8	Stop bleeding; astringent property
Feng Huang Yi	Membrana Follicularis Ovi	21.1	Neutralize excess stomach acid

11.9 逍 遙 丸

Xiao	Yao	Wan
Relieve Liver Stagnation		pills

Source: Tai Ping Hui Min He Ji Ju Fang, (Formulas of the Peoples Welfare Pharmacy), Song Dynasty, 960-1279.

Function: 1. Move Stuck Liver Qi
2. Strengthen Spleen, Nourish Blood

Application: 1. Use to treat Liver Stagnation due to Def. Liver Blood. Symptoms: Hypochondrium pain on both sides, headache, vertigo, dry mouth, dry throat, fatigue, poor appetite, moodiness, possible alternating feeling of hot and cold; possible irregular menstruation, breast distension. The Tongue has a slight red color. The Pulse is Wiry and Empty.

2. Some Western medicine disease applications are listed below: (Note, in order to use this, the patient must also have the above-mentioned symptoms.)

a. Gynecological Disorders: Irregular menstruation, pre-menstrual syndrome with abdominal pain, neurasthenia associated with menopause. When using this medicine with menstrual disorders, it is common to combine it with other Patent Medicines used to treat menstrual disorders, such as 12.12, Wu Ji Bai Feng Wan.

b. Internal Medicine: Chronic hepatitis, pleurisy, cystic hyperplasia of the breast.

Dose: 8 to 10 pills, 3 times a day.

Xiao Yao Wan is produced as "Hsiao Yao Wan, Bupleurum Sedative Pills)" by the Lanzhou Fo Ci Pharmaceutical Factory, Lanzhou, China, in bottles of 200 pills.

A formula similar to this formula is also available in liquid, tincture form as "Relaxed Wanderer," in the Jade Pharmacy product line, available through Crane Enterprises, Plymouth, MA, etc. See bottom of page 343.

Pinyin Name	Pharmaceutical Name	Percent	TCM Function
Chai Hu	Radix Bupleuri	14.28	Clear Heat; Move Stuck Liver Qi
Dang Gui	Radix Angelicae Sinensis	14.28	Tonify Liver Blood; Promote Blood circulation
Bai Zhu	Rhizoma Atractylodis Macrocephalae	14.28	Strengthen Spleen; Dry Spleen Dampness
Bai Shao	Radix Paeoniae Lactiflorae	14.28	Nourish Liver Yin; Strengthen Blood
Fu Ling	Sclerotium Poriae Cocos	14.28	Strengthen Spleen; Calm the spirit
Gan Cao	Radix Glycyrrhizae Uralensis	11.42	Regulate the Middle Warmer Qi; Harmonize other herbs
Sheng Jiang	Rhizoma Zingiberis Officinalis Recens	14.28	Regulate Stomach Qi; Warm the Middle Warmer
Bo He	Herba Menthae	2.85	Smooth Liver; Reduce Liver Wind Heat

Note: 1. Clinical research in China in 1960 with 253 cases of chronic hepatitis, with symptoms such as distending pain in the hypochondrium, swelling in the liver and/or spleen, fatigue, vertigo, insomnia, nightmares, palpitations, shortness of breath, irregular bowel movements, lumbago, low-grade fever; showed that the liver test returned to normal in 36 cases and improved in 139 cases. The overall "effective rate" was 68.8%. Guang Dong Zhong Yi, (Traditional Chinese Medicine Journal), Canton Province, 1960, No. 8.

2. Case Report: A six year old boy was hyperactive in the classroom and at home. An acupuncturist advised his mother to give him 4 pills of Xiao Yao Wan, 2 times a day. Within 2 days, the teacher noticed his behavior at school was much improved. The mother also felt that there was improvement at home.

3. Case Report: A 56 year old women was seen in October, 1990, for treatment of two problems: 1) chronic asthma (greater than 7 years duration) and 2) elevated liver enzymes. The elevated SGOT and SGPT were thought to be secondary to two possible sources: a) a history of hepatitis in 1987 (liver tests had been normal in 1989) or 2) use of antihistamines including Seldane in March, 1990.

The asthma was characterized by a tight, dry cough, with problems breathing in and out. She was using inhalation aerosol treatments several times a day. For this type of Def. Lung Yin asthma, she was given the patent medicines #3.13, Li Fei; and #3.12, Yang Yin Qing Fei Tang Jiang. After 3 weeks of using these two formulas, she no longer had any problems with asthma, was no longer using any inhalants, and her physician reported complete absence of wheezing in the lungs.

For the elevated liver enzymes, she was given the patent medicine, #11.9, Xiao Yao Wan; she took 10 pills, 3 times a day for 3 months (October, November, and December, 1990), after which time, additional blood tests were performed. The elevated liver enzyme levels were reduced for the first time in over 10 months; they are reported below:

	Normal Lab Values	Before use of Herbs March, 1990	Before use of Herbs June, 1990	After 3-month use of Herbs January 2, 1991
SGOT	12 - 45	67	66	43
SGPT	7 - 40	75	107	63

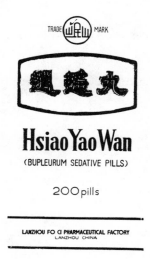

Chapter 12. Regulate Blood

Section A. **Promote Blood Circulation and Remove Blood Stasis**

Section B. **Stop Bleeding**

Section C. **Regulate Menstruation**

12.1 複 方 丹 參 片

Fu	Fang	Dan	Shen	Pian
----------compound--------		-----------Salviae----------		tablets

Function: 1. Promote Blood circulation; Remove Stasis of Blood
2. Eliminate uneasiness; Tranquilize

Application: 1. Use to treat Blood Stasis in coronary heart (artery) disease. Symptoms: Fixed, stabbing, strong sharp pain, possibly worse at night; heart palpitations may be present; dark purple Tongue; deep, choppy Pulse.

2. Use to treat Blood Stasis in dysmenorrhea or amenorrhea.

3. Use to treat Blood Stasis in bruises

Fu Fang Dan Shen Pian is produced as "Danshen Tabletco" by the Tai Zhou Pharmaceutical Factory, Zhe Jiang, China, in bottles of 60 tablets.

Dose: 2 tablets, 3 times a day

Pinyin Name	Pharmaceutical Name	Percent	TCM Function
Dan Shen	Radix Salviae Miltiorrhizae	100	Invigorate the Blood and break up Congealed Blood; Tranquilize

Notes: 1. Laboratory research in China has shown that this medicine is able to improve the muscle contractions of the heart and distend the coronary arteries. Thus, the blood supply to the heart is increased and the heart rate is decreased. The cardiac function is thus improved.

2. Clinical research in China has observed that 80% of cases with heart diease who took this medicine for one month had remission of symptoms such as chest fullness and angina. The EKG was improved in 30-50% of the cases who took this medicine for one month. The EKG was improved in a higher percentage after taking the medicine for one year.

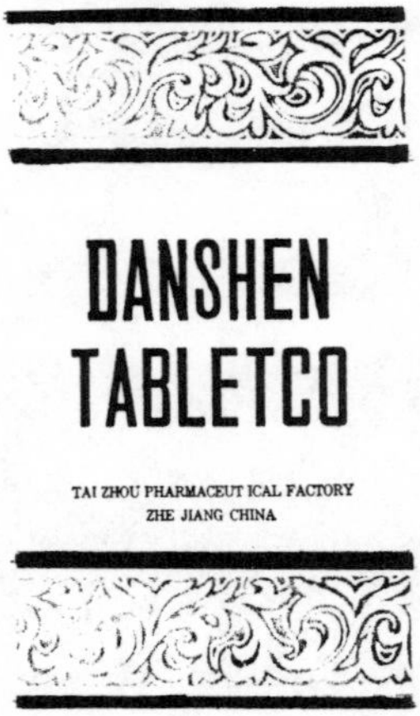

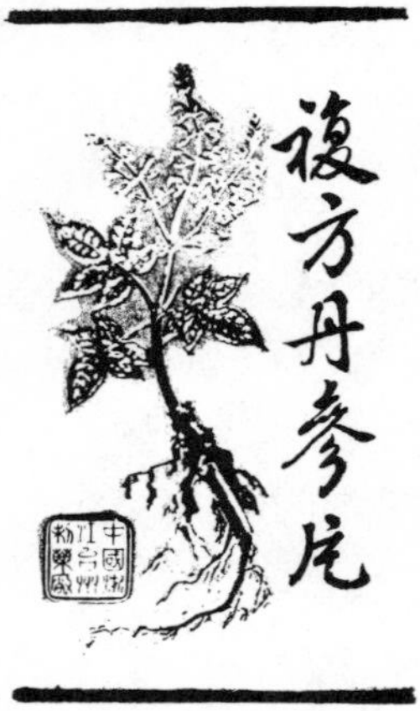

12.2 延 胡 索 止 痛 片

Yan	Hu	Su	Zhi	Tong	Pian
----------Yan Hu Extract----------			stop	pain	tablets

Function: 1. Promote Blood Circulation; Stop pain
2. Relax smooth and striated muscle spasms

Application: 1. Use to treat pain due to Stagnation of Blood and Qi including dysmenorrhea, post-partum uterine pain and other gynecological disorders with pain; stomach ache, including gastric or duodenal ulcer; abdominal pain; hypochondrium pain which may be associated with hepatitis or gall bladder problems; chest pain which may be associated with angina; pain due to rheumatism or injury. This is especially good to treat dull pain.

2. Use to treat uneasiness, agitation, and insomnia especially caused by pain. This has a mild tranquilizing effect; it inhibits the reticular activating system but does not act directly on the cortex or on the periaqueductal grey matter (Bensky and Gamble, 1986).

3. This medicine is effective in relaxing striated muscle spasms and is thus useful in relaxing tremors and spasms. The most effective ingredient in Yan Hu Su, tetrahydropalmatine ($C_{21} H_{25} O_4 N$), has a synergistic effect with Dilantin in reducing seizures. ("Pharmacological Research on Yan Hu Su: The Effect of Tetrahydropalmatine on The Central Nervous System," Sheng Li Xue Bao, Physiology Journal, 1960, Vol. 24, No. 2, pp. 110-120.)

4. Use to treat chronic headache especially associated with insomnia.

Dose: For pain, take 1-2 tablets, 2 or 3 times a day. For insomnia, take 1 - 3 tablets before bedtime. Each tablet contains 50 mg. of the extract, tetrahydropalmatine

Yan Hu Su Zhi Tong Pian is produced as "Coryanalgine Tetrahydropalmatini Sulfas" by the Sing-Kyn Drug House, Guangzhou, China, in vials containing 12 tablets.

Pinyin Name	Pharmaceutical Name	Percent	TCM Function
Yan Hu Suo	Corydalis bulbosa Dc.	100	See above

Note: 1. There is another Patent Medicine with a similar name, Yan Hu Suo Zhi Tong Pian, produced by the Chongqing Chinese Medicine Factory, Chongqing, Szechuan, China. In addition to the herb Yan Hu Suo, that formula contains Bai Zhi and also can be used to treat headache caused by Wind-Cold. Yan Hu Suo Zhi Tong Pian contains only herbs; Yan Hu Su Zhi Tong Pian contains the extract from the Yan Hu Suo herb, tetrahydropalmatine. The prepared formula Yan Hu Suo Zhi Tong Pian is produced as "Corydalis Yanhusus Analgesic Tablets" by the Chongqing Chinese Medicine Factory, Szechuan, China, in vials containing 24 tablets.

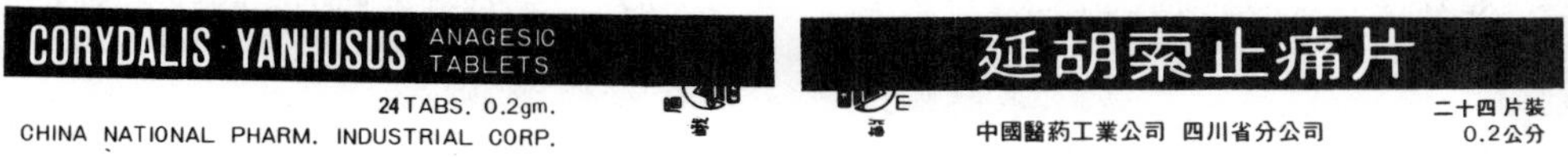

12.3 七 厘 散

七	厘	散
Qi	**Li**	**San**
seven	unit of measure	powder

Source: Liang Fang Ji Ye, (Collection of Fine Formulas), Qing Dynasty, 1644-1911.

Function: 1. Promote Blood circulation; Remove Blood Stagnation
2. Decrease swelling; Stop pain

Application: 1. Use to treat sports injuries and other traumatic injuries including open wounds, broken bones, and soft tissue injuries such as sprains, strains, and bruises.

2. Use to treat skin infections including carbuncles and sores; ulcers with or without infection; first or second degree burns caused by fire or hot water; herpes zoster (shingles).

3. Because this medicine is able to Disperse Blood Stagnation, Open Orifices and Stop pain, some researchers have begun to use it to treat coronary heart disease and myocarditis.

4. Use to treat severe liver region pain due to Stagnation of Blood in chronic hepatitis patients.

Contraindication: Do not use with pregnant women.

Dose: For use with Applications #1 and #2, the powder can either be used externally or internally, or both.

External Use: For external contusions, fractures, sprains, strains, bruises, and burns, make a paste with Qi Li San powder and white wine; apply this paste to the affected area. Cover with sterile dressing and re-apply once a day. For open wounds, sprinkle the powder over the open wound, cover with a sterile dressing and re-apply once a day.

Internal Use: Take 0.2 to 0.9 grams with warm water or wine, 1 to 3 times a day. The powder may also be placed into gelatin capsules and swallowed.

For use with Applications #3 and #4, use internally, only.

Qi Li San is produced by the Tung Jen Tang pharmacy, Beijing, China, in powder form in small glasss vials; each vial contains 1.5 grams.

The ingredients are listed below in 5 groups according to function.

Pinyin Name	Pharmaceutical Name	Percent	TCM Function
Group 1			
Xue Jie	Sanguis Draconis	52.4	Promote Blood circulation;
Hong Hua	Flos Carthami Tinctorii	8.7	Remove Stagnation
Group 2			
Ru Xiang	Gummi Olibanum	8.7	Remove Stagnation of Qi and Blood;
Mo Yao	Myrrha	8.7	Decrease swelling; Stop pain

Group 3			
She Xiang	Secretio Moschus moschiferi	0.7	Promote Circulation of Qi and Blood;
Bing Pian	Borneol	0.7	Open Orifices; Clear Meridians; Stop pain
Group 4			
Zhu Sha	Cinnabaris	7.0	Tranquilize Heart; Calm the Spirit
Group 5			
Er Cha	Acacia seu Uncaria	13.1	Clear Heat; Stop Bleeding

Notes: 1. The Patent Medicine, Jin Gu Die Shang Wan is similar to Qi Li San. This formula has San Qi (Radix Pseudoginseng) as an ingredient which has the effect to stop bleeding. Thus, Jin Gu Die Shang Wan may be better for the traumatic injury with bleeding.

2. The Patent Medicine, Die Da Yao Jing is similar to Qi Li San.

12.4 麝 香 跌 打 膏

She	Xiang	Die	Da	Gao
------------Musk-------------		--------contusion-------		plaster

Function: 1. Promote Blood circulation; Remove Blood Stagnation
2. Stop pain

Application: 1. Use to treat contusions, sprains, strains, sports and other traumatic injuries. This formula is especially effective in decreasing swelling and stopping pain. It will help the injured tissue to regenerate.

Contraindication: Do not use with pregnant women.

How to use the Plaster: Wash the area first with gentle soap and warm water. The plaster will be especially effective if applied after a warm bath. Peel the plaster from the cellophane and place over the affected area. Use as many plasters as necessary, to completely cover the area. The plaster may be left in place for 2 days; keep the plaster dry. If redness, itching, or allergic skin reaction develops, do not use the plaster.

She Xiang Die Da Gao is produced as "Musk Anti-contusion Plasters" by the Tianjin Drug Manufactory, Tianjin, China, in boxes with 6 plasters.

Only the major 7 ingredients are listed below; the percents are not available.

Pinyin Name	Pharmaceutical Name	TCM Function
She Xiang	Secretio Moschus moschiferi	Move Blood Stagnation; Stop pain
Ru Xiang	Gummi Olibanum	Promote Blood circulation; Stop pain
Mo Yao	Myrrha	Promote Blood circulation; Stop pain
Hong Hua	Flos Carthami Tinctorii	Promote Blood circulation; Remove Blood Stagnation
Ding Xiang	Flos Caryophylli	Move Stuck Qi; Stop pain
Chuan Xiong	Radix Ligustici Wallichii	Promote Blood circulation; Remove Stuck Qi
Long Bao	Borneol	Decrease swelling; Stop pain

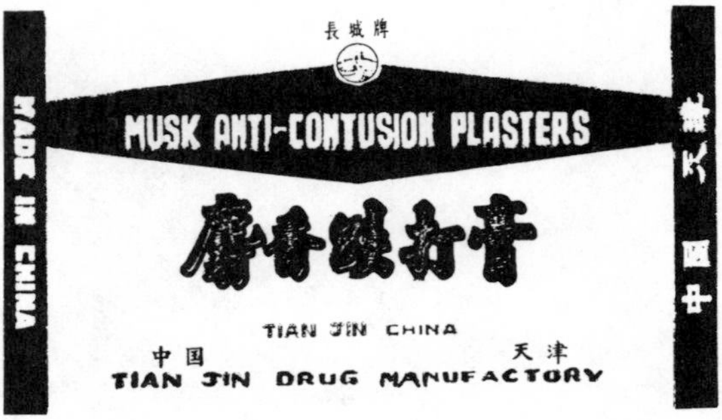

12.5 跌 打 止 痛 膏

跌	打	止	痛	膏
Die	**Da**	**Zhi**	**Tong**	**Gao**
--------contusion-------		stop	pain	plaster

Function: 1. Promote Blood circulation; Relax tendons and muscles
2. Remove Blood Stagnation; Stop pain

Application: 1. Use to treat sports or traumatic injuries with bruising and swelling. Also use to treat sprains and fractures.

2. Use to treat back ache in the lumbar area due to over-exertion.

3. Use to treat neuralgia and chronic arthritis.

Contraindication: Do not use with pregnant women. Do not use on an open wound.

How to use this Plaster: This herbal plaster is 10 cm x 28 cm in size; it is one of the larger plasters produced. The plaster is a dark brown color on the inside and contains many herbs. Either use the whole plaster or cut the plaster to the appropriate size to cover the area. Press the plaster firmly into place; the plaster must form a tight seal with the skin. If the plaster does not stick tightly to the skin, especially in the winter-time, use gauze or tape to secure the plaster in place. This herbal plaster will be effective for 2 days. Keep the plaster dry, if possible.

If redness or itching or allergic skin reaction occurs, discontinue use.

Die Da Zhi Tong Gao is produced as "Plaster for Bruise and Analgesic" by the United Pharmaceutical Manufactory, Guangzhou, China, in boxes containing 10 plasters.

The ingredients are listed below in 4 groups below, according to function.

Pinyin Name	Pharmaceutical Name	Percent	TCM Function
Group 1			
Hong Hua	Flos Carthami Tinctorii	9.17	Promote Blood circulation;
Mo Yao	Myrrha	6.25	Remove Stagnation;
Xue Jie	Sanguis Draconis	4.17	Stop pain
Er Cha	Acacia seu Uncaria	6.25	
Tu Bie Chong	Eupolyphagae seu Opisthoplatiae	10.42	
Group 2			
Xu Duan	Radix Dipsaci	4.17	Promote Blood circulation;
Gu Sui Bu	Drynaria fortunei	4.17	Stop pain;
Long Gu	Os Draconis	10.42	Promote healing of broken bones;
			Relax tendons and muscles
Group 3			
Da Huang	Rhizoma Rhei	8.33	Remove Blood Stagnation;
Pu Gong Ying	Herba Taraxaci Mongolici cum Radice	8.33	Clear Heat; Decrease swelling
Group 4			
Bo He	Herba Menthae	20.0	Move Stuck Qi; Stop pain
Dong Qing Yu	Wintergreen oil	8.32	

10片庄(10X28CM)

IN BOXES OF 10 PIECES
(10X28 CM)

羊城牌
YANG CHENG BRAND

跌打止痛膏

Plaster for Bruise

AND
ANALGESIC

[redacted]

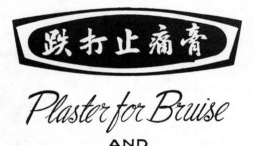

12.6 正 骨 水

Zheng	**Gu**	**Shui**
-------setting-bone-------		solution

Function: 1. Promote Blood circulation; Decrease swelling; Stop pain
2. Promote regeneration of broken bone tissue; Promote healing of fractures

Application: 1. Use to treat fractures and dislocated joints due to sports or other traumatic injuries.

Cautions: 1. This solution is for external use only. Keep away from children.

2. Apply this solution on a daily basis only after the bone has been set, or the dislocation has been re-positioned.

3. When using this solution with children, the duration of time which the soaked cotton ball is left in place should be reduced.

4. When using this solution with adults, do not leave the soaked cotton ball in place for more than the indicated period of time.

5. If the patient has a serious skin reaction to the solution (blistering or rash), discontinue use.

6. Do not apply this solution to an open wound.

7. This solution is flammable. Keep the bottle tightly closed and do not use near open fire or flame.

How to use the solution: The fractured bone should be set by a professional in a hospital setting. This solution should be applied to the affected area, however, before the bone is set, because it will stop the pain. After the bone is set, apply a cotton ball soaked with the solution to the affected area. Two or three soaked cotton balls may be used to "surround" the fractured area. Lightly wrap the soaked cotton balls into place with gauze. Leave the soaked cotton balls on the area for 1 hour if the fracture is on an upper limb. Leave the soaked cotton balls on the area for 1 and 1/2 hours if the fracture is on a lower limb. Then remove the cotton balls; they will be dry and there is no need to wipe away the remaining solution. From the next day on, apply this procedure twice a day to the affected area until complete recovery has taken place.

Zheng Gu Shui is produced as "Zheng Gu Shui Analgesic Liniment" by the Yulin Drug Manufactory, Kwangsi, China, in bottles containing 3.4 fl. oz.

The ingredients are lised below in 3 groups according to function.

Pinyin Name	Pharmaceutical Name	Percent	TCM Function
Group 1			
San Qi	Radix Pseudoginseng	25	Remove Blood Stagnation;
Bai Zhi	Radix Angelicae	13	Eliminate bruising; Stop bleeding; Decrease swelling; Stop pain

Group 2			
Ji Gu Xiang	Cinnamomum camphora	15	Move Stuck Qi; Open Orifices;
Bo He Nao	Menthol Extract	3	Stop pain
Zhang Nao	Camphora (crystals)	2	
Group 3			
Wu Ma Xun Cheng	Croton Tiglium	18	Strengthen bones and tendons;
Qian Jin Ba	Moghania Macrophylla	12	Help regeneration of damaged
Da Li Wang	Inula Cappa	12	tissues; Decrease swelling; Stop pain

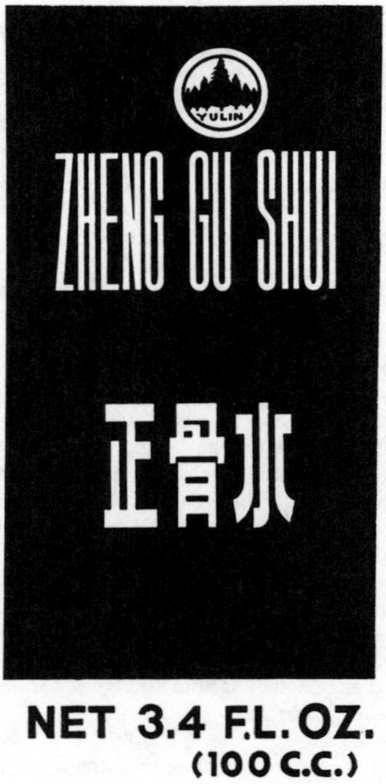

12.7 跌 打 萬 花 油

跌	打	萬	花	油
Die	**Da**	**Wan**	**Hua**	**You**
------sports injury------		10,000	flowers	oil

Function: 1. Promote Blood circulation; Remove Stagnation
2. Decrease swelling; Relax tendons
3. Stop pain; Promote regeneration of damaged tissues

Application: 1. Use to treat sports or traumatic injuries, with or without open wound. Also use to treat sprains and strains of muscles and tendons.

2. Use to treat burns due to flames or hot liquid.

3. Use to treat cuts on the skin with bleeding (including those from martial arts practice).

Caution: For external use only.

How to use this oil: 1. For sports or traumatic injuries without open wound, rub the injured area with a cotton ball soaked with this oil, 2 or 3 times a day.

2. For burns and cuts, place a cotton ball soaked with this oil onto the injured area, and wrap the area with a gauze bandage. Change the soaked cotton ball every day.

Die Da Wan Hua You is produced as "Wan Hua Oil" by the United Pharmaceutical Manufactory, Guangzhou, China, in bottles containing 15 cc.

The major ingredients are listed below in 3 separate groups according to function. The amount of each ingredient is for 100 bottles of the medicine, which is equal to a total of 1500 ml. (Each bottle contains 15cc.)

Pinyin Name	Pharmaceutical Name	Grams	TCM Function
Group 1			
San Qi	Radix Pseudoginseng	15	Stop Bleeding; Remove Blood Stagnation; Strengthen bones and promote regeneration of injured tissues
Gu Sui Bu	Dynaria fortunei (Kunze)	8	
Group 2			
Hong Hua	Flos Carthami Tinctorii	8	Promote Blood circulation; Decrease swelling; Stop pain
Xue Jie	Sanguis Draconis	6	
Ru Xiang	Gummi Olibanum	6	
Mo Yao	Myrrha	6	
Wu Ming Yi	Pyrolusitum	5	
La Mei Hua	Flos Chimonanthus nitens Oliv.	5	
Group 3			
Lu Hui	Herba Aloes	8	Heal burns and wounds

Note: 1. In this formula there are 3 additional herbs (Fu Rong Hua, Huan Hun Cao, Yang Ti Cao); and 3 oils (Hong Hua You, Cha You, Song Jie You).

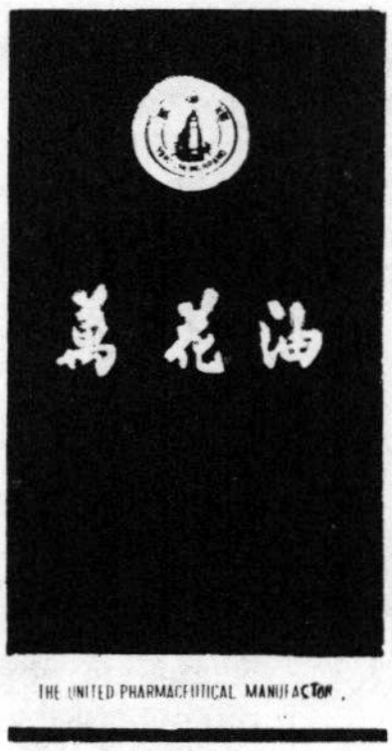
萬花油
THE UNITED PHARMACEUTICAL MANUFACTOR .

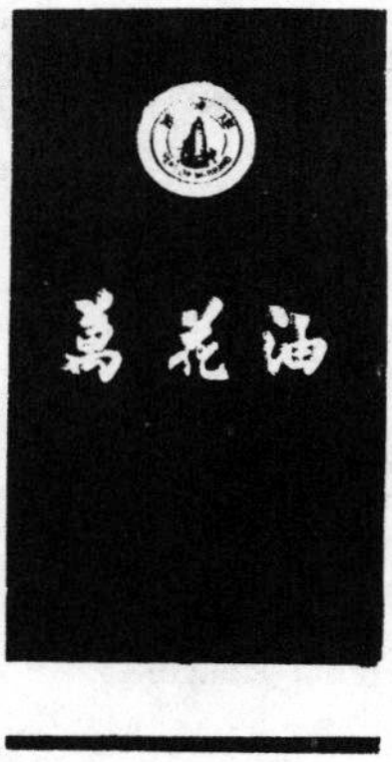
萬花油

12.8 骨 折 挫 伤 散

Gu	Zhe	Cuo	Shang	San
bones	broken	------------bruise-------------		capsules with powder

Function: 1. Promote Blood circulation; Aid regeneration of bone tissue
2. Soothe muscles and tendons; Decrease swelling; Stop pain

Application: 1. Use to aid in the healing of broken bones, bruises, contusions, sprains, strains and other tissue injuries associated with trauma, including sports injuries.

Contraindication: Do not use with pregnant women.

Dose: 7 capsules, 3 times a day, taken with warm water or warm wine. Reduce dosage with children.

Gu Zhe Cuo Shang San is produced as "Fractura Pulvis" by the Kiamusze Chinese Medicine Works, Kiamusze, He Long Jiang Province, China.

The contents are listed below in 4 groups, according to function.

Pinyin Name	Pharmaceutical Name	Percent	TCM Function
Group 1			
Ye Zhu Gu	Wild boar's bone	45.0	Strengthen bones;
Huang Gua Zi	Cucumber seeds	37.0	Aid regeneration of bone tissue
Group 2			
Dang Gui	Radix Angelicae Sinensis	3.0	Nourish Blood; Promote Blood circulation
Group 3			
Hong Hua	Flos Carthami Tinctorii	5.0	Promote Blood circulation;
Xue Jie	Sanguis Draconis	2.0	Remove Blood Stagnation
Da Huang	Rhizoma Rhei	3.0	
Group 4			
Ru Xiang	Gummi Olibanum	2.0	Promote Blood circulation;
Mo Yao	Myrrha	2.0	Remove Blood Stagnation;
Tu Bie Chong	Eupolyphagae seu Opisthoplatiae	1.0	Stop pain; Decrease swelling

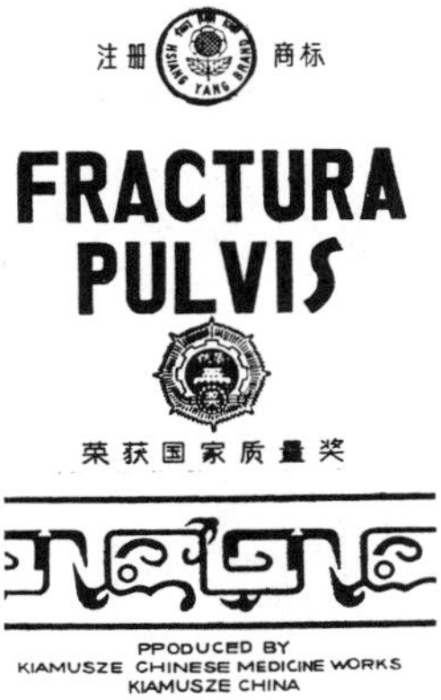

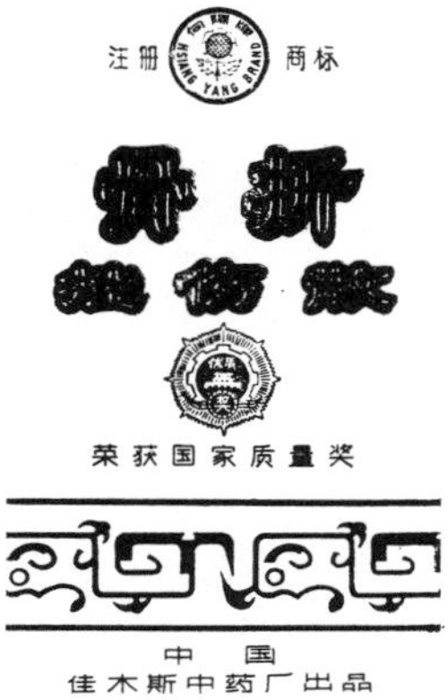

12.9 毛 冬 青

Mao Dong Qing

------------------herb name----------------------

Function: 1. Promote Blood circulation and Remove Blood Stagnation
2. Clear Heat, Detoxify Fire Poison

Application: 1. Use to treat blood vessel disease including cardiac vascular disease, cerebral vascular disease, and peripheral artery disease.

a. Use to treat coronary artery disease, angina pectoris, and other related symptoms associated with coronary artery disease such as headache, dizziness, and limb numbness. It is used to improve the heart function; most patients will notice a positive effect within 1 month; 1 to 3 months is considered one course of treatment. (Observation of 103 Cases of the Treatment of Coronary Artery Cardiac Disease with Mao Dung Qing. Xin Yi Xue, (New Medicine Journal), Vol 5, pp. 12-16, 1972. Zhongshan Medical College, Department of Internal Medicine, Second Teaching Hospital.)

b. Use to treat Buerger's Disease (thromboangiitis obliterans; intravascular clot formation, with inflammation of the vessel wall). The clinical results are better if the patient has local or general Heat signs including swollen, red, painful local symptoms or a general Heat syndrome with feelings of warmth, thirst, constipation, a yellow Tongue coat, and a rapid Pulse.

c. Use to treat patients with a history of transient ischemic attacks and arteriosclerosis. Clinical reports show that this medicine will improve the blood supply to the brain. It is often combined with herbal tea formulas which are designed to improve Blood circulation. (Xin Yi Yao Tong Xun, [New Medicine Report], Vol. 2, p. 37, 1972.)

2. Use to treat infections which may be associated with pharyngitis, tonsillitis, bronchitis.

Contraindication: In most cases this medicine will cause no side effects. In a small percent of cases who use a large dose, slight nausea or abdominal cramps or dizziness or headache may be present. In a small percent of cases, the same side effects observed when taking blood-thiners are present, including bruising easily, increased bleeding, etc. Patients who have a low platelet count or internal bleeding problems (bleeding ulcer) or hypermenorrhea should use this formula with caution.

Dose: 3 capsules, 3 times a day. Take for 7 days, then skip taking the medicine for 3 days, then resume the cycle again.

Mao Dong Qing is produced as "Maodungching Capsules" by the Guangzhou Pharmaceutical Corporation, Guangzhou, China, in bottles of 30 capsules.

Pinyin Name	Pharmaceutical Name	Percent	TCM Function
Mao Dong Qing	Ilex pubescens Hook, et Arn.	100	Promote Blood circulation; Remove Blood Stagnation; Clear Heat, Detoxify Fire Poison

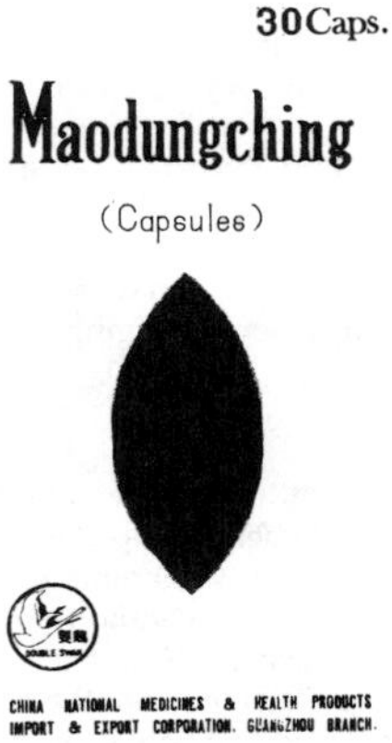

30Caps.
Maodungching
(Capsules)
CHINA NATIONAL MEDICINES & HEALTH PRODUCTS
IMPORT & EXPORT CORPORATION. GUANGZHOU BRANCH.

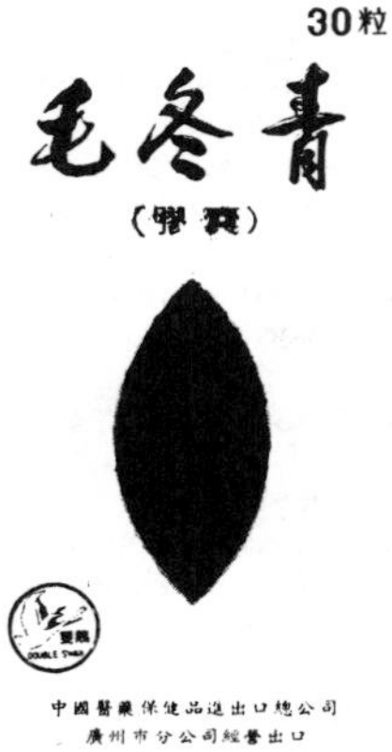

30粒
毛冬青
中國醫藥保健品進出口總公司
廣州市分公司經營出口

12.10 云 南 白 药

Yun	Nan	Bai	Yao
-----Yunnan Province----		white	medicine

Function: 1. Stop bleeding
2. Stop pain (Remove Blood Stagnation)

Application: 1. Use to stop bleeding from an open wound; this includes severe bleeding associated with gunshot wounds.

2. Use to stop internal bleeding.

a. Gastro-Intestinal System Bleeding. This includes serious bleeding associated with vomiting of blood due to stomach ulcer, stomach cancer, or cirrhosis of the liver; and intestinal bleeding with blood in the stools due to colitis, etc.

b. Pulmonary System Bleeding. This includes serious bleeding with coughing up of blood associated with pulmonary tuberculosis, bronchiectasis, lung cancer, etc.

c. Nasal Bleeding (Epistaxis). This includes serious nose bleeding associated with hypertension, leukemia, hemophilia, thrombocytopenia, etc.

3. Use to treat soft tissue sports injuries (internal use) such as sprains and strains of joints and muscles with symptoms such as pain, swelling and bruising.

4. Use to treat gynecological disorders caused by Stagnation of Blood such as dysmenorrhea, amenorrhea, hypermenorrhea, hemorrhaging during postpartum period.

Contraindication: Do not use with pregnant women.

Usage: The medicine comes in loose powder form in a glass bottle; however, at the top of the powder, there is also one small red pill (about the size of a single black peppercorn). This red pill is called Bao Xian Zi, which is translated as "insurance pill for a serious or emergency case." This pill is only used to treat a patient with severe bleeding or injury who is about to go into shock, as a "First Aid" medicine, otherwise do not use the pill. This medicine will help to prevent the patient from going into shock. The contents of the Bao Xian Zi are different from the Yun Nan Bai Yao. The Bao Xian Zi has ingredients to stop pain and Open Orifices to help prevent shock. It will not stop the bleeding. The Yun Nan Bai Yao powder must be swallowed (or if necessary, used locally) to stop the bleeding.

Dose: External Use: Sprinkle the powder on the open wound and apply pressure until bleeding has stopped.

Internal Use: The powder is packaged as 4 grams per glass bottle with 1 Bao Xian Zi.
The capsules are packaged as 16 capsules per package with 1 Bao Xian Zi.

Adults: Powder Form: Take 0.25 to 0.5 grams of powder, 4 times a day. The powder can be swallowed with liquid, or put into gelatin capsules and swallowed with liquid.
Capsule Form: 1 or 2 capsules, 4 times a day

Children: Age 2 to 5 Years: Use one-fourth the adult dose, 4 times a day
Age 5 to 12 Years: Use one-half the adult dose, 4 times a day

1. For injury with bleeding, the powder should be taken with water

2. For injury without bleeding (sprain or strain of joint or muscle), the powder should be taken with wine.

3. For gynecological disorders, the powder should be taken with wine, but if heavy bleeding is present, the powder should be taken with water.

Yun Nan Bai Yao is produced as "Yunnan Paiyao" by the Yunnan Paiyao Factory, Yunnan, China, in small vials containing 4 grams; and in boxes of 80 capsules (0.25 grams per capsule).

Pinyin Name	Pharmaceutical Name	Percent	TCM Function
San Qi	Radix Pseudoginseng	100	Disperse Blood Stagnation; Stop bleeding; Reduce swelling; Stop pain

Notes: 1. The following summary of some recent research with Yun Nan Bai Yao was taken from an article published in the December 30, 1985 issue of the Hong Kong newspaper, South China Morning Post. Dr. James Ma, an organic chemist who specializes in spectroscopy, from the Chemistry Department at Chinese University, Hong Kong, is currently conducting research into the components of Yun Nan Bai Yao. He reports there are 21 components and 4 of these are classified as being active in stopping bleeding. Both in vitro and in vivo studies have been carried out regarding the clotting time for blood when Yun Nan Bai Yao was used. The clotting time for human blood in a test tube was observed to be reduced by 33 per cent. In animal studies where actual body bleeding rate was examined, it was cut by 54 per cent.

During the Vietnam war Yun Nan Bai Yao was often discovered in a tiny bottle on the bodies of Vietcong soldiers. Wounded soldiers sprinkled it on their injuries to halt severe bleeding while waiting for emergency medical treatment.

Other academic work on Yun Nan Bai Yao has been conducted in Taiwan, Japan, India and in Wisconsin, in the U.S. It is grown primarily in Yunnan Province, China, and in Nepal. The Chinese are now also growing it on herb farms.

Dr. Ma states that the herb has a quite different mechanism from anything which is found in Western medicine. He has sent the pure compound to an authority in Sweden who has suggested that it could possibly have anti-cancer properties. Some Chinese medical authorities have also suggested that Yun Nan Bai Yao could be useful in the treatment of leukemia.

2. This medicine is also sometimes called Bai Yao (White Medicine)

云南白药

(胶囊剂)

YUNNAN PAIYAO

(IN CAPSULES)

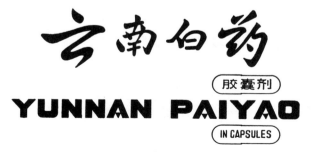

12.11 千 金 止 带 丸

Qian	Jin	Zhi	Dai	Wan
----------woman--------		stop	leukorrhea	pills

Source: Ji Yin Gang Mu, (Compendium of Therapy for Women's Diseases), Qing Dynasty, 1644-1911.

Function: 1. Regulate Qi and Blood
2. Regulate menstruation; Stop leukorrhea

Application: 1. Use to treat Def. Qi and Blood syndrome which has caused leukorrhea. Def. Spleen Qi may cause the body to fail to convert fluid, thus forming Dampness retention, which is the main cause for the production of leukorrhea. Thus, in addition to leukorrhea, the patient should have signs of Dampness including aching in the lumbar area, abdominal distension, fatigue and poor appetite. The Tongue coat is white and greasy; the Pulse is Slippery.

2. Use to treat dysmenorrhea. This formula can be used to treat menstrual cramps because it contains some herbs which Move Stuck Liver Qi as well as some pain killers. This formula can also be used to treat irregular menstruation due to Stagnation of Qi, Stagnation of Blood, or Def. Kidney and Liver

Dose: 10 pills, 1 or 2 times aday.

Qian Jin Zhi Dai Wan is produced as "Chienchin Chih Tai Wan" by the Tientsin Drug Manufactory, Tientsin, China, in bottles of 120 pills.

Only the major 9 ingredients are listed here; an additional 8 ingredients are part of the orginial formula and they are listed under the Notes.)

Pinyin Name	Pharmaceutical Name	Percent	TCM Function
Dang Gui	Radix Angelicae Sinensis	10	Nourish Blood; Promote Blood circulation; Regulate Menstruation
Bai Zhu	Rhizoma Atractylodis Macrocephalae	5	Tonify Spleen; Eliminate Dampness
Xiao Hui Xiang	Fructus Foeniculi Vulgaris	5	Regulate Qi; Warm Yang; Stop pain
Yan Hu Suo	Rhizoma Corydalis Yanhusuo	10	Promote Blood circulation; Stop pain
Mu Xiang	Radix Saussureae seu Vladimiriae	10	Move Stuck Qi; Stop pain
Xu Duan	Radix Dipsaci	10	Strengthen Liver and Kidney; Stop Bleeding; Soothe embryo
Dang Shen	Radix Codonopsis Pilosulae	12	Strengthen Spleen; Tonify Qi
Mu Li	Concha Ostreae (Fired)	12	Stop leukorrhea; Stop hypermenorrhea; astringent
Qing Dai	Indigo Pulverata Levis	16	Clear Damp Heat

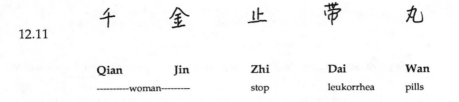

Note: 1. The additional 8 herbs which were in the original formula are as follows:
Xiang Fu, Chun Bai Pi, Ji Guan Hua, Bai Shao, Sha Ren, Bu Gu Zhi, Chuan Xiong, and Du Zhong.

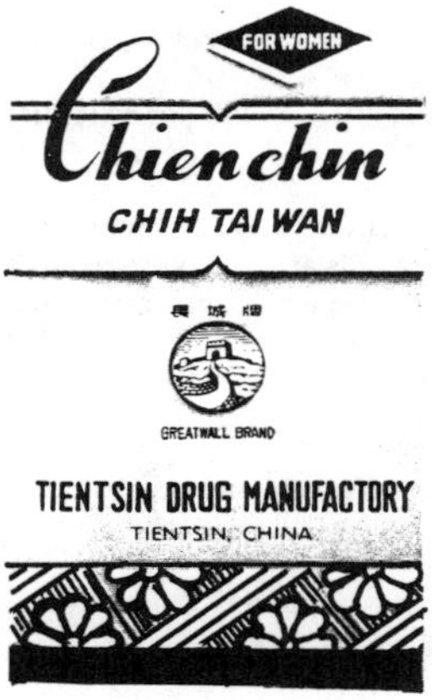

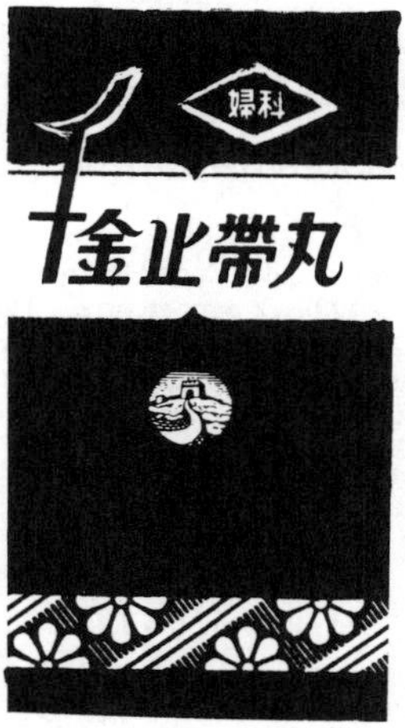

12.12 烏 鷄 白 鳳 丸

Wu	Ji	Bai	Feng	Wan
black	chicken	white	phoenix	pills

Source: Shou Shi Bau Yuan, (Book for Protection of Vital Energy for Long Life), Ming Dynasty, 1368-1644.

Function: 1. Strengthen Qi; Strengthen Blood
2. Regulate menstruation; Stop leukorrhea

Application: 1. Use to treat gynecological disorders due to Def. Qi and Def. Blood.
Symptoms: Irregular menstruation where the period may be early or late, hypermenorrhea or hypomenorrhea, pre-menstrual syndrome, dysmenorrhea or pain with ovulation, leukorrhea, postpartum weakness, postpartum bleeding, fatigue, low-back pain, feeling of weakness in the legs, poor appetite, weight loss or problems gaining weight.

2. Use to treat Def. Qi and Def. Blood syndrome in general. This includes patients with chronic hepatitis (Clinical Research in China has shown this formula to decrease SGPT levels in the blood in chronic hepatitis cases).

Dose: This Patent Medicine is available in two Honey Pill Forms listed below, and in condensed pill form.

1. In one form, the Honey Pill is packaged as one large Honey Pill per cellophane package (inside one wax ball).

2. In a second form, the Honey Pill has already been cut up into 30 or more small, miniature pills (about the size of black peppercorns). The miniature pills are also wrapped as a cluster in a cellophane wrapper (inside one wax ball). These miniature pills are easier to take than the large honey pill listed above, which first must be cut up, or dissolved in water. If the pills are in the miniature pill form, it is indicated on the outside of the box where it is labelled either, "Xiao Min Wan," or "Xiao Wan."

In the honey pill form, the dose is l honey pill (contents inside one wax ball), 2 times a day, every day of the month.

In the condensed pill form, the dose is 5 pills, 3 times a day, every day of the month.

Wu Ji Bai Feng Wan is produced as "Wuchi Paifeng Wan" by the Tientsin Drug Manufactory, Tientsin, China, in 2 formats l) boxes containing 10 honey pills, where each waxed honey pill contains many small honey pills for easier swallowing and 2) bottles of 120 condensed, coated pills. It is also produced by the Beijing Tung Jen Tang pharmacy, in boxes containing 10 honey pills in standard honey pill format as well as waxed honey pills containing many small honey pills.

Only the major ingredients in this Patent Medicine are listed below. In some formulas, there are an additonal 10 ingredients; these are listed in the Notes.

Pinyin Name	Pharmaceutical Name	Percent	TCM Function
Wu Ji	Gaiius Nigrosceus	33.87	Strengthen Liver and Kidney Yin; Tonify Blood
Ren Shen	Radix Ginseng	6.45	Tonify Qi; Strengthen Spleen
Huang Qi	Radix Astragali	1.63	Strengthen Qi; Stop daytime sweating
Dang Gui	Radix Angelicae Sinensis	6.45	Nourish Blood; Promote Blood circulation; Stop bleeding
Bai Shao	Radix Paeoniae Lactiflorae	6.45	Nourish Yin; Strengthen Blood; Stop abdominal pain; Relax smooth muscles
Sheng Di Huang	Radix Rehmanniae Glutinosae	12.90	Strengthen Yin; Clear Empty Heat
Shu Di Huang	Radix Rehmanniae Glutinosae Conquitae	12.90	Nourish Yin; Tonify Blood
Xiang Fu	Rhizoma Cyperi Rotundi	6.45	Regulate Qi and Blood; Stop menstrual cramping
Shan Yao	Radix Dioscoreae Oppositae	6.45	Strengthen Spleen; Stop leukorrhea
Lu Jiao Jiao	Colla Cornu Cervi	6.45	Strengthen Kidney Yang

Notes: 1. In some formulas, there are an additional 10 ingredients. These include the following: Dan Shen, Bie Jia, Yin Chai Hu, Qian Shi, Sang Piao Xiao, Chuan Xiong, Gan Cao, Tian Men Dong, Mu Li, Lu Jiao Shuang.

2. This is one of the most popular and commonly used medicines in China to regulate menstruation. The ingredients will Strengthen Qi and Blood without producing Stagnation, and will Warm the Yang, without producing Dryness.

3. The above-listed formula is the main formula which is commonly used in China to treat gynecological disorders; many women have good results with this formula. More recently, some manufacturers have made some modification in this formula; additional Tonic medicines including Ren Shen (Radix Ginseng) and Lu Rong (Cornu Cervi Parvum), etc. have been added. This type of modification has increased the Tonic function to Strengthen Blood and Qi. The Lu Rong is also Warming and will Warm the Kidney Yang. Some of these altered formulas are available under the names, Shen Rong (herb names) Bai Feng Wan, or Zhen Zhu (pearl) Bai Feng Wan. These will often cost more, double or triple the price, of the main formula, Wu Ji Bai Feng Wan.

4. The Patent Medicine, Bai Feng Wan, is the same as Wu Ji Bai Feng Wan.

5. Some patients may experience a heavier flow (but less, or no menstrual pain). The Patent Medicine #12.10, Yun Nan Bai Yao, may be used at the time of the heavier flow, to help reduce it. The dose is 2 capsules of Yun Nan Bai Yao, every 4 to 6 hours during the time of the heavier flow. This will also help to relieve any menstrual pain that may be present.

6. This formula is sometimes combined with 13.24, Ren Shen Lu Rong Wan, with women who have signs of Cold with Def. Kidney Yang, and have problems with fertility.

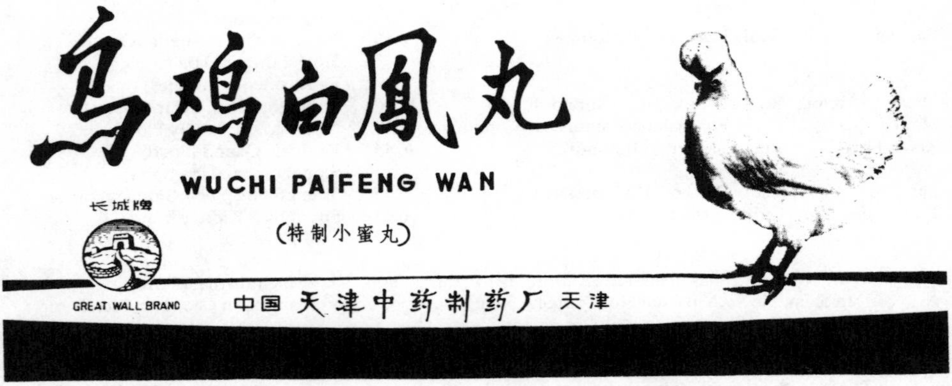

乌鷄白鳳丸
WUCHI PAIFENG WAN
长城牌
GREAT WALL BRAND
(特制小蜜丸)
中国 天津中药制药厂 天津

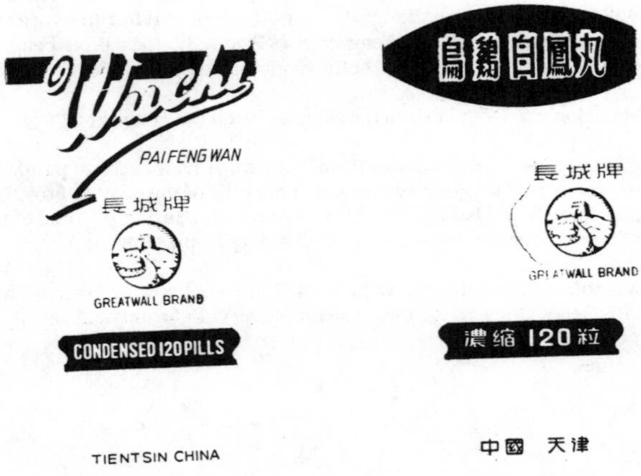

Wuchi
PAIFENG WAN
長城牌
GREATWALL BRAND
CONDENSED 120 PILLS
TIENTSIN CHINA
烏鷄白鳳丸
長城牌
GREATWALL BRAND
濃縮 120粒
中國 天津

12.13 婦 科 烏 金 丸

婦	科	烏	金	丸
Fu	**Ke**	**Wu**	**Jin**	**Wan**
-------gynecology-------		black	gold	pills

Source: Zhong Guo Yi Xue Da Ci Dian, (Complete Glossary of Traditional Chinese Medicine), 1924.

Function: 1. Promote Blood circulation; Remove Stuck Qi
2. Regulate menstruation; Stop pain

Application: 1. Use to treat symptoms due to Stuck Qi and Blood Stagnation which may cause sharp pain in the hypochondrium, dysmenorrhea, amenorrhea, or pain in the lower abdomen during the postpartum period; it may be used to help expel a retained placenta. The patient may also have symptoms such as a pale face, fatigue, low-grade afternoon fever, dry skin,

2. Use to treat endometriosis with the above-mentioned symptoms.

Contraindication: Do not use with pregnant women. This formula contains strong herbs to Move Qi and Move Blood circulation and could cause a miscarriage.

Dose: 1 honey pill, 2 times a day.

Fu Ke Wu Jin Wan is produced by the Chan Li Chai Medical Factory, Hong Kong; 10 honey pills/box.

The contents in this formula are listed below in 5 groups according to function.

Pinyin Name	Pharmaceutical Name	Percent	TCM Function
Group 1			
Yi Mu Cao	Herba Leonuri Heterophylli	38.4	Promote Blood circulation;
San Leng	Rhizoma Sparganii	2.4	Disperse Stagnation of Blood
E Zhu	Rhizoma Curcumae Zedoariae	2.4	
Group 2			
Xiang Fu	Rhizoma Cyperi Rotundi	14.4	Move Stuck Liver Qi;
Yan Hu Suo	Rhizoma Corydalis Yanhusuo	7.2	Stop pain
Wu Zhu Yu	Fructus Evodiae Rutaecarpae	2.4	
Xiao Hui Xiang	Fructus Foeniculi Vulgaris	2.4	
Mu Xiang	Radix Saussureae seu Vladimiriae	2.4	
Group 3			
Bai Shao	Radix Paeoniae Lactiflorae	7.2	Nourish Blood;
Chuan Xiong	Radix Ligustici Wallichii	7.2	Promote Blood circulation;
Dang Gui	Radix Angelicae Sinensis	2.4	Regulate menstruation
Shou Di Huang	Radix Rehmanniae Glutinosae Conquitae	2.4	
Group 4			
Bu Gu Zhi	Fructus Psoraleae Corylifoliae	2.4	Strengthen Kidney Yang; Warm Spleen
Group 5			
Pu Huang	Pollen Typhae	2.4	Regulate menstruation;
Ai Ye Tan	Folium Artemisiae (Carbonized)	2.4	Stop bleeding

Note: 1. The above-listed formula is the original formula for Wu Jin Wan. Different manufactories produce different formulas, but use the same name as that used in the original formula, Wu Jin Wan. A formula manufactured in Hong Kong, Fu Ke Wu Jin Wan (Gynecology Black Gold Pills) has twelve ingredients: Liu Ji Nu, Xiang Fu, E Zhu, Qing Pi, Zhi Qiao, Pu Huang, Ai Ye, Dang Gui, Huang Qin, Chi Gui (Rou Gui), Bai Zhu, and Gan Jiang.

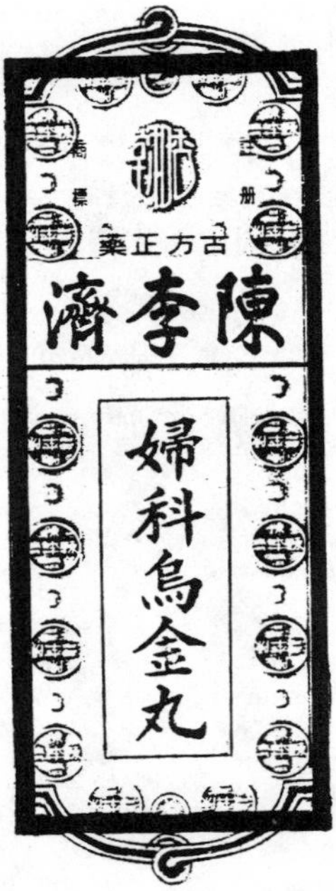

12.14 當 歸 素

Dang Gui Su

---------Angelica--------- extract

Function: 1. Nourish Blood; Regulate menstruation
2. Promote Blood circulation; Stop pain

Application: 1. Use to treat Def. Blood syndrome related to gynecological disorders. It is primarily used to Regulate menstruation; and stop menstrual cramping (dysmenorrhea). Symptoms: Delayed menstruation, hypomenorrhea or hypermenorrhea with blood pale in color, or amenorrhea. May also be used to treat post-partum abdominal pain.

2. Use to treat Def. Blood syndromes related to the following Internal Medicine disorders:

a. Def. Heart Blood Syndrome. Symptoms: Palpitations, poor memory, insomnia, uneasiness.

b. Def. Spleen Blood Syndrome. Symptoms: Fatigue, pale face, poor appetite.

c. Def. Liver Blood Syndrome. Symptoms: Dizziness, vertigo, tinnitus, tremor.

3. Some Western medicine disease applications include the following: Sports injuries; chronic carbuncles which have failed to heal properly; anemia (Laboratory Research in China has observed this to gradually increase the red blood cell count.); coronary heart disease (Laboratory Research in China has observed this to gradually increase the blood supply to the heart.).

Dose: 6 pills, 3 times a day.

Dang Gui Su is produced as "Tangkuisu" by the Lanzhou Chinese Medicine Works, Lanzhou, China, in bottles of 100 pills.

Pinyin Name	Pharmaceutical Name	Percent	TCM Function
Dang Gui	Radix Angelicae Sinensis	100	Nourish Blood; Promote Blood circulation

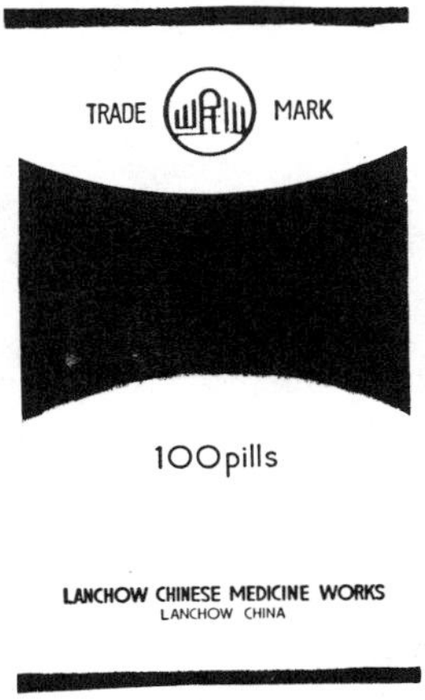

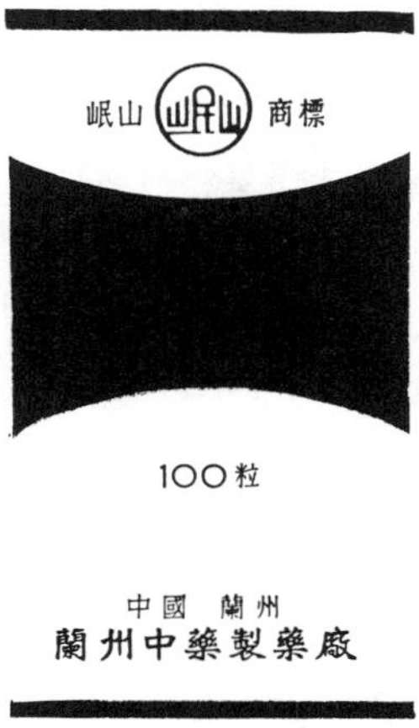

12.15 婦 科 種 子 丸

Fu	Ke	Zhong	Zi	Wan
-------gynecology-------		--------pregnancy-------		pills

Source: Tong Shou Lu, (Longevity Book), Qing Dynasty, 1644 -1911.

Function: 1. Regulate menstruation; Nourish Blood
2. Remove Stuck Qi; Disperse Blood Stagnation

Application: 1. Use to treat irregular menstruation (the period may be early or late), dysmenorrhea, abdominal pain, menstrual bleeding which is dark and where clots are sometimes present; feeling of fullness in the chest or abdomen; Stagnation of Blood in the abdomen. (This may include abdominal mass which may subside spontaneously.) All of these conditions are caused by Stagnation of Qi and Stagnation of Blood.

2. Use to treat Stagnation of Qi and Blood in the abdomen which has caused uterine tumor or endometriosis.

3. Use to treat infertility due to Stagnation of Qi and Blood in the abdomen.

Contraindication: Do not use with pregnant women; it could cause a miscarriage.

Dose: 8 pills, 3 times a day.

Fu Ke Zhong Zi Wan is produced by the Lanzhou Chinese Medicine Works, Lanzhou, China in bottles of 100 pills.

Pinyin Name	Pharmaceutical Name	Percent	TCM Function
Yi Mu Cao	Herba Leonuri Heterophylli	50	Promote Blood circulation; Remove Blood Stasis;
Dang Gui	Radix Angelicae Sinensis	17	Nourish Blood; Promote Blood circulation; Regulate menstruation
Bai Shao	Radix Paeoniae Lactiflorae	17	Strengthen Yin; Nourish Blood; Stop abdominal pain; Relax smooth muscle spasms
Chai Hu	Radix Bupleuri	8	Move Stuck Liver Qi
Mu Xiang	Radix Saussureae seu Vladimiriae	4	Move Stuck Qi in the abdomen; Stop pain; Disperse abdominal mass
Chuan Xiong	Radix Ligustici Wallichii	4	Promote Blood circulation; Remove Blood Stagnation; Stop pain

Note: 1. This formula, Fu Ke Zhong Zi Wan, is also called Zhong Zi Wan or De Sheng Dan; these formulas commonly appear in Chinese herbal medicine books.

12.16 補 血 調 经 片

Bu	**Xue**	**Tiao**	**Jing**	**Pian**
nourish	Blood	regulate	menstruation	tablets

Function: 1. Nourish Blood, Regulate Qi, Normalize menstruation

Application: 1. Use to treat menstrual disorder due to Def. Blood. Symptoms: Fatigue, a pale face; Pre-menstrual syndrome signs including menstrual cramps, insomnia, headache, moodiness, and emotional disorders associated with PMS; amenorrhea, hypomenorrhea, hypermenorrhea, dysmenorrhea.

2. Use to treat leukorrhea due to Def. Spleen (often seen with Def. Qi and Def. Yang) and Dampness Retention.

Contraindication: Do not take during the early stage of a common cold or the flu when fever is present.

Dose: 3 tablets, 2 or 3 times a day, taken with warm water.

Bu Xue Tiao Jing Pian is produced as "Butiao Tablets, A Blood Tonic for Menstrual Disorders," by the United Pharmaceutical Manufactory, Guangzhou, China, in bottles of 100 coated tablets.

There are 18 ingredients; the major 13 ingredients are listed below in 5 groups according to function.

Pinyin Name	Pharmaceutical Name	Percent	TCM Function
Group 1			
Dang Shen	Radix Codonopsis Pilosulae	2.7	Strengthen Qi; Strengthen Spleen
Gan Cao	Radix Glycyrrhizae Uralensis	0.9	
Group 2			
Ji Xue Teng	Radix Millettiae Reticulatae	9.04	Nourish Blood;
Sang Ji Sheng	Ramus Loranthi seu Visci	9.4	Regulate Blood circulation;
A Jiao	Gelatinum Asini	0.54	Stop Bleeding
Da Ji	Herba Cirsii Japonici	3.6	
Group 3			
Rou Gui	Cortex Cinnamomi Cassiae	0.46	Strengthen Yang; Warm meridians;
Gao Liang Jiang	Rhizoma Alpiniae Officinari	6.33	Expel Cold; Stop pain
Ai Ye	Folium Artemisiae	4.52	
Group 4			
Xiang Fu	Rhizoma Cyperi Rotundi	9.4	Regulate circulation of Qi and
Yi Mu Cao	Herba Leonuri Heterophylli	6.33	Blood; Remove Blood Stagnation;
			Regulate menstruation
Group 5			
Cang Zhu	Rhizoma Atractylodis	2.3	Dry Dampness; Stop leukorrhea
Jin Ying Zi	Fructus Rosae Laevigatae	9.04	

Note: 1. The remaining 5 ingredients include Qian Jin Ba (9.04%), Dou Chi Qiang (9.04%), Bai Pu Ye (4.52%), Wu Zhao Long (4.52%), and Gang Shen Ci (9.04%).

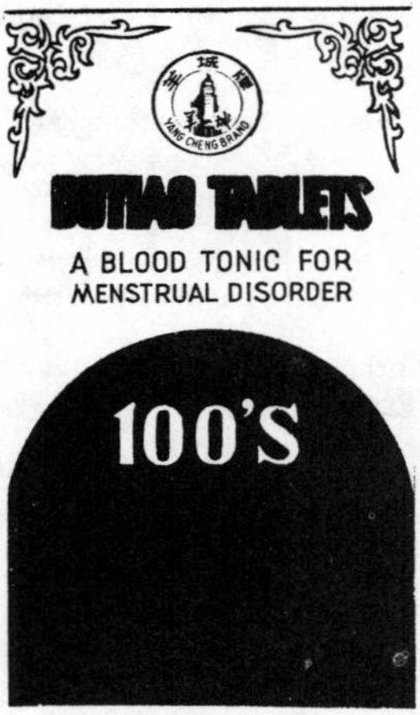
YANG CHENG BRAND
BUTIAO TABLETS
A BLOOD TONIC FOR
MENSTRUAL DISORDER
100'S

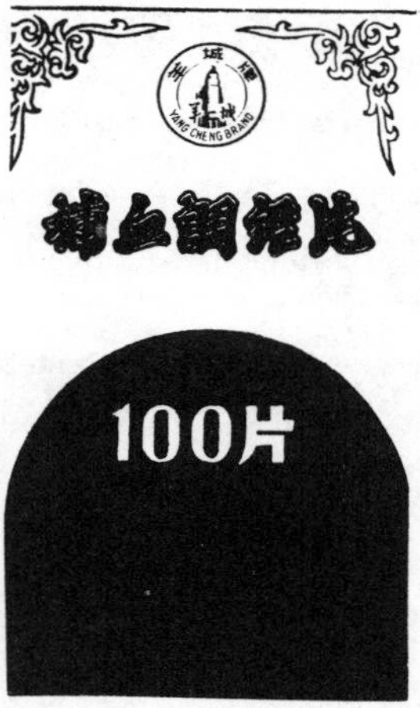
YANG CHENG BRAND
補血調經片
100片

Chapter 13. Tonics

(Includes Kidney and Lung Tonics; Tonics used to Strengthen Qi, Blood, Yin and Yang)

Section A. **Strengthen Qi, Nourish Blood**

Section B. **Nourish Yin, Strengthen Yang**

Note: In general, it is advised that patients stop taking Tonics during the acute phase of an infectious process, such as the common cold, or flu. If only the Tonics are taken during this time, the condition may worsen.

13.1

荔	枝	蜂	王	浆
Ling	**Zhi**	**Feng**	**Wang**	**Jiang**
-Ganoderma Lucidum-		queen bee	royal	essence

Function: 1. General Tonic to Strengthen Qi and Blood

Application: 1. Use as an assistant medicine to help strengthen the body in consumptive diseases such as chronic hepatitis, chronic tuberculosis and cancer. It is also used to help strengthen patients with neurasthenia, weakness associated with aging, diabetes, gastric ulcer and malnutrition in children.

Dose: 1 10cc vial of liquid per day, taken in the morning upon arising. It may be taken indefinitely.

Ling Zhi Feng Wang Jiang is produced as "Lingzhifengwangjiang" in 10cc vials by several manufacturers including the Beijing Dietetic Preparation Manufactory; the Tientsin Native Produce Branch; and the Third Pharmaceutical Manufactory, Harbin, China.

The percents of each ingredient are not available.

Pinyin Name	Pharmaceutical Name	TCM Function
Ling Zhi	Ganoderma Lucidum	Tonify Qi and Blood; Nourish Heart; Tranquilize Spirit
Feng Wang Jing	Royal Jelly	Tonify Qi and Blood; Strengthen Liver and Spleen
Dang Shen	Radix Codonopsis Pilosulae	Tonify Qi
Gou Qi Zi	Fructus Lycii Chinensis	Strengthen Liver and Kidney

Notes: 1. There are several Patent Medicines which also contain Royal Jelly. Some are listed below:

a. Ren Shen Feng Wang Jiang (Royal Jelly made with Ginseng) is especially good for the patient with Def. Qi and Def. Yang. For more research information on Royal Jelly and Ginseng, see Research Note under #13.12, Shuang Bao Su.

b. Feng Ru Jiang (Royal Jelly made with Huang Qi and Dang Shen) is also especially good for patients with Def. Qi and Def. Yang. It is available in liquid or capsule form.

c. Bei Jing Feng Wang Jing (Royal Jelly only) is used with patients to Tonify Qi and Blood, and Strengthen Liver and Spleen.

d. Lu Wei Ba Jing is similar to Ling Zhi Feng Wang Jing, but Lu Wei Ba Jing is made with Royal Jelly which is modified with Lu Wei Ba (deer testes and penis). This medicine has an effect similar to Royal Jelly, but also has the effect of Lu Wei Ba which strengthens Kidney Yang. It is used to increase sexual function and treat impotence. The medicine is in liquid form in 10 cc vials.

e. Bei Qi Jing has a similar Tonic effect to Ling Zhi Feng Wang Jing.

Case Report: A 55 year old man who had had diabetes for several years (non-insulin dependant) had suffered a stroke producing a left-sided paralysis. After 6 months, he was able to return to work as a late night radio host. He found drinking 1 vial of Ren Shen Feng Wang Jiang before working enabled him to work from 11 p.m. to 5 a.m. without being so tired. It did not affect his diabetes in any adverse way, even though it contains honey. The Radix Ginseng (Ren Shen) can cause a decrease in glycosuria, and a reduction in blood glucose by 40-50mg% in mild cases of diabetes (Bensky & Gamble, 1986, p 453).

Note: A liquid ginseng formula called "Active Herbal," was formulated in 1984 in preparation for the Los Angeles Olympic Trials and Olympic Games. This formula contains Siberian Ginseng Root (Eleutherococcus senticosus), American Ginseng Root (Panax quinquefolium), Astragalus, Ginkgo, Codonopsis, Fo-Ti, and Licorice. The herbs are extracted in distilled water and grain alcohol. The dose is 1 teaspoon, 1 - 3 times a day, and each dose is combined with #13.19, Liu Wei Di Huang Wan and #11.1, Shu Kan Wan. It is available through McZand Herbal, Inc., Santa Monica, CA; see bottom of page 343.

Case Report: A 56 year old woman who had had diabetes for several years was using Diabinese to control the blood glucose; the lowest level was 178. After using Active Herbal, Liu Wei Di Huang Wan and Shu Kan Wan twice a day for one week, the blood glucose level dropped to 129. She continues to use both the Diabinese and the herbs, and reports having more energy and generally feeling better. The Radix Ginseng (Ren Shen) can cause a decrease in glycosuria, and a reduction in blood glucose by 40-50mg% in mild cases of diabetes (Bensky & Gamble, 1986, p 453).

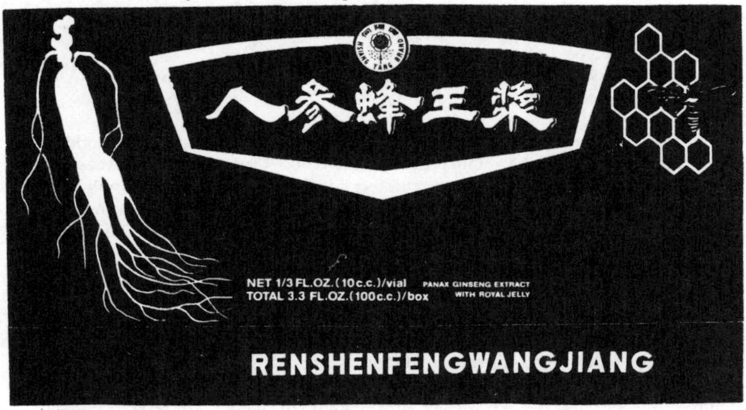
人参蜂王浆
NET 1/3 FL.OZ.(10c.c.)/vial
TOTAL 3.3 FL.OZ.(100c.c.)/box
PANAX GINSENG EXTRACT
WITH ROYAL JELLY
RENSHENFENGWANGJIANG

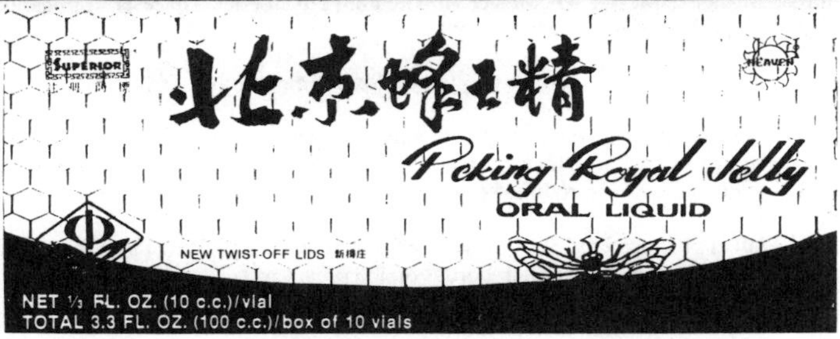
SUPERIOR
北京蜂王精
Peking Royal Jelly
ORAL LIQUID
NEW TWIST-OFF LIDS
NET ⅓ FL. OZ. (10 c.c.)/vial
TOTAL 3.3 FL. OZ. (100 c.c.)/box of 10 vials

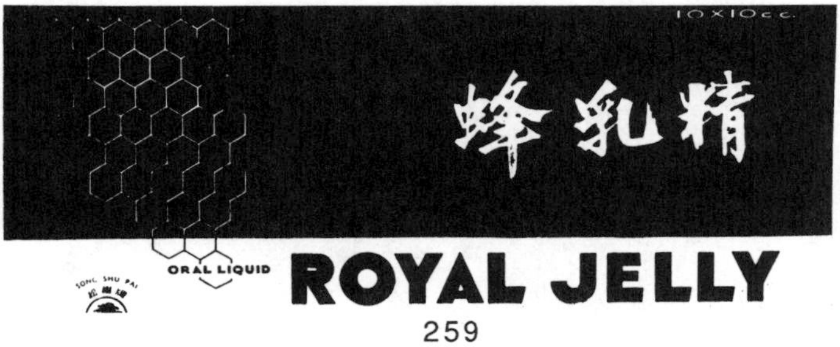

13.2 十 全 大 補 丸

十	全	大	補	丸
Shi	**Quan**	**Da**	**Bu**	**Wan**
ten	complete	big	supplement	pills

Source: Tai Ping Hui Min He Ji Ju Fang, (Formulas of the People's Welfare Pharmacy), Song Dynasty, 960-1279.

Function: 1. Supplement Qi and Blood

Application: 1. Use to treat Def. Qi and general debility following a long illness or surgery. In TCM, any chronic disease will eventually lead to Deficiency.
Symptoms: Weakness, shortness of breath, cold limbs, a pale face (all signs of Def. Qi); palpitations, insomnia, dizziness (all signs of Def. Blood).

2. Use to adjust menstruation in women with excess bleeding due to Def. Blood and Def. Qi, where the Blood and Qi have failed to Hold the Blood, thus resulting in excess bleeding. If the excess bleeding is due to Heat, do not use this Patent Medicine. This will help to stop the bleeding and stop the pain. If the result is not satisfacoty, the patient should also combine this with 12.12, Wu Ji Bai Feng Wan. (See also 12.10, Yun Nan Bai Yao.)

3. Use to treat spermatorrhea due to Def. Qi and Def. Blood.

4. Use internally to help treat chronic, subcutaneous skin ulcers (bedsores, skin breakdown) which may be deep-rooted, and long-standing, possibly a year or more. Low-energy laser is also helpful when applied directly to the sore.

(Source: Mester E, Mester AF, Mester A: The biomedical effects of laser application. Lasers in Surgery and Medicine 1985; 5: 31-39.)

Dose: Honey Pills: 1 pill, 2 times a day. Smaller Pills: 8 pills, 3 times a day.

In China, it is common to take this Tonic for several years. It is recommended that after taking it for 3 months, to stop for 1 week, then resume taking it again. Once the desired effect has been obtained, the medicine can be reduced or stopped.

Shi Quan Da Bu Wan is produced as "Shih Chuan Ta Pu Wan (General Tonic Pills)" by the Lanzhou Fo Ci Pharmaceutical Factory, Lanzhou, China, in bottles of 200 pills.

Pinyin Name	Pharmaceutical Name	Percent	TCM Function
Dang Shen	Radix Codonopsis Pilosulae	10.54	Strengthen Qi; Strengthen Spleen
Huang Qi	Radix Astragali	10.53	Strengthen Qi; Treat chronic carbuncles
Bai Shao	Radix Paeoniae Lactiflorae	10.53	Nourish Yin; Strengthen Blood; Stop abdominal pain
Bai Zhu	Rhizoma Atractylodis Macrocephalae	10.53	Strengthen Spleen; Eliminate Dampness
Fu Ling	Sclerotium Poriae Cocos	10.53	Strengthen Spleen; Promote urination; Tranquilize
Shu Di Huang	Radix Rehmanniae Glutinosae Conquitae	15.78	Nourish Yin; Strengthen Blood
Dang Gui	Radix Angelice Sinensis	15.78	Nourish Yin; Strengthen Blood
Rou Gui	Cortex Cinnamomi Cassiae	5.26	Warm the Yang
Chuan Xiong	Radix Ligustici Wallichii	5.26	Promote Blood circulation
Gan Cao	Radix Glycyrrhizae Uralensis	5.26	Strengthen the Middle Warmer Qi

TRADE MARK

十全大補丸

SHIH CHUAN TA PU WAN

(General Tonic Pills)

LANZHOU FO CI PHARMACEUTICAL FACTORY
LANZHOU CHINA

13.3 胎 盘 糖 衣 片

Tai	Pan	Tang	Yi	Pian
---------placenta--------		------sugar-coated-----		tablets

Function: 1. Strengthen Congenital Jing and Kidney Yang
2. Nourish Blood; Tonify Qi

Application: 1. Use to treat Def. Kidney Yang Syndrome. Symptoms: Infertility, impotence, spermatorrhea, tinnitus, dizziness; cold in the extremities.

2. Use to treat general debility, fatigue, weakness following long illness - e.g. chronic cough, problems breathing due to Def. Lung syndrome.

3. Use to treat Def. Spleen syndrome. - e.g. poor appetite, loose stools.

4. Use to treat nursing mothers with insufficient milk supply.

5. Some Western medicine disease applications include the following: Pulmonary tuberculosis patients with Def. Lung Qi Syndrome - e.g. difficult breathing, weak cough; neurasthenia patients or weaker patients who need Tonification; anemia cases.

Dose: 5 tablets, 3 times a day. With applications 2, 3, and 4, this formula may also be combined with other Tonifying formulas or Strengthen-Spleen formulas.

Tai Pan Tang Yi Pian is produced as "Sugar-Coated Placaenta Tablets" by the Central Medical Manufactory & Co., Tientsin, China, in bottles of 100 coated tablets.

Pinyin Name	Pharmaceutical Name	Percent	TCM Function
Tai Pan	Placenta Hominis	100	Strengthen Congenital Jing and Kidney Yang

Notes. 1: The fresh placenta may be processed at home and used as a General Tonic. The procedure is given below:

1. After the umbiliicus has been cut, wash the placenta and remove the blood.

2. Soak the cleaned-off placenta in fresh water and repeat this at least three times, until no "fish" odor is left.

3. Put the placenta in a non-metal (glass or clay) pot, cover it with water and boil it until the placenta is floating on the top, then stop the cooking.

4. Remove the placenta from the pot, and flatten it out on a flat surface.

5. Bake it in an oven, at very low heat (the lower, the better). This heat (approximately 150° F) can be used over night, if necessary, to completely dry the placenta.

6. Store the placenta in a dry place. When ready to use, grind the placenta into a powder. Also store the powder in a dry place.

Normal Dose: 3-4 grams, 2 or 3 times a day.

Large Dose: 6-9 grams, 3 times a day. The large dose, for example, is used in cases with hypoplastic anemia.

2. The major ingredients of the placenta are the following:
    1. Ovarian hormone
    2. Luteal hormone
    3. Acetylglucosamine $C_6H_{13}O_5N$
    4. Mannitose
    5. Amino acids

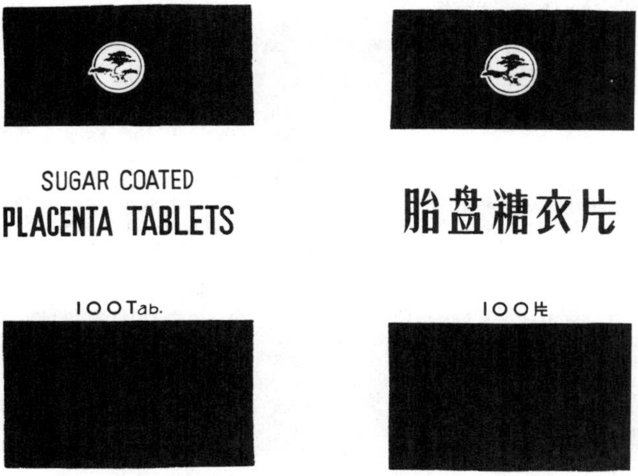

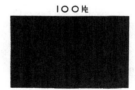

13.4 蛤 蚧 大 補 丸

Ge	Jie	Da	Bu	Wan
----------Gecko----------		great	nourishment	pills

Function: 1. Strengthen Kidney, Liver and Spleen
2. Treat chronic rheumatism

Application: 1. Use to treat weakness associated with chronic illnesses. Use to treat Kidney, Liver and/or Spleen syndromes. Symptoms: Weakness, shortness of breath, fatigue, dizziness, vertigo, tinnitus, frequent urination, lumbago, cold limbs, pain and stiffness in the joints or limbs, problems walking, poor appetite. It is also often used by older people to help maintain good health.

2. Some Western medicine disease applications include the following: (This formula will strengthen both Kidney Yin and Kidney Yang, therefore, neither Def. Kidney Yin nor Def. Kidney Yang has to be predominant.) Anemia, chronic rheumatism, neurasthenia, and Meniere's disease.

Dose: 3-5 capsules, 2 times a day, after meals.

Ge Jie Da Bu Wan is produced as "Gejie Da Bu Wan" by the Yulin Drug Manufactory, Kwangsi, China, in bottles of 50 capsules.

Pinyin Name	Pharmaceutical Name	Percent	TCM Function
Ge Jie	Gecko	21.5	Tonify Kidney Yang; Tonify Lung Yin
Dang Shen	Radix Codonopsis Pilosulae	4.3	Tonify Qi; Strengthen Spleen
Huang Qi	Radix Astragali	4.3	Strengthen Qi; Strengthen Yang
Gou Qi Zi	Fructus Lycii Chinensis	4.1	Strengthen Kidney and Liver Yang
Dang Gui	Radix Angelica Sinensis	3.8	Tonify Blood; Promote Blood circulation
Fu Ling	Sclerotium Poriae Cocos	5	Strengthen Spleen Qi; Remove Dampness
Shu Di Huang	Radix Rehmanniae Glutinosae Conquitae	6.8	Nourish Yin; Tonify Blood
Nu Zhen Zi	Fructus Ligustri Lucidi	5.2	Strengthen Liver and Kidney
Gan Cao	Radix Glycyrrhizae Uralensis	2.8	Warm the Middle Warmer, Strengthen Spleen
Shan Yao	Radix Dioscoreae Oppositae	5.3	Strengthen Spleen/Stomach
Mu Gua	Fructus Chaenomelis Lagenariae	4.7	Nourish Liver, Kidney; Strengthen legs; Stop Rheumatic Pain
Gou Ji	Rhizoma Cibotii Barometz	4.8	Tonify Liver and Kidney; Strengthen tendons and bones
Ba Ji Tian	Radix Morindae Officinalis	4.3	Strengthen Kidney Yang; Strengthen tendons and bones; Treat rheumatism
Bai Zhu	Rhizoma Atractylodis Macrocephalae	4.3	Tonify Spleen; Dry Dampness
Xu Duan	Radix Dipsaci	4.8	Tonify Liver and Kidney; Strengthen tendons and bones
Du Zhong	Cortex Eucommiae	4.3	Tonify Liver and Kidney; Treat lumbago; Strengthen limbs

Huang Jing	Rhizoma Polygonati	5.7	Nourish Yin; Strengthen Spleen and Lung
Gu Sui Bu	Drynaria fortunei	4.0	Strengthen Kidney; Promote healing of broken bones

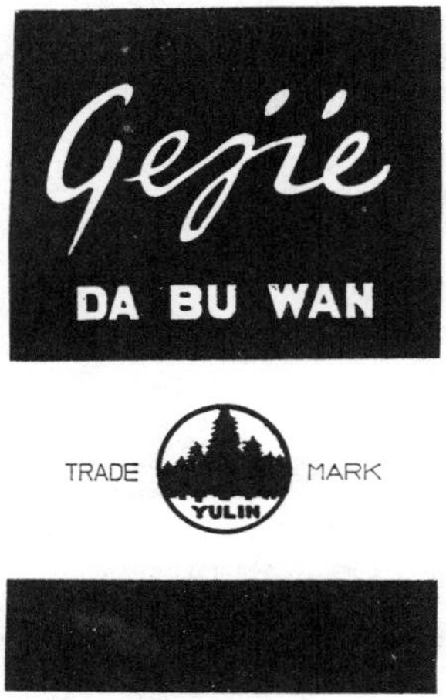

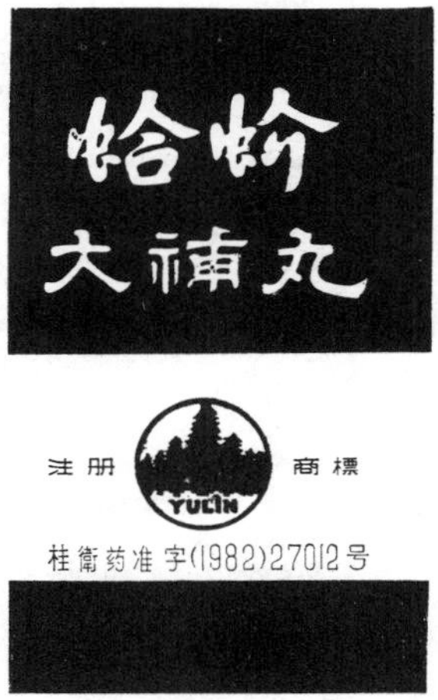

13.5 人 參 養 營 丸

Ren	Shen	Yang	Rong	Wan
----------Ginseng----------		----------healthy----------		pills

Source: Tai Ping Hui Min He Ji Ju Fang, (Formulas of the People's Welfare Pharmacy), Song Dynasty, 960-1279.

Function: 1. Strengthen Qi and Blood
2. Calm the Spirit; Improve memory

Application: 1. Use to treat Def. Heart/Spleen syndrome (Def. Blood and Def. Qi syndrome). Symptoms: Fatigue, low energy, poor appetite, loose stools, poor memory, palpitations, excessive daytime sweating, shortness of breath, general weakness following long or chronic illness.

2. Use to treat Def. Yang in Spleen or Kidney. Symptoms: Patient complains of feeling cold, having chills, cold limbs, early morning diarrhea, lumbago, weakness in knees.

3. Some Western medicine disease applications include the following: (Use with cases who have Def. Qi and Def. Blood symptomatology.) Anemia, hypothyroidism, muscle spasms due to hypocalcemia (including leg cramps at night), boils or skin ulcers that have not healed (internal use).

Dose: 7 pills, 3 times a day, taken with warm water, before meals.

Ren Shen Yang Rong Wan is manufactured as "Yang Rong Wan (Ginseng Tonic Pills)" by the Lanzhou Fo Ci Pharmaceutical Factory, Lanzhou, China in bottles of 200 pills.

Pinyin Name	Pharmaceutical Name	Percent	TCM Function
Ren Shen	Radix Ginseng	9	Tonify Qi; Strengthen Spleen
Bai Zhu	Rhizoma Atractylodis Macrocephalae	9	Strengthen Spleen; Eliminate Dampness
Huang Qi	Radix Astragali	9	Strengthen Qi; Stop sweating; Heal boil on the skin
Chen Pi	Pericarpium Citri Reticulatae	9	Strengthen Spleen; Move Stuck Spleen Qi; Dry Dampness
Shu Di Huang	Radix Rehmanniae Glutinosae Conquitae	6.8	Nourish Yin; Strengthen Blood
Wu Wei Zi	Fructus Schisandrae Chinensis	6.8	Strengthen Qi; Strengthen Kidney; Nourish Heart; Stop sweating
Fu Ling	Sclerotium Poriae Cocos	6.8	Strengthen Spleen; Promote urination; Tranquilize
Da Zao	Fructus Zizyphi Jujubae	13.5	Strengthen Spleen; Nourish Blood; Tranquilize the Spirit
Bai Shao	Radix Paeoniae Lactiflorae	9	Nourish Yin; Strengthen Blood; Stop abdominal pain; Stop muscle spasms (smooth or striated muscle)
Yuan Zhi	Radix Polygalae Tenuifoliae	4.5	Calm the Spirit; Pacify the Heart
Rou Gui	Cortex Cinnamomi Cassiae	2.25	Strengthen Yang; Warm the Middle Warmer; Expel Cold; Stop pain
Sheng Jiang	Rhizoma Zingiberis Officinalis Recens	4.5	Warm the Stomach; Stop vomiting

Gan Cao	Radix Glycyrrhizae Uralensis	9	Warm the Middle Warmer; Harmonize other herbs

Note: 1. There is another Patent Medicine, Ren Shen Yang Ying Wan, which is similar to the formula Ren Shen Yang Rong Wan, and therefore used for similar applications. Some Patent Medicines with the name, Ren Shen Yang Ying Wan, however, may not contain Rou Gui, Sheng Jiang, or Gan Cao (cooked); herbs with Hot or Warming properties. Therefore, it is best to read the contents on the box. Ren Shen Yang Ying Wan is produced as "Ren Shen Yang Ying Wan Ginseng Tonic Pills" by the Lanzhou Chinese Medicine Works, Lanzhou, China, in bottles of 200 pills.

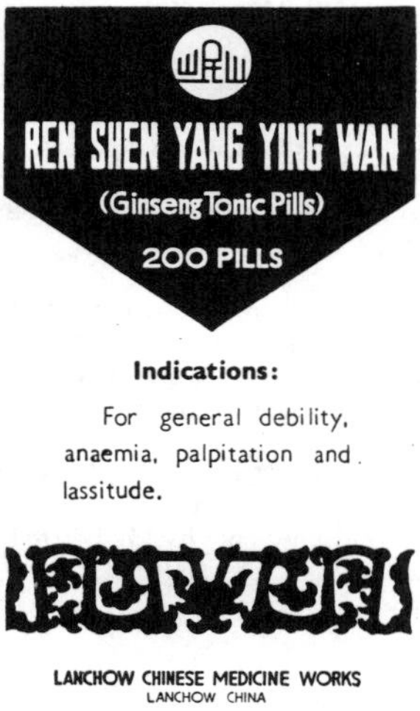

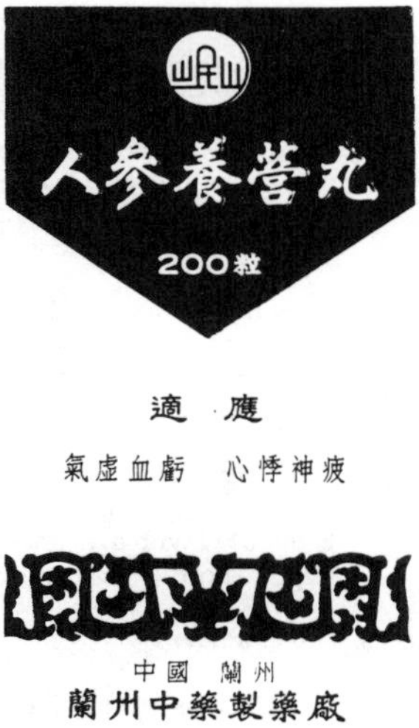
人參養營丸
200粒
適應
氣虛血虧 心悸神疲
中國 蘭州
蘭州中藥製藥廠

13.6 補 中 益 氣 丸

Bu	**Zhong**	**Yi**	**Qi**	**Wan**
nourish	Middle Warmer	strengthen	Qi	pills

Source: Pi Wei Lun, (Treatise on The Spleen and Stomach), Li Gao, 1249.

Function: 1. Strengthen Qi; Cause Yang Qi to ascend
2. Regulate Function of Spleen/Stomach

Application: 1. Use to treat Def. Qi in Spleen and Stomach (Def. Qi in the Middle Warmer). Symptoms: Fatigue, shortness of breath, headache, general feeling of coldness and sensitivity to cold, the patient likes to drink warm liquids, daytime sweating, poor appetite, chronic diarrhea or loose stools.

2. Use to raise up the Middle Warmer Vital Qi and treat organ prolapse.

3. Use to Clear Heat where the Heat is due to Def. Qi in the Middle Warmer; this is a special circumstance in TCM. Symptoms: Chronic low grade fever plus Def. Qi symptoms listed above; also, the patient feels thirsty but likes to drink warm liquids (sign which shows that the fever is due to Def. Middle Warmer Qi). In this special circumstance, the treatment is unusual because herbs which have Warm properties and a Sweet taste (instead of Cold properties and a Bitter taste) are used to Clear the Heat.

4. Some Western medicine disease applications include the following: (Cases treated with this formula must have Def. Middle Warmer Qi symptoms listed above under Application #1.) Chronic gastroenteritis, chronic diarrhea, chronic dysentery. Use to treat organ prolapse such as gastroptosis, anal prolapse, or uterine prolapse.

Use to treat drooping of upper eyelids. In the book, Zhong Yao Cheng Yao Xue, (A Textbook of Patent Medicines), by Liu De-Yi, Tianjing, 1984, this herbal formula is listed as being used with myasthenia gravis cases; Bell's Palsy was not listed. Use to treat hypomenorrhea or hypermenorrhea (each can be due to Def. Spleen Qi).

Dose: 8 pills, 3 times a day.

Bu Zhong Yi Qi Wan is produced by the Lanzhou Fo Ci Pharmaceutical Factory, Lanzhou, China, in bottles of 100 pills.

Pinyin Name	Pharmaceutical Name	Percent	TCM Function
Huang Qi	Radix Astragali	27.78	Strengthen Qi; Stop sweating
Dang Shen	Radix Codonopsis Pilosulae	8.33	Tonify Qi; Strengthen Spleen
Gan Cao	Radix Glycyrrhizae Uralensis	13.89	Warm the Middle Warmer; Harmonize other herbs
Bai Zhu	Rhizoma Atractylodis Macrocephalae	8.33	Strengthen Spleen; Eliminate Dampness
Dang Gui	Radix Angelicae Sinensis	8.33	Tonify Blood; Promote Blood circulation
Chen Pi	Pericarpium Citri Reticulatae	8.3	Strengthen Spleen; Move Stuck Spleen Qi; Dry Dampness

Sheng Ma	Rhizoma Cimicifugae	8.33	Cause Yang Qi to ascend; Treat prolapse
Chai Hu	Radix Bupleuri	8.33	Cause Yang Qi to ascend; Smooth Liver Qi
Sheng Jiang	Rhizoma Zingiberis Officinalis Recens	2.78	Warm the Middle Warmer; Stop nausea and vomiting
Da Zao	Fructus Zizyphi Jujubae	5.57	Strengthen Spleen; Nourish Blood

<u>Notes</u>: 1. The original formula does not contain the last two herbs, Sheng Jiang and Da Zao.

2. A study was reported in China in 1974, where 103 cases with gastroptosis were treated with the herbal formula listed here. The diagnosis of gastroptosis was made with barium-swallow X-ray. The herbal formula was administered in the herbal tea form, not the pill form. Prior to treatment, these patients had symptoms such as nausea, poor appetite, stomach ache, and constipation. After treatment, 54 cases recovered, 25 cases had obvious improvement, and 22 cases had some improvment. Twenty-one of the 54 cases with recovery were followed up for two years. None of these cases had recurrence of the gastroptosis. Source: <u>Xin Yi Yao Xue Za Zhi</u>, <u>(The New Medicine Journal)</u>, No. 11, 1974.

3. A study was reported in China in 1960, where 23 cases of uterine prolapse were treated with this herbal formula. The herbal formula was administered in the herbal tea form, not the pill form. Prior to treatment, these patients had symptoms such as fatigue, shortness of breath, low-back pain, sensation of the pulling-down in the lower abdomen; Thin and Empty Pulse. The patients took the herbal tea every day for two weeks. Two patients did not complete the first two-week course. Of the remaining 21 cases, 76.2% recovered; 6.5% improved; and 14.3% showed no response. <u>Tian Jin Yi Yao Za Zhi</u>, (<u>Tianjin Medical Journal)</u>, January, 1980.

4. A formula similar to this formula is also available in liquid, tincture form as "Arouse Vigor," in the Jade Pharmacy product line, available through Crane Enterprises, Plymouth, MA, etc. See bottom of page 343.

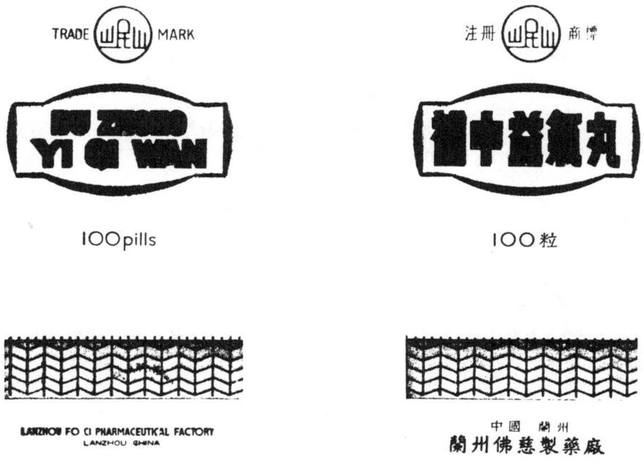

13.7 参 苓 白 术 丸

Shen	Ling	Bai	Zhu	Wan
Codonopsis	Poriae	-------Atractylodis--------		pills

Source: Tai Ping Hui Min He Ji Ju Fang, (Formulas of the People's Welfare Pharmacy), Song Dynasty, 960-1279.

Function: 1. Strengthen Spleen; Tonify Qi
2. Harmonize Stomach function; Eliminate Dampness

Application: 1. Use to treat Def. Spleen and Stomach Qi syndrome: Symptoms: Fatigue, indigestion, nausea, full sensation in the chest or Middle Warmer, loose stools or diarrhea, a pale face; the Tongue is pale, the Pulse is empty. The herbs used in this formula are Warming, but not Drying; it is a commonly used and popular formula which is particularly gentle in treating digestive disorders (even in children) by Strengthening the Spleen; Tonifying Qi and Eliminating Dampness.

2. Some Western medicine disease applications include the following: (These are all gastric system-related disorders, with symptoms such as indigestion, poor appetite, loose stools, fatigue.) Chronic gastroenteritis, anemia, pulmonary tuberculosis, chronic nephritis, and other chronic consumptive diseases.

3. Use in children to treat diarrhea with passage of undigested food (lienteric diarrhea). Additional Symptoms: Abdominal pain which is relieved somewhat when the abdomen is touched (Def. type of pain), the child is thin, under-weight and may appear malnourished.

Dose: Adults: 12 pills, 2 times aday, before meals. Take with warm water or with Jujubae broth.

Jujubae broth is made with the loose herb, Jujubae (Fructus Zizyphi Jujubae, Da Zao). The function of the Jujubae is to Strengthen the Spleen, and Tonify the Blood. Jujubae is a very small (grape-size) dry red fruit, which has a sweet taste. To make 1 cup of broth, take 10 pieces of Jujubae, cut the 10 pieces into halves and put them into a pot; add 1 and 1/2 cups of cold water. Bring to a boil, reduce the heat and cook it down until the liquid is reduced to only 1 cup. Strain off the liquid (squeeze additional broth from the remaining pieces); drink the broth while it is still warm.

Children: 5 - 12 Years: 5 pills, 2 times a day. Under 5 Years: 3 pills, 2 times aday. Dissolve the pills in warm water, if necessary. The pills do not have a bitter taste.

Shen Ling Bai Zhu Wan is produced as "Shenling Baizhupian" by the Sian Chinese Drug Pharmaceutical Works, Sian, China, in bottles of 150 coated tablets.

Pinyin Name	Pharmaceutical Name	Percent	TCM Function
Dang Shen	Radix Codonopsis Pilosulae	11.22	Strengthen Spleen; Tonify Qi
Fu Ling	Sclerotium Poriae Cocos	11.22	Strengthen Spleen; Stop diarrhea; Eliminate Dampness
Bai Zhu	Rhizoma Atractylodis Macrocephalae	11.22	Strengthen Spleen; Eliminate Dampness
Jie Geng	Radix Platycodi Grandiflori	6.12	Open Lung Qi; Guide other herbs upwards
Shan Yao	Radix Dioscoreae Oppositae	11.22	Strengthen Spleen

Chen Pi	Pericarpium Citri Reticulatae	11.22	Strengthen Spleen; Move Stuck Spleen Qi; Dry Dampness
Sha Ren	Fructus seu Semen Amomi	6.12	Move the Middle Warmer Qi; Strengthen the Stomach; Transform Dampness; Stop vomiting
Lian Zi Rou	Semen Nelumbinis Nuciferae	6.12	Strengthen Spleen; Stop diarrhea
Bai Bian Dou	Semen Dolichoris Lablab	8.17	Strengthen Spleen; Stop diarrhea
Yi Yi Ren	Semen Coicis Lachryma-jobi	6.12	Strengthen Spleen; Stop diarrhea; Eliminate Dampness; Promote urination
Gan Cao (cooked)	Radix Glycyrrhizae Uralensis	11.22	Warm the Middle Warmer; Harmonize other herbs

Note: 1. The Patent Medicine, Zi Sheng Wan, is a modification of the formula used in Shen Ling Bai Zhu Wan. Zi Sheng Wan contains more herbs which help digestion and Move Stuck Food. The additional herbs also help Eliminate Dampness and Stop Diarrhea.

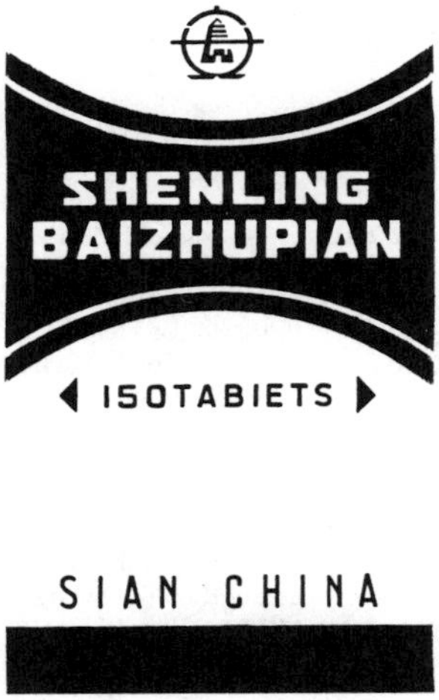

13.8 歸 脾 丸

Gui	**Pi**	**Wan**
nourish	Spleen	pills

Source: Ji Sheng Fang, (Treatment Formulas to Promote Life), Song Dynasty, 960-1279.

Function:
1. Strengthen Qi; Nourish Blood
2. Tonify Spleen; Nourish Heart

Application:

1. Use to treat Def. Heart/Spleen Syndrome due to Overthinking. Symptoms: Insomnia, poor memory, nightmares, palpitations, restlessness, agitation, dizziness, Def. type of headache, fatigue, a pale face, poor appetite, a pale Tongue with thin white moss; an Empty Pulse (thin, weak). Also use to treat neurasthenia.

2. Use to treat the following gynecological problems: Irregular menstrual cycle due to Def. Blood, hypermenorrhea with light red blood due to Def. Spleen, and leukorrhea due to Def. Spleen.

3. Use to treat chronic bleeding which may be associated with gastric ulcer; functional uterine bleeding; bleeding due to thrombocytopenia; aplastic anemia.

Dose: 8-10 pills, 3 times a day.

Gui Pi Wan is produced as "Kwei Be Wan" by the Lanzhou Chinese Medicine Works, Lanzhou, China, in bottles of 200 pills.

Pinyin Name	Pharmaceutical Name	Percent	TCM Function
Dang Shen	Radix Codonopsis Pilosulae	13.8	Strengthen Spleen; Tonify Qi
Fu Shen	Sclerotium Poriae Cocos Pararadicis	13.8	Calm the Spirit
Suan Zao Ren	Semen Ziziphi Spinosae	13.8	Nourish the Heart; Calm the Spirit
Yuan Zhi	Radix Polygalae Tenuifoliae	6.9	Calm the Spirit; Pacify the Heart
Dang Gui	Radix Angelicae Sinensis	6.9	Nourish Blood
Mu Xiang	Radix Saussureae seu Vladimiriae	3.5	Move Stuck Qi
Bai Zhu	Rhizoma Atractylodis Macrocephalae	13.8	Strengthen Spleen; Eliminate Dampness
Gan Cao	Radix Glycyrrhizae Uralensis	3.5	Strengthen the Middle Warmer; Harmonize other herbs
Long Yan Rou	Arillus Euphoriae Longanae	13.8	Strengthen the Heart; Nourish Blood
Huang Qi	Radix Astragali	10.2	Strengthen Qi

Notes: 1. The symptoms listed here under the Applications are all due to Def. Blood. In Traditional Chinese Medicine Theory, the Spleen Governs the Blood (retains the Blood in the Blood Vessels) and the Heart Rules and Moves the Blood. Thus, Def. Blood affects both the Spleen and the Heart. When the patient has Overthinking, this will affect the Spleen and the Spleen will fail to properly Retain the Blood in the Blood Vessels and bleeding will develop. This will then cause an insufficient Blood supply to the Heart and in turn, the Def. Heart/Spleen syndrome will develop, as listed in Application #1.

2. This same formula is sometimes labelled with a different name, Ren Shen Gui Pi Wan. There is another Patent Medicine with a different formula which is called Jian Pi Wan (or Ren Shen Jian Pi Wan). The name of this latter formula differs by only one Chinese character from Gui Pi Wan, but the Function and Applications are different. Jian Pi Wan (or Ren Shen Jian Pi Wan) is used primarily for gastric disorders due to Def. Spleen. It is important to use the appropriate name and formula with the appropriate disorder.

3. A formula similar to this formula is also available in liquid, tincture form as "Gather Vitality," in the Jade Pharmacy product line, available through Crane Enterprises, Plymouth, MA, etc. See bottom of page 343.

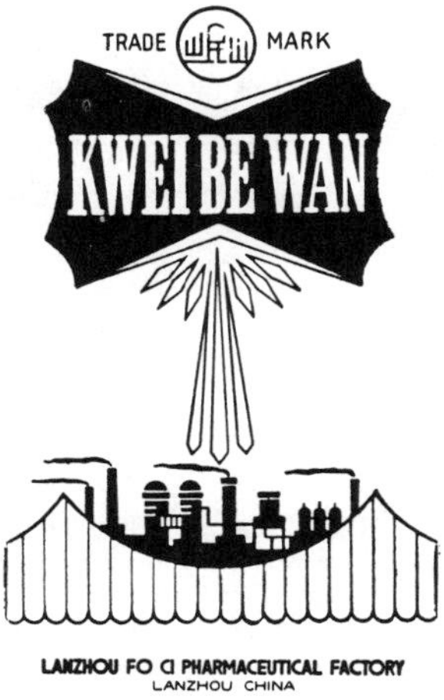

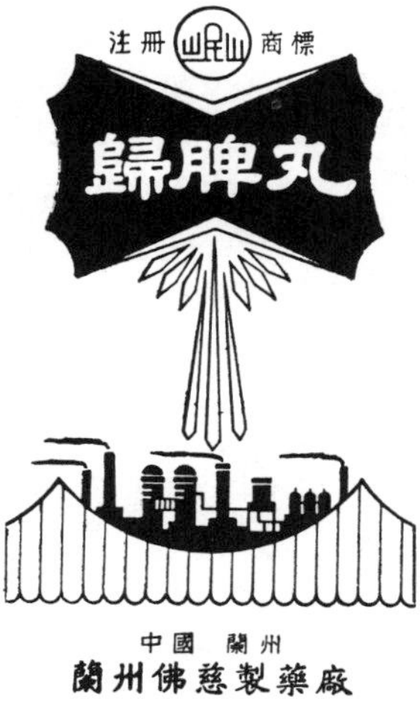

13.9 神 经 衰 弱 丸

Shen	Jing	Shuai	Ruo	Wan
----------nerve------------		--------weakness---------		pills
-----------------------------neurasthenia--------------------------------				

Source: Dr. Shi Jin-Mo, from Beijing, one of the four most famous 20th century physicians of Traditional Chinese Medicine.

Function:
1. Strengthen Qi and Blood; Improve mental health
2. Strengthen Kidney Yin; Tranquilize and Calm the Spirit

Application:
1. Use to treat Heart Empty Fire due to Def. Kidney Yin and Def. Heart Yin.
Symptoms: Fatigue, insomnia, nightmares, night sweats, poor memory, poor concentration, dizziness, tinnitus, palpitations, restlessness, agitation.

2. Some Western medicine disease applications include the following: (In order to use this formula with a case, the patient must also have the Heart Empty Fire symptoms listed above.) Neurosis, neurasthenia, panic attacks and other mental problems with the above-mentioned symptoms.

Dose: 20 pills, 2 times a day. Note, it is common that the patient will need to take this formula for one or two weeks before it will begin to be effective.

Shen Jing Shuai Ruo Wan is produced as "Shen Ching Shuai Jao Wan" by the Tung Jen Tang pharmacy, Beijing, China, in bottles of 200 pills.

Pinyin Name	Pharmaceutical Name	Percent	TCM Function
Dang Gui	Radix Angelicae Sinensis	3	Nourish Heart Blood
Zi He Che	Placenta Hominis	12	
	Strengthen Kidney; Tonfiy Qi; Nourish Blood		
Huang Lian	Rhizoma Coptidis	6	
	Clear Heart Heat		
			(Cold Property, Bitter Taste herb)
He Shou Wu	Radix Polygoni Multiflori	6	Tonify Kidney; Strengthen Blood
Fu Ling	Sclerotium Poriae Cocos	3	Tranquilize the Spirit; Strengthen Spleen
Suan Zao Ren	Semen Ziziphi Spinosae	12	Nourish Liver Blood; Tranquilize the Heart; Calm the Spirit
A Jiao	Gelatinum Asini	6	Nourish Blood and Yin
Mai Men Dong	Tuber Ophiopogonis Japonici	6	Nourish Heart Yin; Tranquilize the Spirit
Ren Shen	Radix Ginseng	15	Strengthen Spleen Qi; Improve Energy
Zi Bei Chi	Concha Cypraeae	6	Calm the Spirit; Tranquilize
Wu Wei Zi	Fructus Schisandrae Chinensis	6	Nourish Kidney Yin; Nourish Heart Yin; Calm the Heart; Stop nightsweats
Huang Qi	Radix Astragali	19	Strengthen Qi; Stop sweats

Note: 1. This herbal formula is able to extinguish the Empty Heart Fire in three ways: 1) It will Nourish Kidney Yin. 2) It will Nourish Heart Blood (Yin). 3) It contains a "Cold Property, Bitter Taste" herb (Huang Lian, Rhizoma Coptidis) which will directly Cool the Heart Empty Fire.

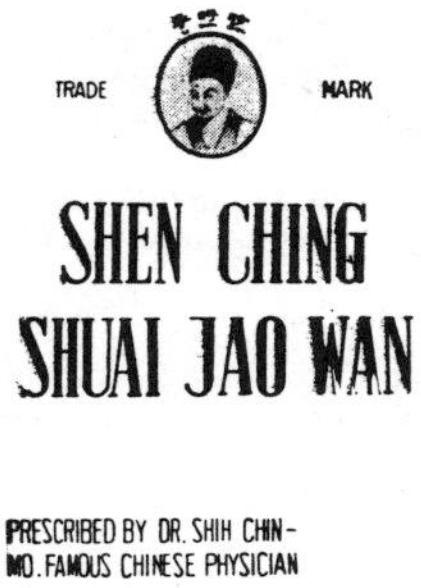
TRADE MARK
SHEN CHING
SHUAI JAO WAN
PRESCRIBED BY DR. SHIH CHIN-MO. FAMOUS CHINESE PHYSICIAN

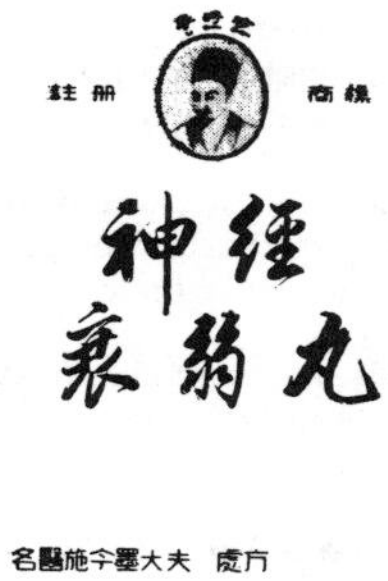
註册 商標
神经
衰弱丸
名醫施今墨大夫 處方

13.10 妇 科 八 珍 丸

Fu	Ke	Ba	Zhen	Wan
-------gynecology-------		eight	values	pills

Source: Rui Zhu Tang Jing Yan Fang, (Formulas from Experience of the Rui Zhu Tang Pharmacy), Yuan Dynasty, 1279-1368.

Function: 1. Supplement Qi; Nourish Blood

Application: 1. Use to treat gynecological disorders with Def. Qi and Def. Blood syndrome. The Def. Qi and Def. Blood syndrome is often due to blood loss. Symptoms: The patient feels fatigued, has a pale face, dizziness, vertigo, shortness of breath; irregular menstruation, hypermenorrhea, hypomenorrhea, dysmenorrhea; general deficiency during pregnancy, or general deficiency in the post-partum period (including fatigue with low-grade fever, not due to infection).

2. Use to treat Def. Qi and Def. Blood due to Def. Spleen. Symptoms: Fatigue, a pale face, weight loss, dizziness, poor appetite, palpitations, low-grade fever with uneasiness due to exhaustion.

3. Some Western medicine disease applications include the following: (Note, the patient must have the above-mentioned Def. Qi and Def. Blood symptoms.) Anemia, hypoglycemia, optic atrophy.

3. Use to treat stubborn skin ulcers that have not healed (bedsores, skin breakdown). The area around the ulcer should be flat, and not red or swollen. Low energy laser is also helpful, see 13.2.

Dose: 8-10 pills, 3 times a day.

Fu Ke Ba Zhen Wan is produced as "Precious Pills (Women's Precious Pills)" by the Lanzhou Fo Ci Pharmaceutical Factory, Lanzhou, China, in bottles of 200 pills.

Pinyin Name	Pharmaceutical Name	Percent	TCM Function
Dang Shen	Radix Codonopsis Pilosulae	12.12	Strengthen Spleen; Tonify Qi
Fu Ling	Sclerotium Poriae Cocos	12.12	Tonify Spleen; Discharge Dampness
Bai Zhu	Rhizoma Atractylodis Macrocephalae	12.12	Strengthen Spleen; Dry Dampness
Dang Gui	Radix Angelicae Sinensis	18.18	Nourish Blood; Promote Blood circulation; Regulate menstruation
Chuan Xiong	Radix Ligustici Wallichii	9.10	Promote Blood circulation; Regulate Qi; Regulate menstruation
Bai Shao	Radix Paeoniae Lactiflorae	12.12	Nourish Blood; Nourish Yin; Stop pain; Relax smooth muscle spasms
Shou Di Huang	Radix Conquitae Rehmanniae Glutinosae	18.18	Nourish Yin; Nourish Blood
Gan Cao	Radix Glycyrrhizae Uralensis	6.06	Warm the Middle Warmer; Strengthen Spleen; Harmonize other herbs

Notes: 1. This formula consists of two basic formulas. 1) Si Jun Zi Tang which is a basic formula to strengthen Qi; and 2) Si Wu Tang which is a basic formula to Strengthen Blood. Therefore, this combination, Fu Ke Ba Zhen Wan, is used to Tonify both Qi and Blood. In TCM theory, all gynecological disorders are due to Blood disorders, and most of them are due to Def. Blood. Therefore, the principle treatment in gynecology is to Strengthen the Blood. Also, in TCM theory, because the Blood is visible, it cannot be Tonified immediately. Thus, because the Qi is the leader of the Blood, and because the Qi (not visible) can be Tonified immediately, it is necessary to Tonify the Qi and the Blood at the same time. This formula uses herbs to both Tonify Qi and Tonify Blood at the same time, thus Strengthening the Blood to treat the gynecological disorder.

2. There is a modification of this formula which is called Tai Shan Pan Shi San. This modified formula has the function to Strengthen Qi, Tonify Blood and Soothe the embryo. It is commonly used to treat excess fetal movement and help prevent miscarriage in Def. Qi and Def. Blood cases. The difference between the original formula and this modified formula is the following: 1) The Fu Ling in the original formula is replaced with 4 other herbs. 2) These additional herbs include Huang Qi, Xu Duan, Huang Qin, and Sha Ren. This modified formula, however, is not available in the Patent Medicine form.

3. In Laboratory research in China, when this formula was used in decoction form with humans, the formula was able to promote regeneration of red blood cells in acute anemia cases. Source: Zhong Yao Cheng Yao Xue (Traditional Chinese Patent Medicines Text). Tianjin: Tianjin Science and Technology Press, 1984, p. 214.

4. The Patent Medicine in liquid form, Dang Gui Ji Jin (Essence of Chicken with Tangkwei), is similar to Fu Ke Ba Zhen Wan. It is a modification of Fu Ke Ba Zhen Wan made with chicken meat. It has a greater effect to Strengthen the Blood because it contains the protein from chicken meat. It is especially good for patients with Def. Qi and Def. Blood, including those with anemia or post-partum weakness. Stir one bottle into an equal amount of warm water. The dose is one bottle per day.

5. The Patent Medicine in liquid form, Ren Shen Ji Jin, is similar to Dang Gui Ji Jin, in that both are made from chicken broth, but in the Ren Shen Ji Jin, Ginseng has been added instead of Dang Gui. Therefore, Ren Shen Ji Jin especially Tonifies Qi; stronger Qi, in turn, will help to Strengthen the Blood.

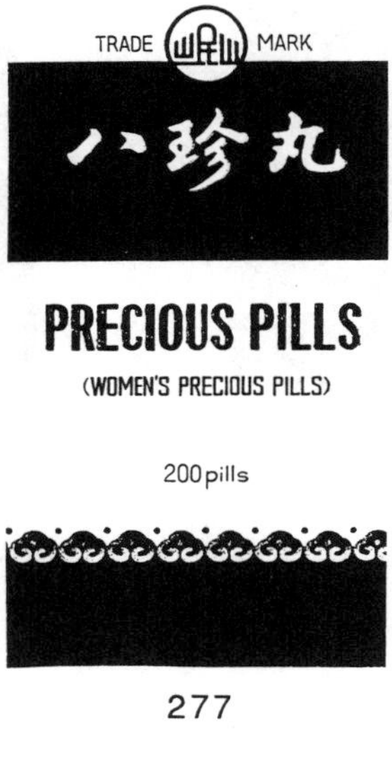

13.11 當 歸 片

Dang	Gui	Pian
---------Angelicae---------		tablets

Function: 1. Nourish Blood; Tonify Qi

Application: 1. Use to treat Def. Blood during post-partum period. Symptoms: Extended uterine bleeding following childbirth, pale face, dizziness, vertigo, palpitations, spontaneous sweating (day or night), feeling of cold in the limbs; an Empty Pulse. This Def. Blood condition may have been caused by the following: 1. Prior to childbirth, the Def. Blood condition was already present, and following childbirth, the condition worsened. 2) During childbirth, there was excess loss of blood.

Dose: 5 tablets, 3 times a day

Dang Gui Pian is produced as "Angelicae Tablets" by the Lanzhou Chinese Medicine Works, Lanzhou, China, in bottles of 100 coated tablets.

Pinyin Name	Pharmaceutical Name	Percent	TCM Function
Dang Gui	Radix Angelicae Sinensis	70	Nourish Blood; Promote Blood circulation
Chuan Xiong	Radix Ligustici Wallichii	10	Promote Blood Circulation; Move Stuck Qi; Stop pain
Bai Zhu	Rhizoma Atractylodis Macrocephalae	10	Strengthen Spleen; Dry Dampness
Da Zao	Fructus Zizyphi Jujubae	10	Strengthen Spleen; Nourish Blood due to Def. Spleen Qi and Def. Liver Blood

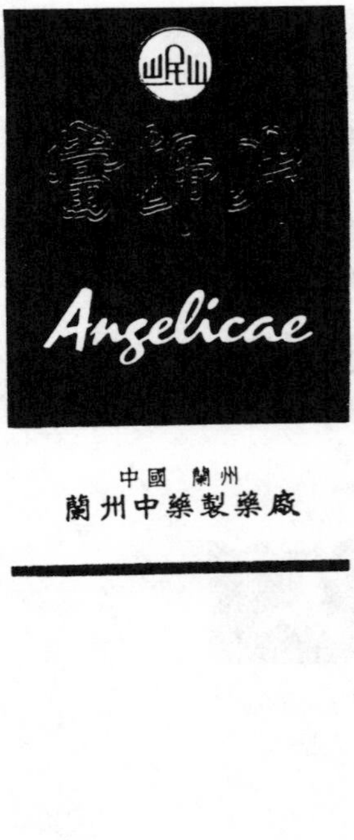

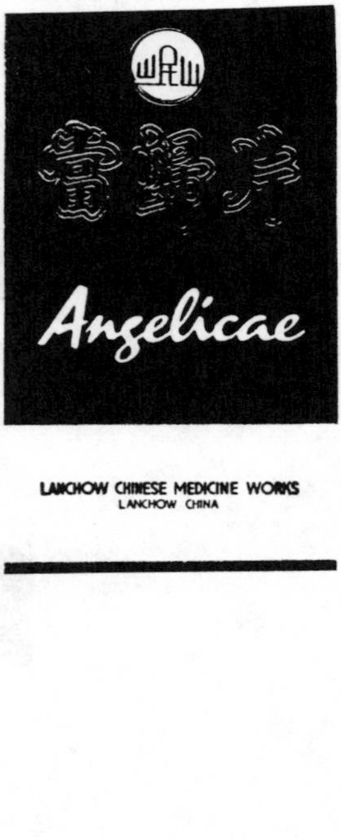

13.12 雙寶素口服液

Shuang	Bao	Su	Kou	Fu	Ye
double	precious	extract	mouth	drink	liquid

Function: 1. Use to Strengthen Vital Qi, Nourish Liver; Tonify Spleen

Application: 1. This is a general Tonic Patent Medicine. Use it to treat general weakness. It is also useful as an assistant medicine with some chronic diseases such as coronary artery disease, chronic hepatitis, neurasthenia, rheumatoid arthritis, chronic gastritis, stomach or duodenal ulcer, hair loss due to weakness (alopecia), and impotence.

Dose: Capsule Form: 1 or 2 capsules, 3 times a day. Liquid Form: 1 vial, once a day, in the morning.

Shuang Bao Su is produced as "Ginseng Extract and Fresh Royal Jelly Mixture" by the Hangzhou Second Traditional Chinese Pharmaceutical Works, Hangzhou, China, in vials of 10 cc (10 vials per box) and in bottles of 30 capsules.

The percents for each ingredient are not available. The function is the same for all 3 ingredients.

Pinyin Name	**Pharmaceutical Name**	**TCM Function**
Feng Wang Jiang	Royal Jelly (Bee Milk)	Strengthen Qi and Blood
Ren Shen	Radix Ginseng	
	Glucose	

Notes: 1. The name of this Patent Medicine, "Shuang Bao (double precious) Su (extract)" reflects the fact that the two main ingredients, Royal Jelly and Ginseng, are considered to be two valuable medicines. Research in China has suggested that each of these ingredients strengthens the immune system; results from one study are summarized, below.

In a pharmacological study in China, rats were divided into 2 groups. The experimental group was given standard Royal Jelly plus Ginseng; the control group was given none. Both groups were given standard food and water. After several days, the rats in each group were subjected to various adverse conditions (cold environment, reduced oxygen levels, no water, no food, or hepatitis induced by carbon tetrachloride injection). After a fixed period of time, there was a greater number of survivors in the experimental group. The Royal Jelly plus Ginseng is believed to increase immune system function and is used to improve the function of bone marrow in blood production. Source: Zhong Yao Cheng Yao Xue, (Textbook of Traditional Chinese Medicine Patent Medicines), Liu De-Yi, Tianjin Science and Technology Publishing House, March, 1984, p. 217.

2. Another Patent Medicine, Qing Chun Bao, is similar to Shuang Bao Su. The Qing Chun Bao formula is from the Imperial Hospital during the Ming Dynasty, 1368-1644, and was intended for use only by the emperor. This formula is reported to be important in strengthening the immune system and slowing the aging process.

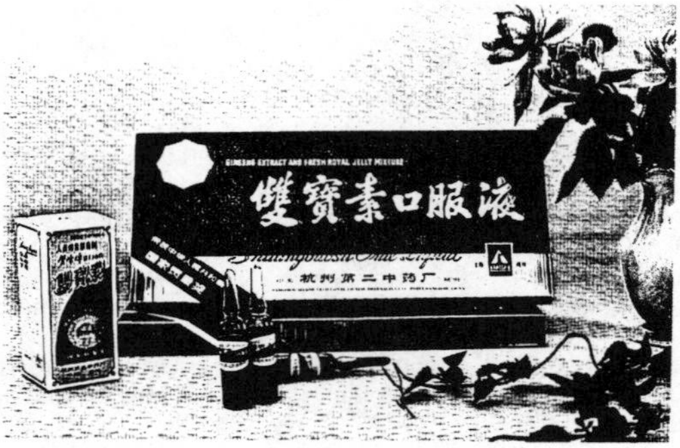
GINSENG EXTRACT AND FRESH ROYAL JELLY MIXTURE
雙寶素口服液
杭州第二中药厂

雙寶素

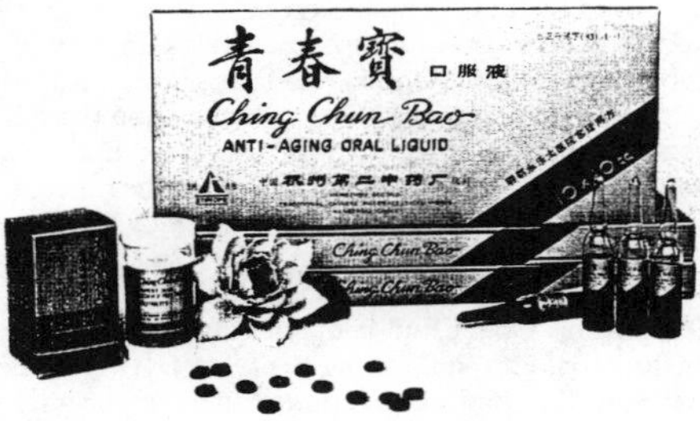
青春寶 口服液
Ching Chun Bao
ANTI-AGING ORAL LIQUID
杭州第二中药厂
Ching Chun Bao

13.13 安 胎 丸

An	Tai	Wan
soothe	embryo	pills

Source: Chan Hou Bian, (Post-Partum Volume), Ming Dynasty, 1368-1644.

Function:
1. Nourish Qi and Blood
2. Soothe embryo
3. Regulate Stomach Qi

Application:

1. Use to treat overactive movement of the embryo due to Def. Qi and Blood in the mother. Use to help treat lumbago or leg pain in the mother.

2. Use to help prevent miscarriage or premature delivery by stopping bleeding from the uterus. In addition to bleeding, the symptoms may include pulling pain in the lower abdomen.

Dose: 7 pills, 3 times a day.

An Tai Wan is produced by the United Pharmaceutical Manufactory, Guangzhou, Guangdong, China, in bottles of 100 pills.

The 16 herbs are listed below in 8 groups, according to function.

Pinyin Name	Pharmaceutical Name	Percent	TCM Function
Group 1			
Dang Gui	Radix Angelicae Sinenesis	8.5	Strengthen Blood;
Shou Di Huang	Radix Rehmanniae Glutinosae Conquitae	6.8	Nourish Yin
Bai Shao	Radix Paeoniae Lactiflorae	8.5	
Chuan Xiong	Radix Ligustici Wallichii	6.8	
Group 2			
Huang Qi	Radix Astragali	5.1	Strengthen Qi; Nourish Spleen
Bai Zhu	Rhizoma Atractylodis Macrocephalae	6.8	
Gan Cao	Radix Glycyrrhizae Uralensis	5.1	
Group 3			
Tu Si Zi	Semen Cuscutae	6.8	Strengthen Liver and Kidney;
Ai Ye	Carbonized Folium Artemisiae	4.3	Stop bleeding; Soothe embryo
Group 4			
Huang Qin	Radix Scutellariae Baicalensis	5.1	Clear Heat; Soothe embryo
Group 5			
Sha Ren	Fructus seu Semen Amomi	4.3	Regulate Spleen Qi; Soothe embryo
Group 6			
Qiang Huo	Rhizoma et Radix Notopterygii	2.6	Eliminate Wind; Stop pain
Jing Jie	Herba seu Flos Schizonepetae Tenuifoliae	5.1	

<u>Group 7</u>			
Zhi Qiao	Fructus Citri seu Ponciri	6.8	Regulate Stomach Qi;
Hou Po	Cortex Magnoliae Officinalis (Cooked)	4.3	Stop pain
<u>Group 8</u>			
Chuan Bei Mu	Bulbus Fritillariae Cirrhosae	8.5	Clear Heat; Reduce Phlegm

<u>Note</u>: 1. The original name of this formula, Bao Chan Wu Yu Ying, first appeared in the sourcebook <u>Chan Hou Bian</u>, during the Ming Dynasty, 1368-1644. After that time, several modifications were made, including An Tai Wan, and these were put into the Patent Medicine form. Some of these modified formulas are called Bao Tai Wan, Shi San Tai Bao Wan, or Bao Chan Wu Yu Wan.

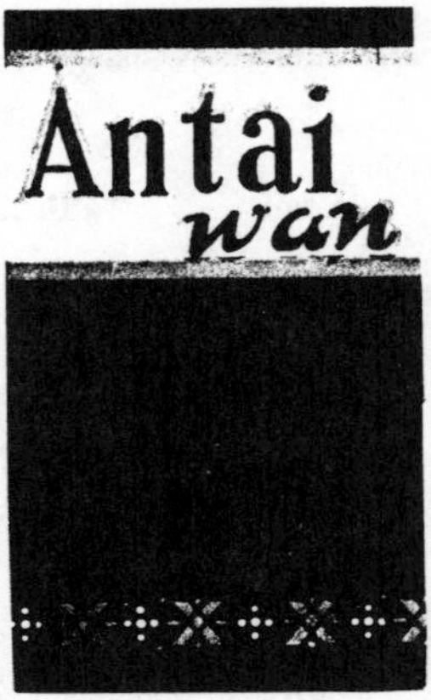

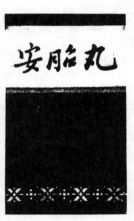

13.14 當 歸 養 血 膏

當	歸	養	血	膏
Dang	**Gui**	**Yang**	**Xue**	**Gao**
---------Angelicae--------		nourish	Blood	syrup

Function: 1. Nourish Qi and Blood

Application: 1. Use to treat Def. Blood syndrome. Symptoms: dizziness, palpitations, poor memory, fatigue, anemia. Specific symptoms related to gynecological disorders include irregular menstruation with pale blood, amenorrhea or hypomenorrhea; and postpartum weakness due to excess blood loss.

Dose: Drink 1 or 2 tablespoons dissolved in warm water or tea, 2 times a day.

Dang Gui Yang Xue Gao is produced as "Tankwe Gin for Tea" by the Zhong Lian Manufacturing Co., Wuhan, China, in bottles of 150 cc.

The contents are listed below in 4 groups, according to function.

Pinyin Name	Pharmaceutical Name	Percent	TCM Function
Group 1			
Dang Gui	Radix Angelicae Sinensis	69.0	Nourish Blood; Nourish Yin;
Shou Di Huang	Radix Rehmanniae Glutinosae Conquitae	4.5	Regulate menstruation
Bai Shao	Radix Paeoniae Lactiflorae	4.5	
Group 2			
Dang Shen	Radix Codonopsis Pilosulae	4.5	Strengthen Spleen; Tonify Qi
Huang Qi	Radix Astragali	4.5	
Fu Ling	Sclerotium Poriae Cocos	4.5	
Gan Cao	Radix Glycyrrhizae Uralensis	2.0	
Group 3			
Chuan Xiong	Radix Ligustici Wallichii	2.0	Strengthen Blood; Promote Blood circulation to prevent possible Blood Stagnation due to large amounts of herbs which Nourish the Blood
Group 4			
A Jiao	Gelatinum Asini	4.5	Strengthen Blood; Nourish Yin; Stop bleeding

Note: 1. The Patent Medicine, Dang Gui Jin Gao, is the same as Dang Gui Yang Xue Gao.

TRADE
MARK
TanKwe
Gin
FOR TEA
NET 7 FL,
EXPORTERS
CHINA NATIONAL NATIVE PROD
BY-PRODUCTS IMP. &
HUPEH PROVINCIAL
5 TIANJIN RO
HANKOU, HUPEH,

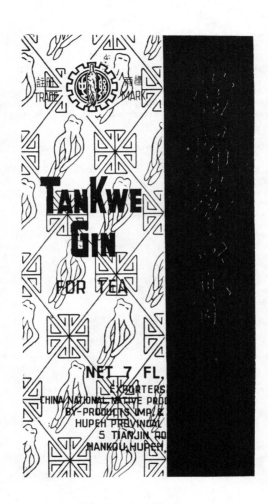

13.15 刺 五 加 片

Ci	Wu	Jia	Pian
---------Acanthopanax senticosus---------			tablets

Function: 1. Strengthen Vital Qi and Tonify Kidney Jing.
2. Calm the Spirit; Improve brain function.

Application: 1. Use to treat Def. Vital Qi. Symptoms: Fatigue, dizziness, insomnia, poor appetite, migraine headaches.

2. Use to treat sexual dysfunction with spermatorrhea, impotence, or impaired sexual desire.

3. Some Western medicine disease applications include the following:

Research in China has suggested that the only herb in this Patent Medicine, Ciwujia, is especially effective in relieving fatigue. It has a greater stimulating effect than Ginseng; but it can also calm the patient and reduce anxiety. It also strengthens the immune system. It is useful in protecting the body from damage due to radiation. It decreases inflammation. It also normalizes blood pressure. If the blood pressure is too high, it will lower the blood pressure; if it is too low, it will raise the blood pressure.

Research in China has also suggested that this herb, Ciwujia, has the effect of increasing endocrine function (ovaries, testes, adrenal glands). It will increase insulin, and decrease blood sugar if it is excessively high. It has an antidiuretic property and will help prevent the patient from producing excess urine.

Research in China has also suggested that this herb, Ciwujia can be helpful in treating cancer. In experiments with rats, the rats treated wtih this herb were able to get rid of SSK sarcoma. In addition, this herb prevented the spread of the sarcoma to other parts of the body. In China, the use of this herb, Ciwujia, with cancer patients is preferable to the use of Ginseng.

Dose: 3 tablets, 2 or 3 times a day. Each tablet contains 0.150 grams of the herb.

Ci Wu Jia is produced as "Ciwujia Tablet" by the Harbin Sixth Pharmacy Factory, Harbin, China, in bottles with 100 coated tablets.

Pinyin Name	Pharmaceutical Name	Percent	TCM Function
Ciwujia	*Acanthopanax senticosus* Harms	100	See "Application" above.

13.16 參 蓍 大 補 丸

Shen	Qi	Da	Bu	Wan
Codonopsis	Astragalus	great	supplement	pills

Function: 1. Tonify Qi, Strengthen Spleen

Application: 1. Use to treat Def. Qi syndrome due to long illness, blood loss, or post-partum weakness. Symptoms: Spontaneous sweating (especially in the daytime), fatigue, excess thirst, poor appetite, weight loss. Also useful to help patients with diabetes mellitus.

Dose: 8-10 pills, 3 times a day.

Shen Qi Da Bu Wan is produced as "Shen Qi Da Bu Wan (Shenqi Tonic Pills)" by the Lanzhou Fo Ci Pharmaceutical Factory, Lanzhou, China, in bottles of 100 pills.

Pinyin Name	Pharmaceutical Name	Percent	TCM Function
Huang Qi	Radix Astragali	50	Strengthen Vital Qi, Stop sweating
Dang Shen	Radix Pilosulae Codonopsis	50	Strengthen Spleen Qi

Note: 1. Originally, this formula was made into a syrup called Shen Qi Gao. The function is the same. The syrup form is easier for the weaker patient and the elderly patient to absorb. There is also a form available called Shen Qi Pian, which is a sugar-coated tablet.

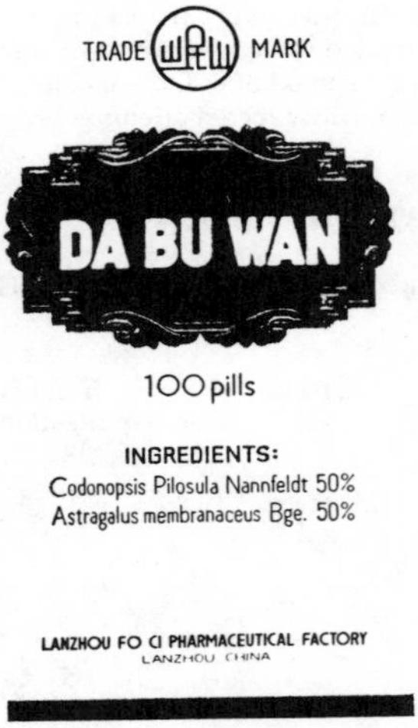
TRADE MARK
DA BU WAN
100 pills
INGREDIENTS:
Codonopsis Pilosula Nannfeldt 50%
Astragalus membranaceus Bge. 50%
LANZHOU FO CI PHARMACEUTICAL FACTORY
LANZHOU CHINA

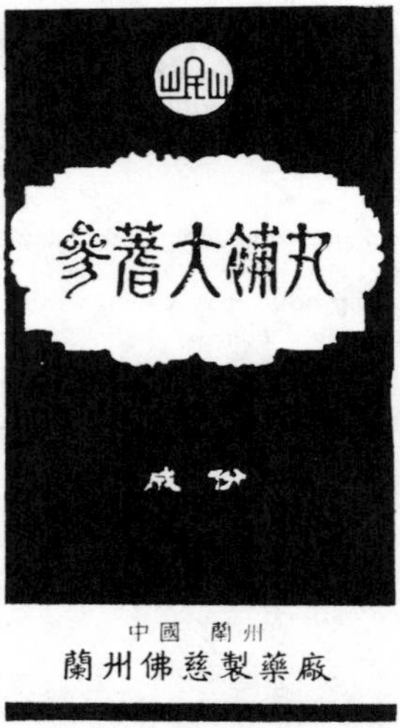

13.17 河 車 大 造 丸

He	Che	Da	Zao	Wan
-----human placenta-----		big	nourishment	pills

Source: Jing Yue Quan Shu, (Jing Yue's Complete Works), Ming Dynzsty, 1368 - 1644.

Function: 1. Nourish Liver and Kidney; Tonify Def. Yin

Application: 1. Use this to treat disorders associated with Def. Liver and Def. Kidney.
Symptoms: Dizziness, tinnitus, the legs are weak and tired with aching in the lower back or waist; low-grade fever in the afternoon; fatigue, red cheeks or hot flushed face; spermatorrhea. The spermatorrhea here is the Def. Yin type - i.e. the semen is usually lost at night, during a dream.

2. Some Western medicine disease applications include the following: Any type of hypertension with Def. Yin symptomatology (headache, dizziness, restlessness, etc., see above); later stages of tuberculosis with Def. Yin symptomatology (dry cough, expectoration of blood may or may not be present); any consumptive disease which is accompanied by Def. Yin syndrome - i.e. cancer, chronic hepatitis, chronic hyperthyroidism, chronic diabetes, chronic nephritis, chronic bronchitis. (This formula will only treat the Def.Yin symptoms.)

Dose: 8 pills, 3 times a day In China, cases with def. Yin symptomatology have used this formula for several months or years, as necessary; it is alright to use this medicine for a long period of time, as long as necessary.

He Che Da Zao Wan is produced as "Placenta Compound Restorative Pills" by the Lanzhou Chinese Medicine Works, Lanzhou, China, in bottles of 100 pills.

Pinyin Name	Pharmaceutical Name	Percent	TCM Function
Gui Ban	Plastrum Testudinis	15	Nourish Yin and Settle the Yang; Lower Empty Fire
Shou Di Huang	Radix Rehmanniae Glutinosae Conquitae	15	Supplement Blood; Nourish Yin
Dang Shen	Radix Codonopsis Pilosulae	11	Tonify Qi
Huang Bai	Cortex Phillodendri	11	Settle Ascending Kidney Fire
Du Zhong	Cortex Eucommiae Ulmoidis	11	Tonify Liver and Kidney; Strengthen tendons and bones; Lower blood pressure
Zi He Che	Placenta Hominis	8	Tonify Kidney Qi; Strengthen Blood
Niu Xi	Radix Achyranthis	8	Promote Blood circulation; Remove Blood Stasis; Induce downward movement of Blood; Lower blood pressure; Tonfiy Liver and Kidney; Strengthen tendons and bones.
Tian Men dong	Tuber Asparagi Cochinchinensis	8	Nourish Yin; Clear Heat; Tonify Kidney and Lung Yin
Mai Men Dong	Tuber Ophiopogonis Japonici	8	Nourish Yin; Clear Heat; Moisten Lung; Tranquilize and Clear Heart Heat; Strengthen Stomach Yin

Fu Ling	Sclerotium Poriae Cocos	3.5	Strengthen Spleen; Tranquilize Heart and Spirit
Sha Ren	Fructus seu Semen Amomi	1.5	Regulate Stomach Qi to prevent Stagnation of Qi in the Stoamch after taking the medicine

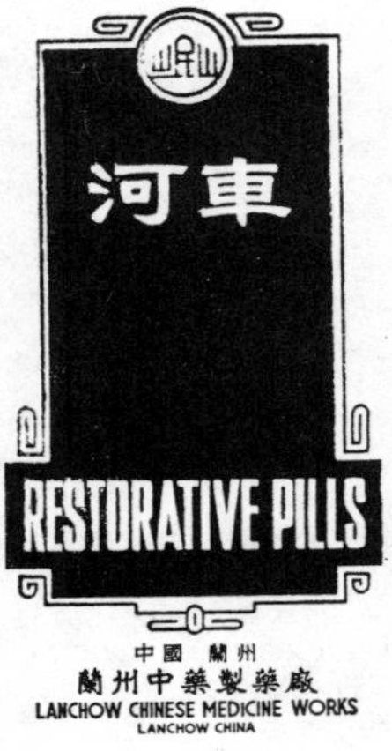

13.18 健 步 虎 潛 丸

健	步	虎	潛	丸
Jian	**Bu**	**Hu**	**Qian**	**Wan**
healthy	steps	tiger	stealthily	pills

Source: Dan Xi Xin Fa, (Methodology of Dan Xi), Yuan Dynasty, 1279 - 1368.

Function: 1. Strengthen Yin; Clear Empty Fire
2. Strengthen tendons and bones

Application: 1. Use to treat Def. congenital Jing in Kidney and Def. congenital Blood in Liver. Symptoms: Weakness and stiffness in the lumbar area, weak limbs, debility in walking. The Tongue may be red, with less Tongue coat. The Pulse may be Thin and Empty.

2. Use to treat Wei syndrome due to Def. Liver and Kidney Yin. Symptoms: Limbs which are flaccid and without strength, inability to stand up or even to make a fist. In serious cases, muscle atrophy may be present and there is little or no muscle function, especially in the legs, where inability to walk may be present.

3. Some Western medicine disease applications include the following: Sequelae of poliomyelitis in children, i.e., flaccid paralysis of limbs, muscle atrophy, etc. This is more effective when combined with acupuncture treatments. Sequelae of tuberculosis in the knee joints in patients with Def. Yin and Empty Heat signs.

Dose: Adults: 20 pills, 2 or 3 times a day.
Children: Under 5 Years: 5 pills, 2 or 3 times a day. 5 to 12 Years: 10 pills, 2 or 3 times a day.
Dissolve the pills in warm water, and drink.

Jian Bu Hu Qian Wan is produced as "Chen Pu Hu Chien Wen" by the Beijing Tung Jen Tang pharmacy, Beijing, China, in bottles of 200 pills.

Pinyin Name	Pharmaceutical Name	Grams	TCM Function
Hu Gu	Os Tigris	10	Strengthen bones and tendons
Niu Xi	Radix Acyranthis Bidentatae	35	Strengthen Liver and Kidney; Nourish Yin
Dang Gui	Radix Angelicae Sinensis	10	Tonify Blood; NourishYin
Zhi Mu	Radix Anemarrhenae Asphodeloidis	20	Clear Heat; Nourish Yin
Huang Bai	Cortex Phellodendri	40	Clear Heat in the Lower Warmer
Shou Di Huang	Radix Rehmanniae Glutinose Conquitae	20	Nourish Yin; Strengthen Blood
Gui Ban	Plastrum Testudinis	40	Clear Empty Heat; Nourish Yin
Bai Shao	Radix Paeoniae Lactiflorae	15	Nourish Yin; Strengthen Liver
Suo Yang	Herba Cynomorii Songarici	10	Strengthen Kidney Yang and Kidney Jing
Chen Pi	Pericarpium Citri Reticulatae	7.5	Regulate Qi; Regulate Stomach

Note: 1. The Patent Medicine, Du Zhong Feng Shi Wan, is similar to Jian Bu Hu Qian Wan.

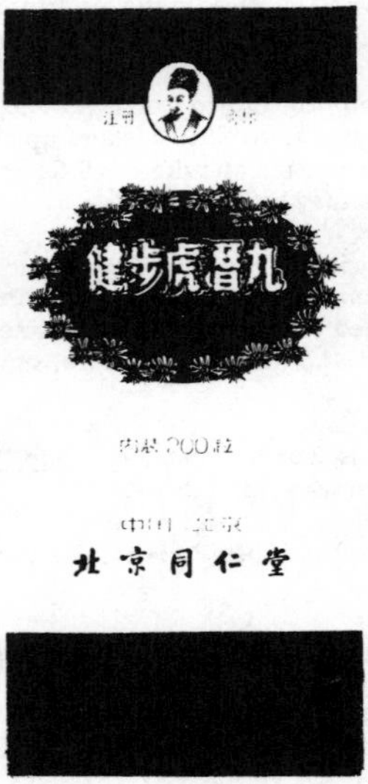

13.19 六 味 地 黃 丸

Liu	**Wei**	**Di**	**Huang**	**Wan**
six	herb	---------Rehmannia---------		pills

Source: Xiao Er Yao Zheng Zhi Jue, (Pediatric Pharmaceutics), by Qian Yi, Song Dynasty, 960-1279. This text originally contained herb formulas for children, but now, many of the formulas are used for adults.

Function: 1. Nourish Kidney and Liver. A special formula for Def. Kidney and Liver Yin.
2. Clear Empty Fire.

Applications: 1. This is the primary formula used to treat Def. Yin, especially Def. Kidney and Liver Yin. Symptoms: Headache, dizziness, tinnitus, poor hearing, debility of the lumbar area, lassitude of the legs (the patient cannot stand for a long period of time and wants to sit down), low-grade afternoon fever, "bone steaming" (a term for afternoon fever and night sweating, symptoms of consumptive disease with extreme Def. Yin cases), difficult urination, diabetes, nocturnal emission. The Tongue is a red, and there is less Tongue coating. The Pulse is Thin and rapid.

2. Some Western medicine disease applications include the following:

1) Nephritis. Research in China has shown that this will improve Kidney function; it was studied in a group of patients in their 20's who had glomerulonephritis due to tonsillitis. Research in China has also observed this to decrease the number of fatalities in cases with Kidney infections.

2) Def. Yin type of diabetes, tuberculosis, hyperthyroidism, mild emotional disturbances.

3) Use it to inhibit abnormal cell growth in the esophagus (Epitheliosis, where cells may become potential Cancer cells). Research in China with 46 cases showed 41/46 to improve; 4 cases to remain stable and only 1 case to develop esophageal Cancer. Source: Xin Yi Yao Xue Za Zhi, Issue No. 7, 1977

Dose: Adults: Smaller Pills: 8-10 pills, 3 times a day, taken with warm water.

Condensed Pills: 9-15 pills, 2 times a day, taken with warm water.

Honey Pills (10 grams each): 1 pill, 2 or 3 times a day, taken with warm water.

Children: Reduce proportionately

Liu Wei Di Huang Wan is produced by the Lanzhou Chinese Medicine Works, Lanzhou, China, in bottles of 200 smaller pills. It is produced as "Liu Wei Dihuang Wan" by the Min-Kang Drug Manufactory, I-Chang, China, in bottles of 100 concentrated, smaller pills.

A formula similar to this formula is also available in liquid, tincture form as "Quiet Contemplative," in the Jade Pharmacy product line, available through Crane Enterprises, Plymouth, MA, etc. See bottom of page 343.

Pinyin Name	Pharmaceutical Name	Percent	TCM Function
Shu Di Huang	Radix Rehmanniae Glutinosae Conquitae	32	Nourish Yin; Strengthen Blood
Shan Yao	Radix Dioscoreae Oppositae	16	Tonify Spleen and Stomach
Mu Dan Pi	Cortex Moutan Radicis	12	Clear Blood Heat; Extinguish Liver Fire
Fu Ling	Sclerotium Poriae Cocos	12	Strengthen Spleen; Discharge Dampness; Promote urination
Shan Zhu Yu	Fructus Corni Officinalis	16	Strengthen Liver and Kidney Yin; Stop sweating; Stop spermatorrhea
Ze Xie	Rhizoma Alismatis Plantago-aquaticae	12	Promote urination; Drain Kidney Empty Fire

Notes: 1. This herbal formula is a basic formula to Nourish Yin and Strengthen the Kidney. This formula is special because although three of the ingredients are Tonic herbs and three of the ingredients Drain Empty Fire, the relative percent of the Tonic herbs is greater than the percent of the herbs which Drain Empty Fire. Therefore, this is considered to be a Tonifying herbal formula.

Because this is the basic formula to Strengthen Kidney Yin, there are several variations of this formula which are used to treat other disorders in addition to Def. Kidney Yin. Some of these variations include #13.20, Zhi Bai Di Huang Wan (Clear more Empty Fire); #13.26, Qi Ju Di Huang Wan (Strengthen Liver Yin; Stop Internal Wind; Brighten the Eyes); Gui Shao Di Huang Wan (Strengthen Blood, Soothe Liver); #3.15, Mai Wei Di Huang Wan, also called Ba Xian Chang Shou Wan (Strengthen Def. Yin in both the Lung and Kidney).

2. The physician Qian Yi, who wrote the text, Xiao Er Yao Zheng Zhi Jue (Pediatric Pharmaceutics) Song Dynasty, 960-1279), in which this formula first appeared, used this medicine with children who experienced any of the "Five Delays."

1. Delay in standing up
2. Delay in walking
3. Delay in growth of hair on the head
4. Delay in the development of teeth
5. Delay in speech development

3. Case Report: In 1988, MN had the opportunity to work with a family from Long Island who had a 6 year-old boy with cerebral palsy. They came to Boston for a few acupuncture treatments with a low-energy laser. The laser treatments were used to temporarily release the involuntary muscle spasms which caused the boy's arms and legs to contract up into the midline position. During this visit they were told about the use of Liu Wei Di Huang Wan with children who experience the "Five Delays." This boy, at age six, was still experiencing all of these "Delays," and was unable to sit up by himself, walk or talk, and was very small for his age.

After a week, the family returned to Long Island and began to use the Liu Wei Di Huang Wan. Six weeks later, the mother telephoned MN to tell her that her son was beginning to vocalize more, and had said a few short phrases during a speech therapy session; something he had never previously been able to do. She also reported that her son was "filling out and getting bigger." He had grown a few inches over the summer; he was taking the Liu Wei Di Huang Wan during the last half of the summer. She gave him 1 small pill, 3 times a day for 6 weeks. As of 1989, she continues the herbs, plus laser-acupuncture and acupuncture treatments with continued improvements.

4. Case Report: In 1989, MN used this with a 68 year old stroke patient who was diabetic (non-insulin dependant). The frequent urination at night was decreased from 3 times per night to only once per night after 2 weeks. He also had a history of renal insufficiency and glomerulonephritis.

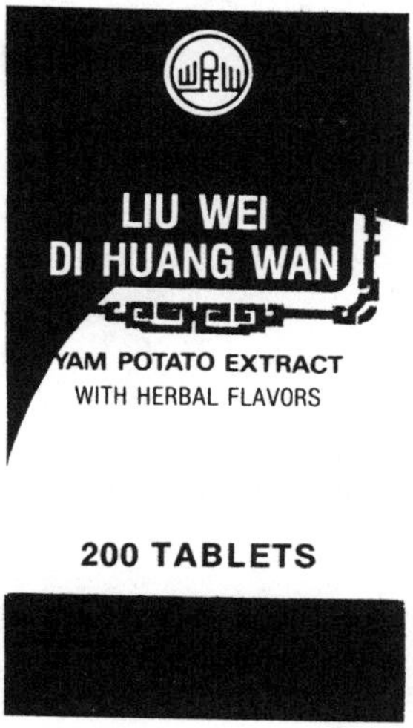
LIU WEI
DI HUANG WAN
YAM POTATO EXTRACT
WITH HERBAL FLAVORS
200 TABLETS

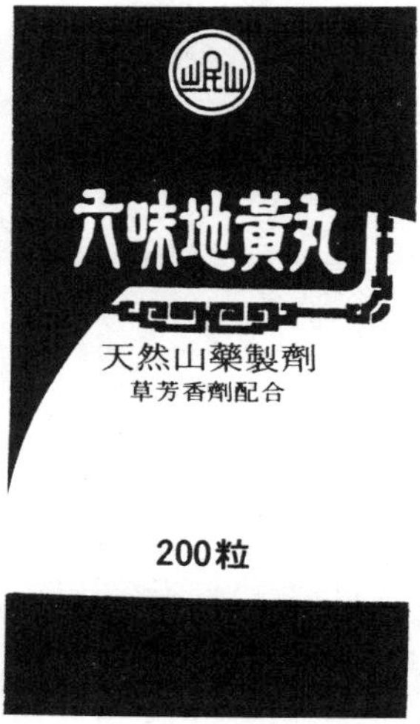
六味地黄丸
天然山藥製劑
草芳香劑配合
200粒

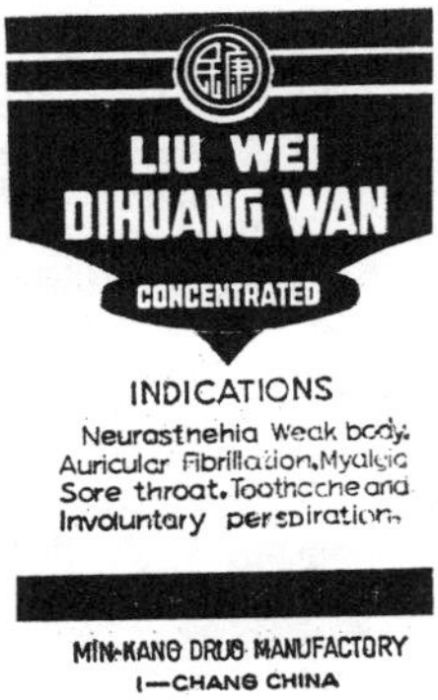
LIU WEI
DIHUANG WAN
CONCENTRATED
INDICATIONS
Neurastnehia Weak body.
Auricular Fibrillation.Myalgic
Sore throat.Toothache and
Involuntary perspiration.
MIN-KANG DRUG MANUFACTORY
I—CHANG CHINA

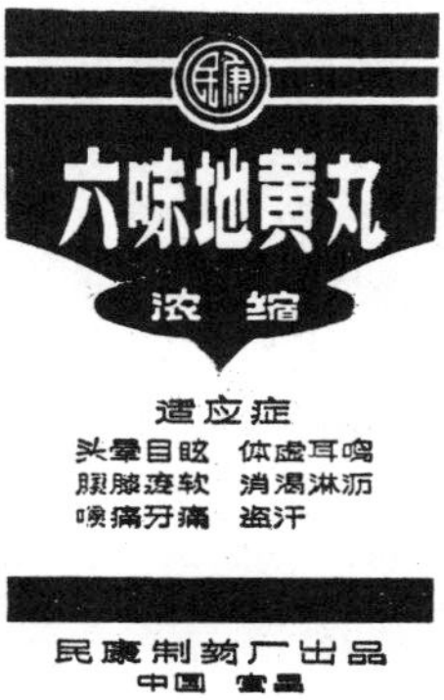
六味地黄丸
浓缩
适应症
头晕目眩 体虚耳鸣
腰膝酸软 消渴淋沥
喉痛牙痛 盗汗
民康制药厂出品
中国

13.20 知 柏 地 黄 丸

Zhi	Bai	Di	Huang	Wan
Anemarrhenae	Phellodendri	----------Rhemannia----------		pills

Source: Yi Zong Jin Jian, (The Golden Mirror of Medicine), Qing Dynasty, 1644-1911.

Function:
1. Moisten Yin
2. Quell ascending Yang (Eliminate Empty Fire)

Application:
1. Use to Quell ascending Yang (Eliminate Fire) in Ming Men (Life Gate) due to Def. Kidney Yin. Symptoms: Low-grade afternoon fever, Heat in the Five Centers, flushed face, red cheeks, uneasiness, night sweat during sleep, nocturnal emission (with dreams); chronic throat pain due to rising Empty Fire; frequent urination of small amounts of concentrated, dark urine (also a sign of Def. Kidney Yin with Empty Fire).

2. Use to treat "hot flashes" associated with menopause.

Dose: Smaller Pills: 8-16 pills, 3 times a day, taken with warm water. Honey Pills: 1 pill, 2 times a day.

Zhi Bai Di Huang Wan is produced as "Chih Pai Di Huang Wan" or "Chih Pai Pa Wei Wan" by the Lanzhou Chinese Medicine Works, Lanzhou, China, in bottles of 200 pills.

A formula similar to this formula is also available in liquid, tincture form as "Temper Fire," in the Jade Pharmacy product line, available through Crane Enterprises, Plymouth, MA, etc. See bottom of p. 343.

Pinyin Name	Pharmaceutical Name	Percent	TCM Function
Shu Di Huang	Radix Rehmanniae Glutinosae Conquitae	27.58	Nourish Yin; Strengthen Blood
Shan Zhu Yu	Fructus Corni Officinalis	13.80	Strengthen Liver and Kidney Yin; Stop sweating; Stop spermatorrhea
Shan Yao	Radix Disocoreae Oppositae	13.80	Tonify Spleen and Stomach
Ze Xie	Rhizoma Alismatis Plantago-aquaticae	10.34	Promote urination; Drain Kidney Empty Fire
Mu Dan Pi	Cortex Moutan Radicis	10.34	Clear Blood Heat; Extinguish Liver Fire
Fu Ling	Sclerotium Poriae Cocos	10.34	Strengthen Spleen; Discharge Dampness; Promote urination
Huang Bai	Cortex Phellodendri	6.90	Clear Heat; Detoxify Fire Poison; Reduce Empty Fire
Zhi Mu	Radix Anemarrhenae Asphodeloidis	6.90	Clear Heat; Reduce Fire; Nourish Yin

Notes:
1. When using this Patent Medicine, Zhi Bai Di Huang Wan, in treating hot flashes during menopause (due to Def. Kidney Yin), it may also be combined with the Patent Medicine, Ren Shen Gu Ben Wan, which will Clear Empty Fire, Nourish Yin and Increase Body Fluids.

2. Another name for this Patent Medicine, Zhi Bai Di Huang Wan, is Zhi Bai Ba Wei Wan.

3. This formula is important to consider for use with patients who have long-term use of steroids (prednisone) or thyroid hormone replacement therapy, because these patients often develop Def. Yin over a period of time. They may develop a red Tongue, which may become swollen. They may also have mouth dryness which can lead to tooth loss due to inadequate amounts of saliva.

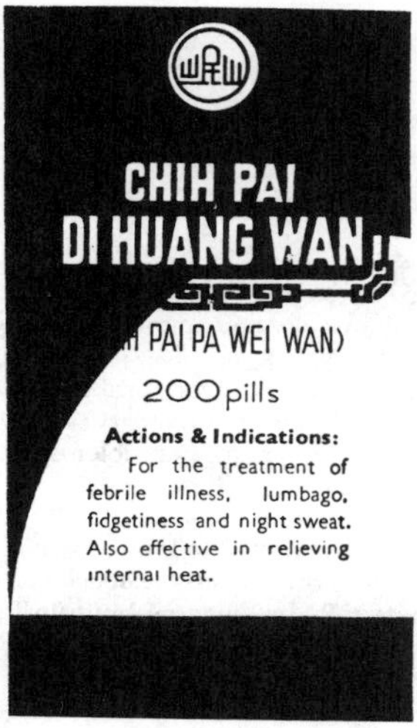
CHIH PAI
DI HUANG WAN
H PAI PA WEI WAN)
200 pills
Actions & Indications:
For the treatment of febrile illness, lumbago, fidgetiness and night sweat. Also effective in relieving internal heat.

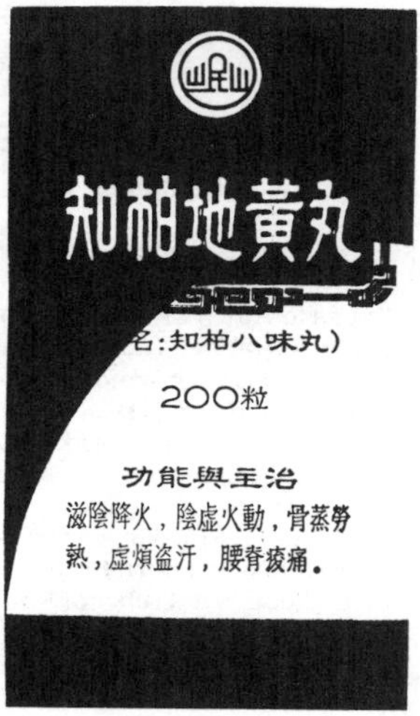

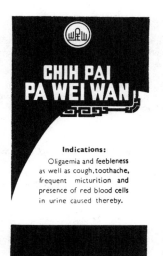
知柏地黃丸
名:知柏八味丸)
200粒
功能與主治
滋陰降火，陰虛火動，骨蒸勞熱，虛煩盜汗，腰脊痠痛。

CHIH PAI
PA WEI WAN
Indications:
Oligaemia and feebleness as well as cough, toothache, frequent micturition and presence of red blood cells in urine caused thereby.

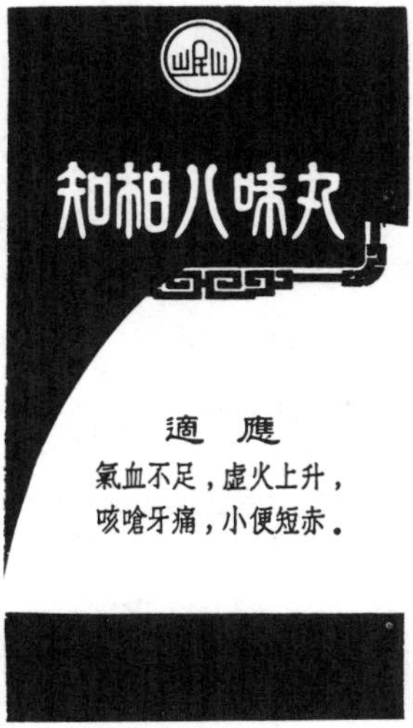
知柏八味丸
適 應
氣血不足，虛火上升，咳嗆牙痛，小便短赤。

13.21 首 烏 片

Shou	Wu	Pian
head	black	tablets

Function: 1. Nourish Liver and Kidney Yin
2. Tonify Blood
3. Strengthen bones and tendons

Applications: 1. Use to enrich Liver and Kidney Yin, including marrow and sperm, especially in older patients with Def. Kidney Yin and Def. Liver Yin. Symptoms: Lassitude of legs where the patient cannot stand for a long period of time (tendons, Liver); problems with eyesight (eyes, Liver); dizziness, headache (Def. Liver Blood has lead to Internal Wind which has lead to dizziness and headache); tinnitus (ears, Kidney); memory problems (brain, sea of marrow, Kidney); spermatorrhea (Kidney).

2. Use to avoid white hair on the head. If the hair has turned to grey or white, this may be used to help return the hair back to the natural color. This is the special function of the herb, "Shou Wu" (Tuber of Multiflower, Knotweed; Radix Polygoni Multiflori). See Note #3, below.

3. Use with alopecia areata cases where low-energy laser treatments are being used to help stimulate new hair growth. See Note #4, below.

4. Use to treat weakness in the lumbar area, weak legs, and weak knees in older people.

5. Use to treat weak bladder control (frequent urination) in older people.

6. Use as a secondary medicine in cases with atherosclerosis who have Def. Kidney Yin. After several months of use, this medicine will help to reduce the high cholesterol levels. (Bensky and Gamble, 1986, p. 473.)

7. Use to treat skin allergy - e.g. Wind Rash from Def. Blood which has caused Internal Wind. In China, research has suggested that this herbal medicine may have some "Cortisone-like" effect in reducing inflammation.

Dose: 5 tablets, 3 times a day.

Shou Wu Pian is produced by the Shanghai Chinese Medicine Works, Shanghai, China, in bottles of 100 tablets.

Pinyin Name	Pharmaceutical Name	Percent	TCM Function
He Shou Wu	Radix Polygoni Multiflori	100	Nourish Liver and Kidney Yin; Tonify Blood; Strengthen bones and tendons

Notes: 1. Most Tonic medicines are somewhat greasy. This Tonic medicine is not greasy, therefore, it will not affect the appetite or the stools.

2. The Patent Medicines, Shou Wu Zhi, and Zhong Guo Shou Wu Zhi, are modifications of Shou Wu Pian; several Tonic medicines have been added. Shou Wu Zhi and Zhong Guo Shou Wu Zhi are in

liquid form; this form is more readily absorbed by the weaker patient than the pill form. The liquid form is especially good for elderly patients or patients who may need to take this medicine for a long time.

3. There is a story related to the discovery of the Kidney Tonic function of the herb, He Shou Wu. At least 1000 years ago, an elderly man, Mr. He, could no longer farm and there was no food during a famine. He had to go into the mountains to search for food. After several months, when he returned to the village, the villagers observed many changes in Mr. He from the time when he left to search for food. For example, his grey hair had turned to black and he appeared much younger. The villagers asked him how these changes had taken place. He told them that he had survived by eating the root (Shou Wu). The villagers concluded that Shou Wu had a Tonic function for the Kidney and they named the herb, "He Shou Wu," in honor of Mr. He.

4. Anecdotal Case Reports: MN has used this in conjunction with low-energy laser acupuncture in the treatment of alopecia areata, sudden patchy hair loss on the scalp associated with an auto-immune disorder where the hair folicle is inflammed against itself. (It is not the same as male pattern baldness.) It occurs in men and women, children and adults.

A 40 year old woman had experienced increasing areas of hair loss on the scalp for over 7 months. During the month of July, 1988, she received 9 low-energy laser treatments (2 per week), with a 20 mW Gallium Aluminum Arsenide diode laser (Uni-laser, Asah Medico, Denmark) which was used for 80 seconds per 1 cm^2 area of hair loss. There were 5 large areas of hair loss. She also took this Patent Medicine, Shou Wu Pian, plus the Patent Medicine, "Alopecia Areata Pill" (see sample picture, below). She also took other Kidney and Blood Tonics including 13.24, Ren Shen Lu Rong Wan and 12.12, Wu Ji Bai Feng Wan, for one month.

After the one-month period, new hair began to grow in on the periphery of all 5 areas where there was previously no hair. During August, while she was on vacation in another state, the new hair on the periphery continued to grow, and new hair also began to grow in the center of the areas which were bald. In the month of September, she received 9 more low-energy laser treatments. By October 1, the hair was 1/4 ro 1/2 inch throughout all areas of patchy hair loss. Eight months later, without any further treatments, the hair was 4 inches long throughout all areas of original hair loss. The relative contribution of the herb Tonics vs. the low-energy laser treatments is not possible to assess.

As of November, 1989, MN has successfully treated 3/3 cases of alopecia areata with low-energy laser in Boston. Hair begins to grow in about 4 weeks, after the first laser treatment. Better results are obtained if the treatments are done 3 times per week, every other day.

The low-energy laser has been used to treat alopecia areata cases in China since 1980, with a 90% success rate in 400 cases. It is 30% successful in cases with alopecia totalis (total baldness). The low-energy laser increases micro-circulation and decreases inflammation. Source: Wei, Xiu-Bing: Laser Treatment of Common Diseases in Surgery and Acupuncture in the People's Republic of China: Preliminary Report. Acupuncture and Electro-Therapeutics Research, International Journal, Vol. 6, 1981, pp. 19-31.

The low-energy laser has been used to treat alopecia areata cases in Spain, since 1986. Reports indicate that treatment with the low-energy laser are helpful in preventing a recurrence of the hair loss. Source: Colls Cruanes, J: Laser Therapy Today, Barcelona, Laser Documentation Centre, S.A., English Edition, 1986.

5. An herbalist in the Boston Area, Stephen Howard, Lic. Ac., has prepared a topical hair tonic consisting of 4 Chinese herbs which are traditionally used in Chinese Medicine with male pattern baldness or other forms of hair loss such as alopecia areata. For more information, he may be reached at Gateway Health Care Associates, 150 Harvard Rd., Stow, MA 01775 (508) 897-5979.

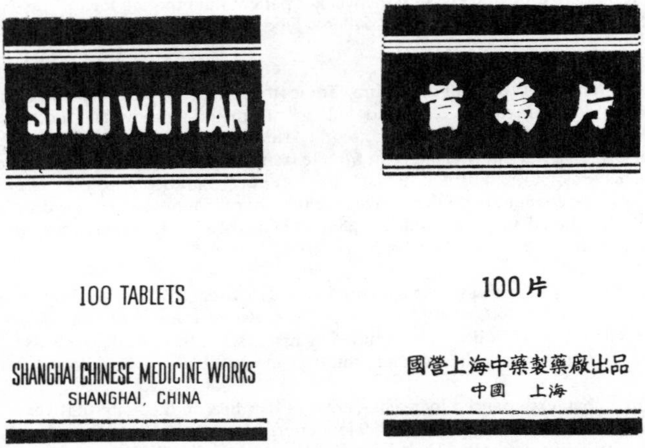

Another Patent Medicine used with alopecia areata is Ban Tu Wan, "Alopecia Areata Pills," shown below. The major ingredient is He Shou Wu. An additional herb, Qiang Huo, is included which guides the effect of the formula toward the head (Governing Vessel). The dose is 4 to 6 pills, 3 times a day.

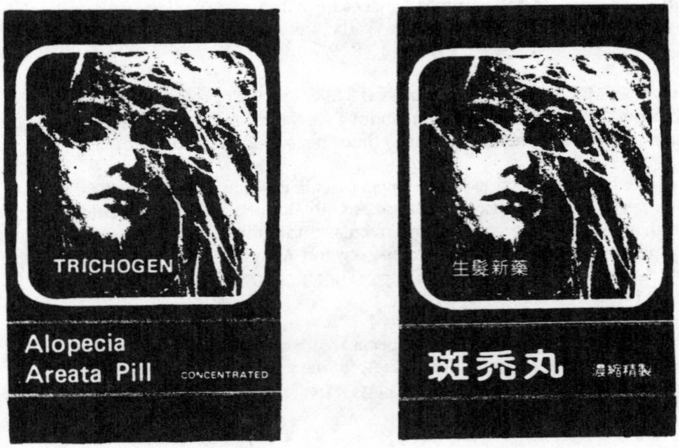

13.22 金匱腎氣丸

金	匱	腎	氣	丸
Jin	**Gui**	**Shen**	**Qi**	**Wan**
golden	box	Kidney	Qi	pills

<u>Source</u>: <u>Jin Gui Yao Lue</u>, by Zhang Zhong Jing, Eastern Han Dynasty, 25-220 A.D. This formula is approximately 2000 years old.

<u>Function</u>: 1. Warm the Kidney; this is especially used in cases with Cold in the Kidney.

<u>Application</u>: 1. Use to treat cases where symptoms are indicative of Cold in Kidney.
<u>Symptoms</u>: Lassitude, legs always tired, low backache, lumbar pain, feeling of cold in the waist area, frequent or difficult urination with clear copious urine; abundant expectoration of sputum. The Tongue has a pale color (not red), and a thin white moss.

2. Some Western medicine disease applications include the following:

Diabetes in cases with the above-mentioned "Cold in the Kidney" syndrome. Additional symptoms may include excess urination and excess thirst.

Chronic nephritis with edema. These cases are weak, the face is pale, anemia may be present, and sometimes there is excess urination, especially at night.

Chronic asthma which is the Def. Kidney type (not Lung Heat type or Spleen Damp type). In these cases the asthma is worse in the winter.

Hypothyroidism in cases where the patient feels cold, has myxedema, a pale face, a weak Pulse, and is always tired and wants to sleep a lot.

Sexual dysfunction due to Def. Kidney Yang.

Ascites. Use this to help expel abdominal fluid retention (ascites) in cases with Cold in the Kidney. The ascites may have developed, for example, as a result of cirrhosis of the liver.

Optic nerve atrophy.

<u>Dose</u>: 8 pills, 3 times a day. It is common to take this for 6 months or more.

Jin Gui Shen Qi Wan is produced as "Sexoton Pills" by the Lanzhou Chinese Medicine Works, Lanzhou, China, in bottles of 200 pills.

A formula similar to this formula is also available in liquid, tincture form as "Dynamic Warrior," in the Jade Pharmacy product line, available through Crane Enterprises, Plymouth, MA, etc. See bottom of page 343.

Pinyin Name	Pharmaceutical Name	Percent	TCM Function
Shu Di Huang	Radix Rehmanniae Glutinosae Conquitae	29.63	Nourish Yin; Strengthen Blood
Shan Yao	Radix Dioscoreae Oppositae	14.81	Tonify Spleen and Stomach
Mu Dan Pi	Cortex Moutan Radicis	11.11	Clear Blood Heat; Extinguish Liver Fire
Fu Ling	Sclerotium Poriae Cocos	11.11	Strengthen Spleen; Discharge Dampness; Promote urination
Shan Zhu Yu	Fructus Corni Officinalis	14.83	Strengthen Liver and Kidney Yin; Stop sweating; Stop spermatorrhea
Ze Xie	Rhizoma Alismatis Plantago-aquaticae	11.11	Promote urination; Drain Kidney Empty Fire
Rou Gui	Cortex Cinnamomi Cassiae	3.70	Warm the Kidney; Strengthen Yang
Fu Zi	Radix Aconiti Carmichaeli Praeparata	3.70	Warm the Yang in the Kidney

Notes: 1. This formula is the same as #13.19, Liu Wei Di Huang Wan, plus 2 herbs that are very warming, Rou Gui and Fu Zi.

2. Jin Gui Shen Qi Wan Tonifies both Yin and Yang, whereas #13.19, Liu Wei Di Huang Wan Tonifies only Yin. The Jin Gui Shen Qi Wan formula is 2000 years old; the Liu Wei Di Huang Wan formula is 1000 years old and is a modification of the Jin Gui Shen Qi Wan formula.

3. Jin Gui Shen Qi Wan is also available as a Patent Medicine under the name, Gui Fu Di Huang Wan. It is also available under two other names, Ba Wei Di Huang Wan and Gui Fu Ba Wei Wan ("Pills containing 8 ingredients including Rou Gui and Fu Zi"). All of these Patent Medicines have the same function and application as Jin Gui Shen Qi Wan. Gui Fu Ba Wei Wan is produced by the Sing Kyn Drug Manufactory, Guangzhou, China.

4. The "Jin Gui" portion of the name for this herbal formula, "Jin Gui Shen Qi Wan," means that this formula is taken form the book, Jin Gui Yao Lue. There is another Patent Medicine named "Shen Qi Wan," which is produced in the Shanghai area. The formula used in Shen Qi Wan is taken from the book, Ji Sheng Fang. Therefore, Shen Qi Wan is also sometimes called Ji Sheng Shen Qi Wan. The difference between Jin Gui Shen Qi Wan and (Ji Sheng) Shen Qi Wan is in the number of herbs used in each. (Ji Sheng) Shen Qi Wan has two additional herbs (Che Qian Zi and Niu Xi), and is more effective in promoting urination.

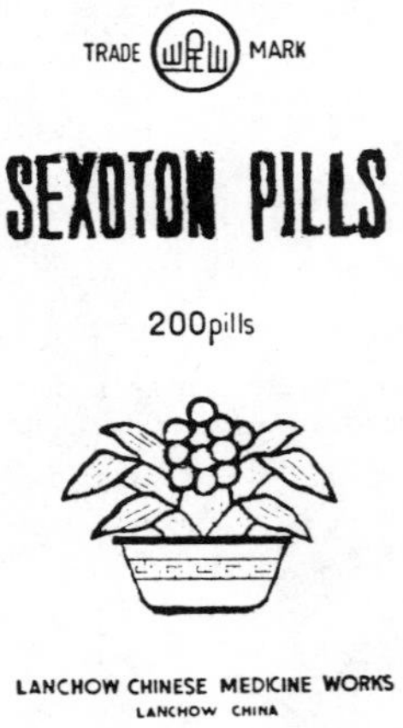

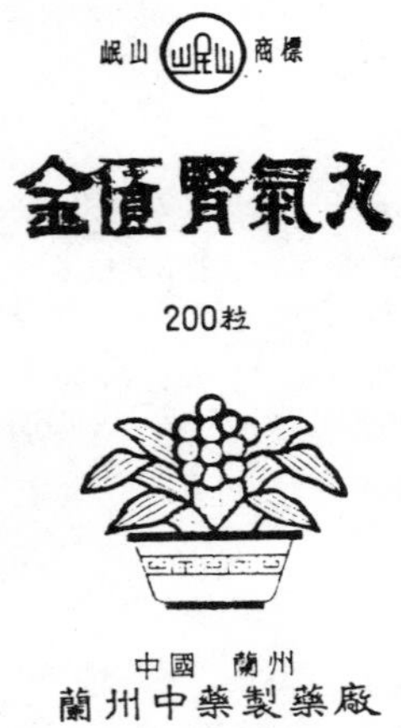

13.23	海	馬	補	腎	丸
	Hai	**Ma**	**Bu**	**Shen**	**Wan**
	sea	horse	supplement	Kidney	pills

Function: 1. Nourish Kidney Yin and Yang
2. Strengthen the lumbar area
3. Strengthen the brain

Application: 1. Use to treat Def. Qi, Def. Blood and Def. Kidney Yang. Symptoms: Low sperm count or weak sperm, impotence, spermatorrhea, debility of limbs, night or day sweating, insomnia, palpitations, soreness and weakness of the lumbar area, poor eyesight (Def. Kidney Yin has lead to Def. Liver Yin), tinnitus, and weariness. This herbal formula will both Nourish Yin and Reinforce Yang, but it will especially Reinforce the Yang.

2. Use to treat neurasthenia, neurosis and other psychological disorders with Def. Kidney.

Dose: 10 pills, 2 times a day before meals. In cases being treated for impotence due to def. Kidney, it is better to avoid excess sexual intercourse while taking this medicine.

Hai Ma Bu Shen Wan is produced as "Sea Horse Genital Tonic Pills, General Tonic and Genital Strengthener" by the Tientsin Drug Manufactory, Tientsin, China, in bottles of 120 pills.

Pinyin Name	Pharmaceutical Name	Percent	TCM Function
Hai Ma	Hippocampus	10	Warm the Kidney Yang
Ren Shen	Radix Ginseng	10	Tonify Qi; Strengthen Spleen
Long Gu	Os Draconis	5	Stop spermatorrhea; Tranquilize; Calm the Spirit
Gou Qi Zi	Fructus Lycii Chinensis	5	Strengthen Liver and Kidney; Strengthen Blood; Brighten the eyes
Hei Lu Shen	Testis et Penis Equus	3	Strengthen Kidney Yang
Lu Jin	Ligament Tumcervi	4	Strengthen the Liver
Bu Gu Zhi	Fructus Psoraleae Coryliforiae	3	Warm the Kidney Yang
Fu Ling	Sclerotium Poriae Cocos	3	Strengthen Spleen; Eliminate Dampness; Promote urination
Huang Qi	Radix Astragali	5	Strengthen Qi; Stop sweating
Hu Tao Ren	Semen Juglandis	3	Tonify Kidney and Liver
Lu Rong	Cornu Cervi Parvum	6	Warm the Kidney Yang
Ge Jie	Gecko	6	Strengthen Kidney Yang
Hau Gou Shen	Testis et Penis Otariae	5	Strengthen Kidney Yang
Hua Lu Shen	Penis Ettes Tiscervi	5	Strengthen Kidney Yang
Hu Gu	Os Tigris	6	Strengthen bones and tendons
Dui Xia	Macrura Spleen.	6	Strengthen Kidney and Liver
Shan Zhu Yu	Fructus Corni Officinalis	3	Strengthen Liver Yin
Dang Gui	Radix Angelicae Sinensis	5	Tonify Blood
Ding Xiang	Fructus Caryophylli	2	Warm the Kidney Yang; Move Cold Stagnation in the Stomach
Shu Di Huang	Radix Rehmanniae Glutinosae Conquitae	5	Nourish Yin; Tonify Blood

<u>Note</u>: 1. The Patent Medicine, Hai Long Bu Wan, is similar to Hai Ma Bu Shen Wan.

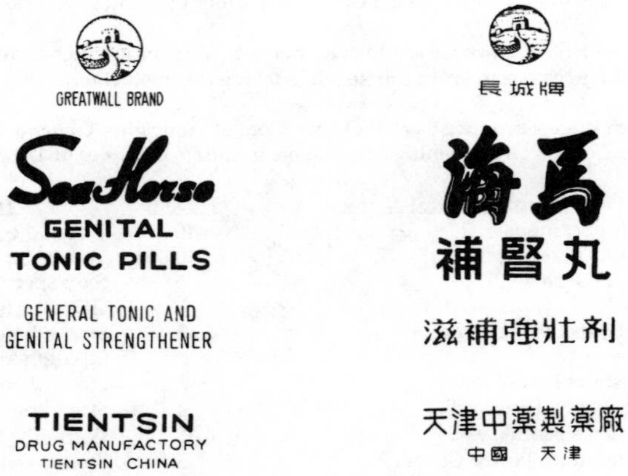

13.24 人 参 鹿 茸 丸

Ren	Shen	Lu	Rong	Wan
----------Ginseng----------		-------hairy deer-horn------		pills

Source: Sheng Ji Zong Lu, (The Complete Record of Holy Benevolence), 1117 A.D., the Imperial Medical Institute.

Function:
1. Supplement Qi, Strengthen Yang
2. Nourish Blood; Promote Congenital Jing

Application:

1. Use to treat Def. Yin and Def. Yang. Symptoms: Fatigue, weariness, shortness of breath, poor hearing, tinnitus, leg weakness, palpitations, insomnia. Use as general Tonic for patients with weakness associated with long illness.

2. Use to Strengthen the Kidney Yang. Symptoms: Feelings of Cold in the limbs, impotence, spermatorrhea, frequent urination.

3. Use to treat gynecological disorders due to Def. Qi and Def. Blood, including amenorrhea, hypomenorrhea, hypermenorrhea, leukorrhea.

4. Some Western medicine disease applications include the following: Neurasthenia, anemia, diabetes mellitus.

Dose: Small pills: 5 pills, 2 times a day. It is better for diabetes patients to use the small coated pills.
Honey Pills: 1 pill, 2 times a day. Each Honey Pill weighs 9 grams.

Ren Shen Lu Rong Wang is produced as "Jen Shen Lu Yung Wan" by the Tientsin Drug Manufactory, Tientsin, China, in bottles of 120 coated pills; and by the Beijing Tung Jen Tang pharmacy in honey pill form, 10 pills per box.

Pinyin Name	Pharmaceutical Name	Percent	TCM Function
Ren Shen	Radix Ginseng	4.7	Strengthen Qi; (Decrease blood sugar levels)
Du Zhong	Cortex Eucommiae Ulmoidis	9.0	Strengthen Kidney Yang; Nourish Liver; Strengthen tendons and bones
Ba Ji Tian	Radix Morindae Officinalis	9.0	Strengthen Kidney Yang
Huang Qi	Radix Astragali	9.0	Strengthen Qi
Lu Rong	Cornu Cervi Parvum	3.8	Tonify Kidney Yang; Strengthen Blood and Congenital Jing; Strengthen tendons and bones
Dang Gui	Radix Angelicae Sinensis	9.0	Strengthen Blood; Regulate menstruation
Niu Xi	Radix Achyranthis Bidentate	9.0	Strengthen Kidney and Liver; Strengthen tendons and bones
Long Yan Rou	Arillus Euphoriae Longanae	9.0	Tonify Spleen and Heart; Nourish Blood; Calm the Spirit

Note: 1. The Patent Medicine, Shen Rong Wei Sheng Wan is similar to Ren Shen Lu Rong Wan.

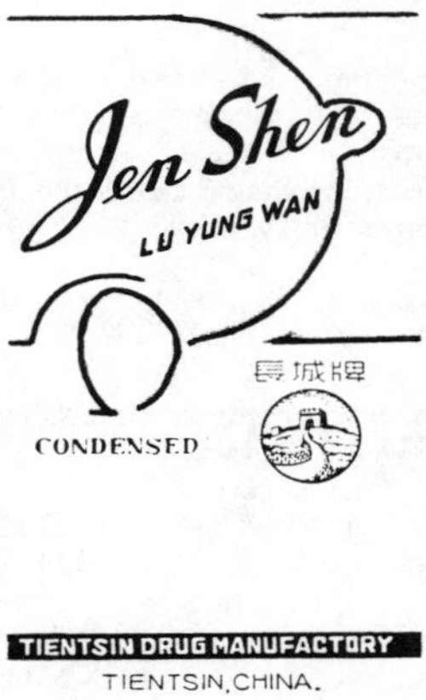

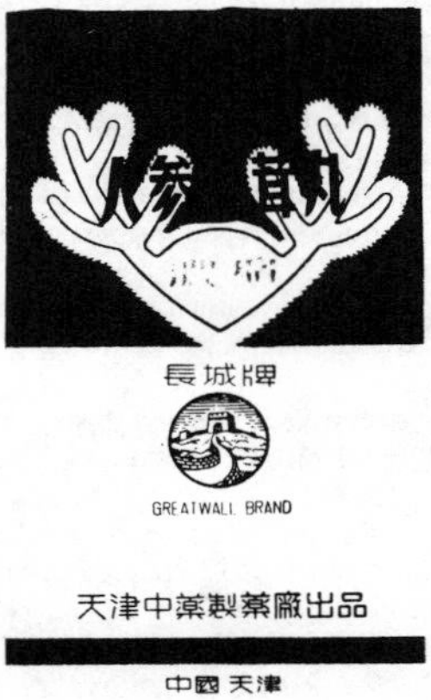

13.25 明 目 地 黄 丸

Ming	Mu	Di	Huang	Wan
brighten	eyes	----------Rehmannia-----------		pills

Source: Wan Bing Hui Chun, (The Recovery of Ten Thousand Diseases), Ming Dynasty, 1368-1644.

Function: 1. Nourish Liver and Kidney Yin; Strengthen vision

Application: 1. Use to treat eye disorders due to Def. Liver and Kidney Yin with Empty Fire. Symptoms: Poor vision, vertigo, photophobia, excess tearing of the eyes, night blindness.

2. Use to treat other disorders associated with Def. Liver and Kidney Yin such as dizziness, dry mouth, dry throat, tinnitus, night sweating, fatigue.

3. Some Western medicine disease applications include the following: Retinitis, optic neuritis, vitreous opacity. (Note: This formula is applicable for use in the following eye disorders only when they are accompanied by Def. Liver and Kidney Yin symptomatology as listed above. If signs of Fire are present, e.g. swollen, red eyes, etc., do not use this formula, instead use Expel Wind Heat formulas or Clear Liver Fire formulas such as Ming Mu Shang Qing Pian or #7.12, Long Dan Xie Gan Wan.)

Dose: 10 pills, 3 times a day.

Ming Mu Di Huang Wan is produced as "Ming Mu Ti Huang Wan" by the Lanzhou Chinese Medicine Works, Lanzhou, China, in bottles of 200 pills.

Pinyin Name	Pharmaceutical Name	Percent	TCM Function
Shu Di Huang	Radix Rehmanniae Glutinosea Conquitae	12.0	Nourish Yin; Tonify Blood
Shan Yao	Radix Dioscoreae Oppositae	6.0	Strengthen Spleen; Nourish Kidney
Mu Dan Pi	Cortex Moutan Radicis	4.5	Clear Empty Fire; Clear Blood Heat
Fu Ling	Sclerotium Poriae Cocos	4.5	Strengthen Spleen
Shan Yu Rou	Fructus Corni Officinalis	6.0	Strengthen Kidney Yin; Smooth Liver
Ze Xie	Rhizoma Alismatis Plantago-aquaticae	4.5	Promote urination; Drain Kidney Fire
Gou Qi Zi	Fructus Lycii Chinensis	25.0	Strengthen Liver and Kidney; Nourish eyes
Shi Jue Ming	Concha Haliotidis	12.5	Calm Liver Fire affecting the eyes
Bai Ji Li	Fructus Tribuli Terrestris	12.5	Extinguish Liver Wind; Brighten the eyes

Note: 1. The original formula contained 3 additional ingredients: Dang Gui (Tonify Blood, Nourish Liver), Bai Shao (Smooth Liver, Strengthen Liver Yin), and Ju Hua (Extinguish Liver Wind, Brighten the eyes).

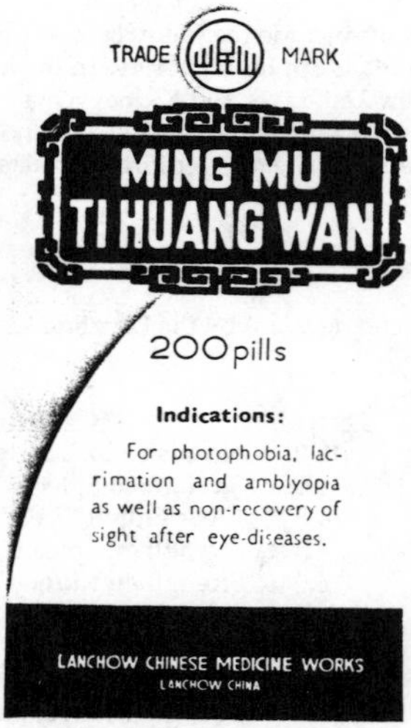
TRADE MARK
MING MU
TI HUANG WAN
200 pills
Indications:
For photophobia, lacrimation and amblyopia as well as non-recovery of sight after eye-diseases.
LANCHOW CHINESE MEDICINE WORKS
LANCHOW CHINA

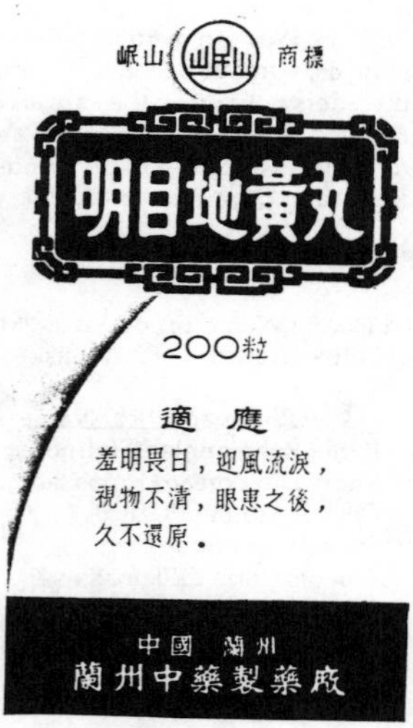
岷山 商標
明目地黃丸
200粒
適應
羞明畏日，迎風流淚，
視物不清，眼患之後，
久不還原。
中國 蘭州
蘭州中藥製藥廠

13.26 杞 菊 地 黄 丸

Qi	Ju	Di	Huang	Wan
Lycium	Chrysanthemum	----------Rehmannia----------		pills

Source: Xiao Er Yao Zheng Zhi Jue, (Pediatric Pharmaceutics), by Qian Yi, Song Dynasty, 960-1279.

Function: 1. Nourish Liver and Kidney Yin
2. Nourish eyes; Strengthen vision

Application: 1. Use to treat Def. Liver and Kidney Yin Syndrome especially with dryness in the eyes and poor vision: Symptoms: Dizziness, vertigo, tinnitus, dryness in the eyes, poor vision.

Dose: 8 pills, 3 times a day.

Qi Ju Di Huang Wan is produced as "Lycium-Rehmannia Pills" by the Lanzhou Fo Ci Pharmaceutical Factory, Lanzhou, China, in bottles of 100 pills.

Pinyin Name	Pharmaceutical Name	Percent	TCM Function
Shu Di Huang	Radix Rehmanniea Glutinosae Conquitae	27.59	Nourish Yin; Tonify Blood
Shan Yao	Radix Dioscoreae Oppositae	13.79	Strengthen Spleen; Nourish Kidney
Mu Dan Pi	Cortex Moutan Radicis	10.35	Clear Empty Fire; Clear Blood Heat
Fu Ling	Sclerotium Poriae Cocos	10.35	Strengthen Spleen
Shan Yu Rou	Fructus Corni Officinalis	13.78	Strengthen Kidney Yin; Smooth Liver
Ze Xie	Rhizoma Alismatis Plantago-aquaticae	10.35	Promote urination; Drain Kidney Fire
Gou Qi Zi	Fructus Lycii Chinensis	6.9	Strengthen Liver and Kidney; Nourish the eyes
Ju Hua	Flos Chrysanthemi Morifloii	6.9	Expel Wind Heat; Brighten the eyes

Note: 1. This formula is a modification of #13.19, Liu Wei Di Huang Wan, the basic formula used to nourish Kidney Yin. The special application of Qi Ju Di Huang Wan is to nourish the eyes.

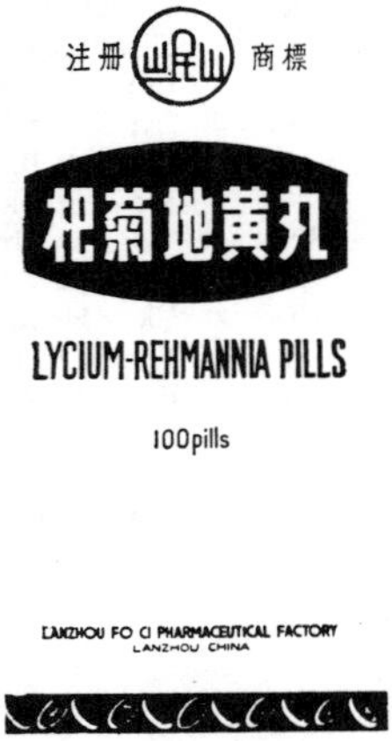

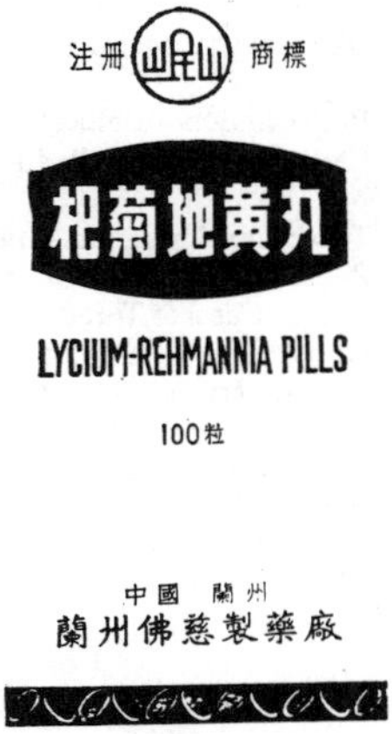

13.27 石 斛 夜 光 丸

Shi	Hu	Ye	Guang	Wan
------Dendrobium------		night	light	pills

Source: Rui Zhu Tang Jing Yan Fang, (Formulas from Experience from the Rui Zhu Tang Pharmacy), Yuan Dynasty, 1279-1368. In this text, the name of this formula is Ye Guang Wan. After the Ming Dynasty (1368-1644), the name of this formula was changed to the present one, Shi Hu Ye Guang Wan.

Function: 1. Nourish Yin; Eliminate Empty Fire
2. Nourish Liver and improve eyesight

Application: 1. Use to treat eye diseases due to Def. Liver and Kidney Yin with signs of Empty Fire. Symptoms: Poor vision, photophobia, feeling of dryness in the eyes. Other Def. Yin signs may also be present such as fatigue, lumbago, insomnia, night sweats.

2. Some Western medicine disease applications include the following: (Use this formula for the eye disorders listed below only when Def. Liver and Kidney Yin with Empty Fire signs are present.) Glaucoma, retinitis, choroiditis, optic neuritis, night blindness.

Dose: 1 honey pill, 2 times a day

Shi Hu Ye Guang Wan is produced as "Dendrobium Moniliforme Night Sight Pills" by the Tientsin Drug Manufctory, Tientsin, China, in boxes of 10 honey pills.

Pinyin Name	Pharmaceutical Name	Percent	TCM Function
Ling Yang Jiao	Cornu Antelopis	4	Clear Liver Heat
Xi Jiao	Cornu Rhinoceri	4	Clear Heart Heat
Shi Hu	Herba Dendrobii	4	Nourish Yin; Clear Heat; Promote Body Fluid
Ren Shen	Radix Ginseng	16	Tonify Qi; Strengthen Spleen
Gou Qi Zi	Fructus Lycii Chinensis	6	Nourish Yin; Strengthen Blood; Smooth Liver; Improve eyesight
Ju Hua	Flos Chrysanthemi Morifolii	6	Clear Heat; Expel Wind Heat; Improve eyesight
Fang Feng	Radix Ledebouriellae Sesloidis	4	Expel Wind
Chuan Xiong	Radix Ligustici Wallichii	4	Promote Blood Circulation Move Stuck Qi; Stop Headache
Mai Men Dong	Tuber Ophiopogonis Japonici	8	Nourish Yin; Clear Heat
Sheng Di Huang	Radix Rehmanniae Glutinosae	8	Nourish Yin; Clear Heat
Jue Ming Zi	Semen Cassiae Torae	6	Clear Heat; Improve vision
Rou Cong Rong	Herba Cistanches	4	Tonify Kidney; Strengthen Yang
Bai Ji Li	Fructus Tribuli Terrestris	4	Extinguish Wind; Brighten the eyes
Niu Xi	Radix Achyranthis Bidentatae	6	Nourish Liver and Kidney
Wu Wei Zi	Fructus Schisandrae Chinensis	4	Strengthen Kidney; Nourish Qi
Zhi Qiao	Fructus Citri seu Ponciri	4	Move Stuck Qi
Qing Xiang Zi	Semen Celosiae Argenteae	4	Clear Heat; Improve vision
Huang Lian	Rhizoma Coptidis	4	Clear Heat; Detoxify Fire Poison

Notes: 1. The original formula contained 7 additional herbs: Fu Ling, Shu Di Huang, Shan Yao, Tu Si Zi, Xing Ren, Tian Men Dong, Gan Cao.

2. The Patent Medicine, Nei Zhang Ming Yan Wan, is similar to Shi Hu Ye Guang Wan.

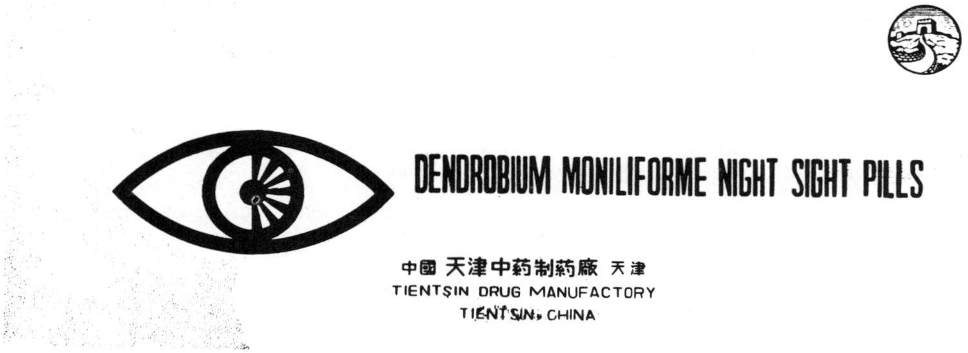

13.28 龟 龄 集

Gui	Ling	Ji
turtle	age	gather-up

Source: This formula is from the Song Dynasty, 960-1279. It was later listed in the book, Liang Fang Ji Yan, (Collection of Effective Formulas), Qing Dynasty, 1644-1911.

Function: 1. Strengthen Kidney Yang

Application: 1. Use to treat the following disorders associated with Def. Kidney Yang:

Def. Kidney Yang disorders with the following symptoms: Impotence, spermatorrhea, lumbago with feeling of coldness in lower lumbar area, frequent urination, dizziness, or tinnitus.

Liver disorders due to Def. Kidney Yang with the following symptoms: Hypermenorrhea or amenorrhea.

Lung disorders due to Def. Kidney Yang with the following symptoms: Chronic asthma (use this to strengthen Lung/Kidney function, thus reducing the severity of future asthmatic attacks); chronic cough (weak cough with thin white phlegm).

Spleen disorders due to Def. Kidney Yang with the following symptoms: Early morning diarrhea, "5 a.m. diarrhea." This formula can also be used to treat leukorrhea.

Heart disorders due to Def. Kidney Yang with the following symptom: Poor memory

2. Some Western medicine disease applications include the following: (All with Def. Kidney Yang symptomatology.) Sexual dysfunction associated with neurasthenia; problems associated with climacteric syndrome in men or women; chronic nephritis.

Contraindications: Do not use with pregnant women. Do not use during the acute phase of OPI Wind Cold or Wind Heat.

Dose: 2 or 3 capsules, once a day.

Gui Ling Ji is produced as "Kwei Ling Chi Super Tonic" by the Shansi Drug Manufactory, Shansi, China, in boxes of 30 capsules.

Pinyin Name	Pharmaceutical Name	Percent	TCM Function
Ren Shen	Radix Ginseng	20	Tonify Qi; Strengthen Spleen
Lu Rong	Cornu Cervi Parvum	25	Warm the Kidney Yang
Hai Ma	Hippocampus	8	Strengthen the Kidney Yang
Gou Qi Zi	Fructus Lycii Chinensis	3	Strengthen Liver and Kidney; Improve vision
Shou Di Huang	Radix Rehmanniae Glutinosae Conquitae	6	Nourish Yin; Strengthen Blood
Que Nao	Brain of Sparrow	2	Use to treat impotence; spermatorrhea

Niu Xi	Radix Achyranthis Bidentatae	3	Strengthen Liver and Kidney; Promote Blood circulation
Suo Yang	Herba Cynomorii Songarici	2	Strengthen Kidney Yang; Use to treat impotence and spermatorrhea
Ding Xiang	Flos Caryophylli	2	Warm the Middle Warmer; Strengthen Kidney Yang
Sha Ren	Fructus seu Semen Amomi	3	Move Stuck Qi; Warm the Spleen; Stop diarrhea
Du Zhong	Cortex Eucommiae Ulmoidis	2	Strengthen Liver and Kidney
Da Qing Yan	Salt	2	Use it to direct other herbs to the Kidney, due to the salty taste.
Rou Cong Rong	Herba Cistanches	6	Strengthen Kidney Yang
Chuan Shan Jia	Squama Manitis Pentadactylae	6	Promote Blood circulation
Tu Si Zi	Semen Cuscutae	2	Strengthen Kidney; Benefit Congenital Jing
Bu Gu Zhi	Fructus Psoraleae Corylifoliae	2	Warm the Kidney Yang
Yin Yang Huo	Herba Epimedii	2	Strengthen Kidney Yang; Strengthen tendons and bones
Gan Cao	Radix Glycyrrhizae Uralensis	2	Harmonize other herbs Strengthen Spleen; Warm the Middle Warmer
Tian Men Dong	Tuber Asparagi Cochinchinensis	1	Nourish Yin; Moisten dryness which could develop from use of several Warm/Dry herbs in this formula
Shi Yan	Fossilia Spiriferis	1	

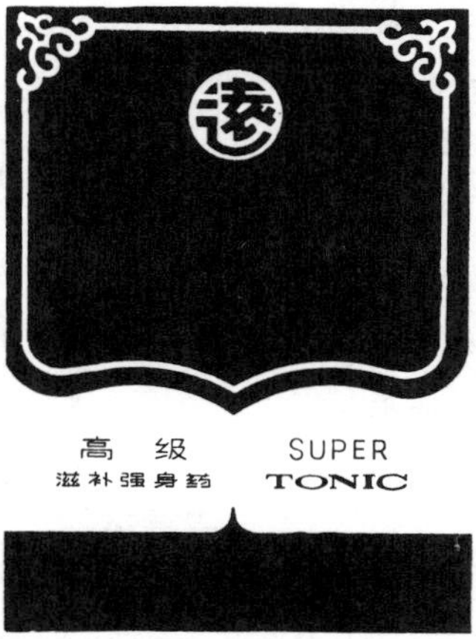

13.29 蛤蚧補腎丸

Ge	Jie	Bu	Shen	Wan
----------Gecko----------		nourish	Kidney	pills

Function: 1. This has the special function to Strengthen Kidney Yang and Congenital Jing.
2. Tonify Lung Yin; Strengthen Qi; Nourish Blood

Application: 1. Use to treat general weakness after long illness or during a chronic disease.

2. Use to treat lumbago due to Def. Kidney and Liver.

3. Use to treat Def. Lung syndrome due to Def. Kidney (Kidney not grasping the Qi which has lead to Def. Lung syndrome). Symptoms: Difficult breathing, chronic cough with or without thin white phlegm. In Def. Kidney type of, asthma there is difficult breathing, especially on inhalation, but without wheezing. (Do not use this formula with Excess Asthma syndrome where thick yellow phlegm is present; this formula contains some Warm property herbs.)

4. Use to treat Def. Kidney Yang syndrome with the following symptoms: Impotence, spermatorrhea, premature ejaculation, frequent urination with clear copious urine (without Heat signs).

Dose: 3 or 4 pills, 2 or 3 times a day, around mealtime.

Ge Jie Bu Shen Wan is produced as "Gejie Nourishing Kidney Pills" by the Yulin Drug Manufactory, Kwangsi, China, in bottles of 50 capsules.

Pinyin Name	Pharmaceutical Name	Percent	TCM Function
Ge Jie	Gecko Gecko	20	Tonify Kidney Yang; Tonify Lung Yin
Lu Rong	Cornu Cervi Parvum	5	Tonify Kidney Yang
Ren Shen	Radix Ginseng	5	Tonify Qi; Strengthen Spleen and Lung Qi; Strengthen Congenital Jing
Huang Qi	Radix Astragali	10	Strengthen Qi; Strengthen Yang
Du Zhong	Cortex Eucommiae	10	Tonify Liver and Kidney
Gou Shen	Testis et Penis Canitis	5	Nourish Kidney Yin and Yang; Nourish Lung Yin
Dong Chong Xia Cao	Cordyceps sinensis	5	Nourish Kidney Yin and Yang; Nourish Lung Yin
Gou Qi Zi	Fructus Lycii Chinensis	10	Strengthen Kidney and Liver Yang
Fu Ling	Poria	17	Strengthen Spleen Qi; Remove Dampness
Bai Zhu	Rhizoma Atractylodis Macrocephalae	13	Tonify Spleen; Dry Dampness

Notes: 1. Anecdotal experience with this formula in Boston has suggested it to be useful in helping cases with hypoglycemia where Def. Kidney Yang symptoms were also present. Taking this medicine around mealtime may be helpful in maintaining blood suger levels for a longer period of time following a meal. Also, if this or other Tonic medicines are taken on an empty stomach, first thing upon arising, and breakfast is then taken 1 hour or so later, the hypoglycemic low 2 hours after breakfast, may not occur.

2. This Patent Medicine, Ge Jie Bu Shen Wan, is used primarily to treat Def. Kidney Yang. There is another Patent Medicine in liquid form, Ge Jie Jin, which is less Warming and not as Drying as Ge Jie Bu Shen Wan. The Ge Jie Jin will treat Def. Kidney Yin and Def. Kidney Yang, as well as Def. Blood and Def. Qi. It is used to treat older or weaker patients; patients with chronic illness; pregnant women who are weak or with weakness post partum. It is also used to treat patients with debility of legs and feet, and lumbar weakness, as well as to help treat pulmonary tuberculosis cases, and cases with neurasthenia, poor memory or excess fatigue. The dose is 1 vial a day, preferably in the morning.

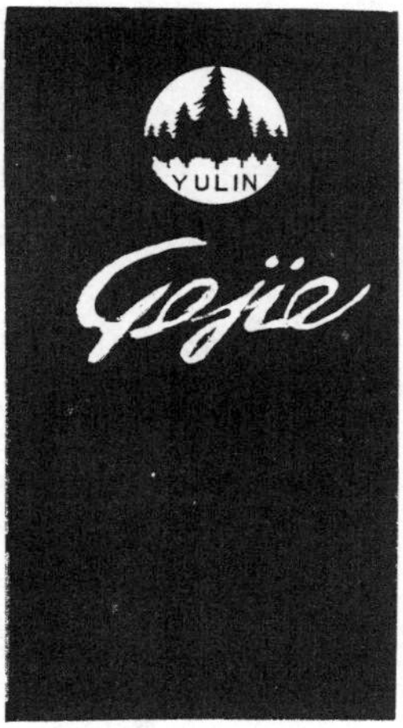

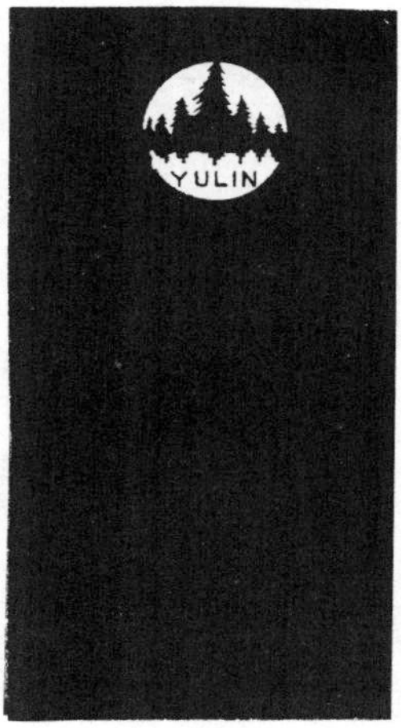

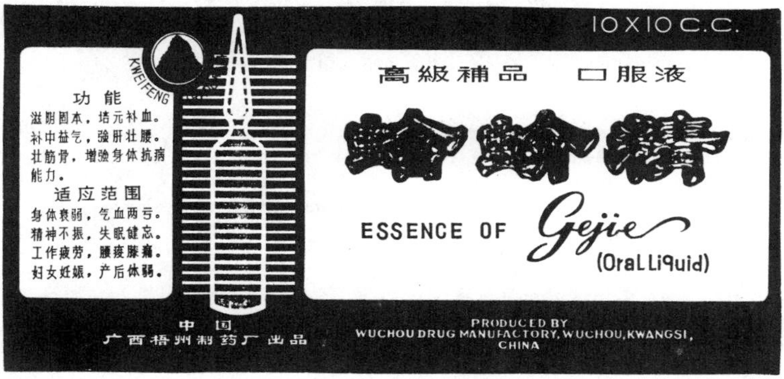

13.30 抗 骨 增 生 片

Kang	Gu	Zeng	Sheng	Pian
against	bone	------bone hyperplasia-----		tablets

Function: 1. Strengthen Liver and Kidney; Improve function of tendons and bones
2. Promote Blood circulation; Regulate Qi; Stop pain

Application: 1. Use to treat joint pain (large or small joints including vertebrae) due to Def. Liver and Kidney. In Western medicine terms, most of these patients will have "bone hyperplasia."

In TCM theory, the Liver controls the tendons, and the Kidney controls the bones. After middle-age, the Liver Blood and Kidney Jing begin to weaken and the Qi and Blood become more Deficient. Therefore, this process affects the tendons and bones, especially when people over-exert themselves or are exposed to OPI Wind-Cold-Dampness. Thus, at this time, joint pain begins to present as a major problem.

In some cases, the joint pain is originally due to chronic over-exertion and the Def. Liver and Kidney condition is not present. However, if the over-exertion continues, and damage to the tendons and bones develops, then eventually a Def. Liver and Kidney condition will also develop. Thus, a cycle is developed where there is damage to the tendons and bones, which in turn weakens the Liver and Kidney, etc. Therefore, Liver symptoms and Kidney symptoms are commonly observed with this syndrome.

Symptoms: Joint pain (dull aching pain) which is temporarily made worse, when the patient initiates movement; joint pain is worse in the morning, for example, when getting out of bed, etc.; joint dysfunction; fatigue, a pale face, feeling of cold in the limbs; the Pulse is thin and deep; the Tongue is pale.

2. Some Western medicine disease applications include the following: (Note, the patient must be over age 40 and have signs of Deficiency to use this formula.) Bone hyperplasia; spondylitis associated with bone hyperplasia; slipped or dislocated intervertebral disc condition after the disc has returned to the original position. This formula can also be used to help prevent future dislocation of the disc.

Caution: Do not use when fever is present or common cold or flu condition is present.

Dose: 6 tablets, 3 times a day. This formula may be taken for a long period of time, i.e. 1 to 3 months, or in some cases, 6 months. The producer of this medicine states that the "Effective Rate" is 90%, where 63.2% of the cases had "Significant improvement" and 27.7% "improved."

Kang Gu Zeng Sheng Pian is produced by the United Pharmaceutical Manufactory, Foshan, Guangdong, China, in bottles of 100 coated tablets.

Pinyin Name	Pharmaceutical Name	Percent	TCM Function
Shu Di Huang	Radix Rehmanniae Glutinosae Conquitae	15	Nourish Kidney Yin; Strengthen Blood
Lu Han Cao	Herba Pyrolae	10	Strengthen tendons and bones; Stop joint pain; Especially good for older people
Lu Lu Tong	Fructus Liquidambaris Taiwanianae	10	Clear Meridians; Stop joint pain
Chuan Shan Long	Rhizoma Dioscoreae Nipponicae	8.2	Promote Blood circulation; Stop joint pain
Lao Guan Cao	Herba Erodii seu Geranii	8	Strengthen tendons and bones; Soothe joints; Stop joint pain
Rou Cong Rong	Herba Cistanches	12.5	Strengthen Liver and Kidney
Chang Chun Teng	Hedera nepalensis	10	Strengthen tendons and bones; Stop joint pain; Especially good for older people
Yin Yang Huo	Herba Epimedii	3.5	Strengthen Kidney Yang; Stop leg pain
Hu Gu	Os Tigris	8	Strengthen bones; Stop joint pain

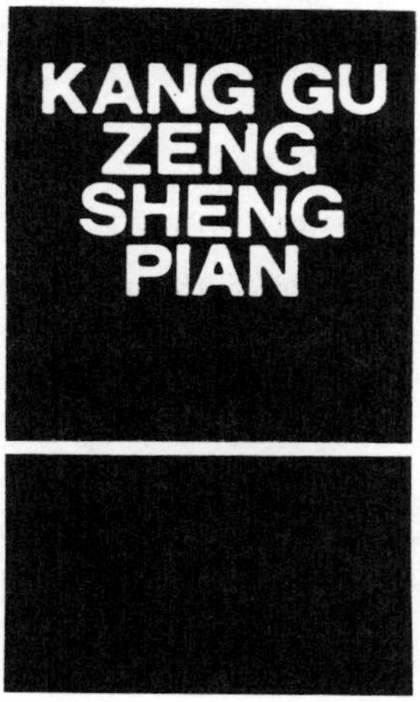

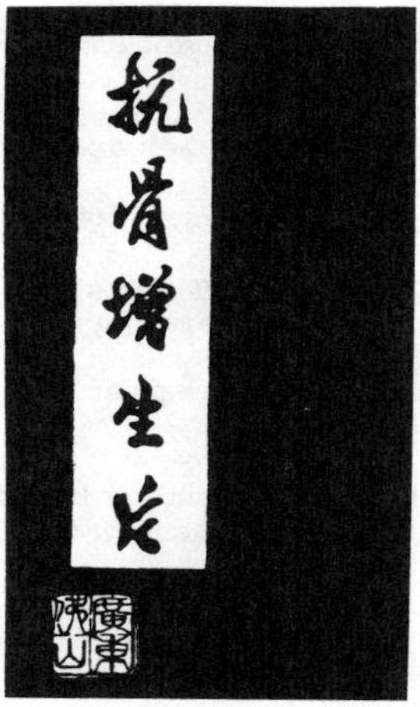

13.31 參 茸 虎 骨 丸

Shen	Rong	Hu	Gu	Wan
Ginseng	Deer Antler	tiger	bone	pills

Function: 1. Strengthen Qi; Nourish Blood; Strengthen tendons and bones
2. Eliminate Wind-Cold and Dampness (Bi); Stop pain

Application: 1. Use to treat weakness of limbs and lumbar area due to Def. Qi and Blood and Def. Kidney Yang. Symptoms: Numbness and pain in the limbs or lumbar area; feeling of cold, especially in the limbs or lumbar area; fatigue.

2. Use to treat chronic arthritis cases (rheumatoid arthritis or osteoarthritis) who have reached the stage where they no longer have sharp pain in the joints, but rather a dull pain or no pain in the joints, but there is joint deformity and joint dysfunction. They also have the above-mentioned symptoms such as feeling of numbness or cold in the limbs or lumbar area plus fatigue.

Cautions: 1. Do not use with pregnant women.

2. Do not use when fever is present.

3. Decrease the dose if feeling of warmth in chest, numbness in limbs, or slight dizzines develops.

4. For use with a cardiac patient, decrease the doseage.

Dose: Adults: 4-6 pills, 2 times a day. Do not increase the dose to more than 8 pills, 2 times a day.

Children: 9 to ll Years: 1 or 2 pills, 2 times a day. 12 to 16 Years: 2 or 3 pills, 2 times a day
Do not increase the dose.

Shen Rong Hu Gu Wan is produced as "Shenyung Huku Wan" by the Fu Song Pharmaceutic Works in bottles of 200 pills.

The contents are listed below in 3 separate groups according to function.

Pinyin Name	Pharmaceutical Name	Percent	TCM Function
Group 1			
Ren Shen	Radix Ginseng	5	Strengthen Qi and Blood;
Lu Rong	Cornu Cervi Parvum	2	Tonify Spleen;
Dang Gui	Radix Angelicae Sinensis	30	Strengthen Kidney Yang
Group 2			
Hu Gu	Os Tigris	5	Strengthen tendons and bones
Group 3			
Guang Fang Ji	Radix Aristolochiae seu Cocculi	25	Expel Wind-Dampness;
Fang Feng	Radix Ledebouriellae Sesloidis	33	Stop joint pain

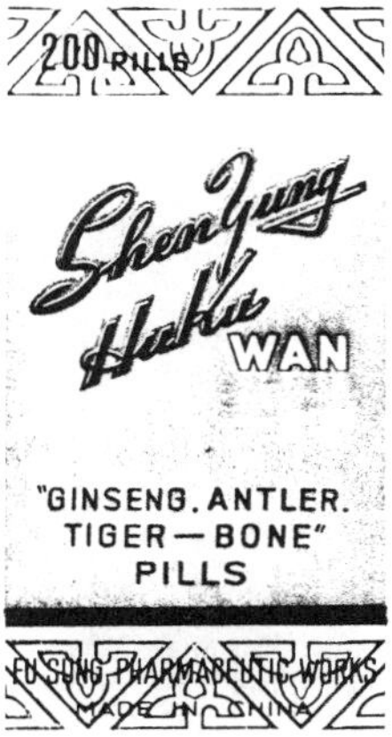
200 PILLS
WAN
"GINSENG. ANTLER.
TIGER—BONE"
PILLS
FU SUNG PHARMACEUTIC WORKS
MADE IN CHINA

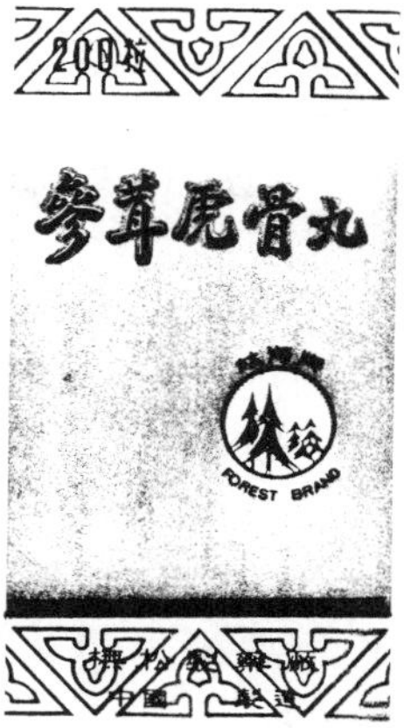
參茸虎骨丸
FOREST BRAND

13.32 耳 鳴 左 慈 丸

Er	Ming	Zuo	Ci	Wan
------------tinnitus----------		left (Kidney Yin)	support	pills

Source: Xiao Er Yao Zheng Zhi Jue, (Pediatric Pharmaceutics), Song Dynasty, 960-1279.

Function: 1. Nourish Yin; Hide the Liver Yang

Application: 1. Use to treat hearing disorders such as tinnitus, and partial but not complete deafness (sensori-neural) which is due to Def. Kidney Yin with relative Excess Yang. In addition, the patient may have related symptoms such as dizziness or vertigo.

2. Use to treat poor vision or blurred vision due to Def. Kidney Yin and Def. Liver Yin.

Dose: 8 pills, 3 times a day, taken with warm water. (Slighty salty water may be used as a Yao Yin.)

Er Ming Zuo Ci Wan is produced as "Tso-Tzu Otic Pills" by the Lanzhou Chinese Medicine Works, Lanzhou, China, in bottles of 200 pills.

Pinyin Name	Pharmaceutical Name	Percent	TCM Function
Shu Di Huang	Radix Rehmanniae Glutinosae Conquitae	30.0	Nourish Yin; Strengthen Blood
Shan Yao	Radix Dioscoreae Oppositae	15.0	Tonify Spleen and Stomach
Mu Dan Pi	Cortex Moutan Radicis	10.5	Clear Blood Heat; Extinguish Liver Fire
Fu Ling	Sclerotium Poriae Cocos	10.5	Strengthen Spleen; Discharge Dampness; Promote urination
Shan Zhu Yu	Fructus Corni Officinalis	15.0	Strengthen Liver and Kidney Yin; Stop sweating; Stop spermatorrhea
Ze Xie	Rhizoma Alismatis Plantago-aquaticae	10.5	Promote urination; Drain Kidney Empty Fire
Ci Shi	Magnetitum	4.0	Eliminate Excess Liver Yang; Improve hearing and vision
Chai Hu	Radix Bupleuri	4.5	Smoothe Liver; Move Stuck Liver Qi

Notes: 1. This formula consists of a total of 8 herbs. The first 6 herbs are those used in #13.19, Liu Wei Di Huang Wan, the major formula used to Nourish Kidney Yin. The 2 additional herbs are Ci Shi and Chai Hu.

2. The name, Er Ming Zuo Ci Wan, contains the term Zuo (left) refering to the Left Kidney; Ming men,"Life Gate," would refer to the Right Kidney. Thus, this formula is designed to Nourish Kidney Yin (Left Kidney), as opposed to Nourishing Kidney Yang (Right Kidney).

3. This formula has different names, according to where it is produced. In Wuhan, it is called Chai Ci Di Huang Wan; in Nanking, it is called Er Ming Wan. In addition, in the current Chinese Pharmacopoeia, (Yao Dian), this formula is named, Er Long Zuo Ci Wan.

TRADE MARK

耳鳴左慈丸

Tso-Tzu Otic
PILLS

200 pills

LANCHOW CHINESE MEDICINE WORKS
LANCHOW CHINA

岷山 商標

耳鳴左慈丸

Tso-Tzu Otic
PILLS

200粒

中國 蘭州
蘭州中藥製藥廠

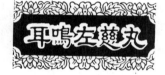

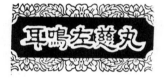

13.33 大 補 銀 丸

大	補	銀	丸
Da	**Bu**	**Yin**	**Wan**
super	supplement	Yin	pills

Source: Dan Xi Xin Fa, Vol. III (The Teachings of Dr. Dan-Xi Zhu's Treatment Methodology), Yuan Dynasty, 1279-1368.

Function: 1. Nourish Kidney Yin; Reduce Empty Fire

Application: 1. Use to treat Def. Kidney Liver Yin Syndrome, especially when the Def. Yin has caused Empty Fire (Empty Heat syndrome) with the following symptoms: Hot flashes, night sweats, spermatorrhea, insomnia, night mares, dizziness, tinnitus, lumbago, knee weakness.

2. Use to stop bleeding where the patient is coughing blood or vomiting blood due to the condition where "Def. Yin fails to balance the Yang," thus causing a Relative Excess Yang syndrome with bleeding due to the Relative Excess Heat.

3. Some Western medicine disease applications include the following: (Note, use this formula with the diagnoses listed below only when the above-mentioned Def. Yin symptoms are also present.) Hyperthyroidism, diabetes mellitus, kidney, lung or bone tuberculosis (acute or chronic)

Dose: 10 pills, 3 times a day.

Da Bu Yin Wan is produced by the Lanzhou Chinese Medicine Works, Lanzhou, China, in bottles of 200 pills.

The contents are listed in 3 groups according to function.

Pinyin Name	Pharmaceutical Name	Percent	TCM Function
Group 1			
Shou Di Huang	Radix Rehmanniae Glutinosae Conquitae	30.0	Nourish Yin; Strengthen Kidney; Nourish Blood
Group 2			
Gui Ban	Plastrum Testudinis	30.0	Nourish Yin; Settle the Yang;
Ju Ji Sui	Pig Spinal Cord (10 spinal cords per 626 grams of the herbal medicine)		Strengthen bones and marrow; Cool the Blood
Group 3			
Zhi Mu	Radix Anemarrhenae Asphodeloidis	20.0	Eliminate Empty Fire by using Cold
Huang Bai	Cortex Phellodendri	20.0	Property herbs; Protect Body Fluid from Empty Fire

Notes: 1. At the time when this formula was developed during the Yuan Dynasty, Dr. Dan-Xi Zhu believed that Yin was almost always Deficient, and Yang was almost always Excess. Therefore, he developed this formula as a model formula to treat Def. Yin and Relative Excess Yang. Dr. Dan-Xi Zhu headed his own successful medical school where this belief was prevalent.

2. In some Drug Manufactories, the pig spinal cord is not used. For example, when this formula is produced by the TianJin Pharmaceutical Works, the pig spinal cord is not used.

13.34 全 鹿 丸

Quan complete · **Lu** deer · **Wan** pills

Source: Jing-Yue Quan Shu, (Jing-Yue's Complete Book), Ming Dynasty, 1368 - 1644.

Function:
1. Strengthen Kidney Yang and Yin
2. Strengthen Vital Qi; Nourish Blood

Application:

1. Use to treat both Def. Yang and Yin with symptoms such as general weakness, fatigue, dizziness, tinnitus, low back pain, knee weakness, poor appetite, weight loss, spontaneous day or night sweating.

2. Use to treat spermatorrhea or impotence due to Def. Kidney Yang or Def. Kidney Yin.

3. Use to treat menstrual disorders including irregular period, hyper- or hypomenorrhea, leukorrhea.

4. Some Western medicine disease applications include the following: Neurasthenia, diabetes (adult), pulmonary tuberculosis, chronic nephritis with symptoms indicated in application #1, above (symptoms due to Def. Qi and Blood).

Dose: Small Pills: 4 pills, 3 times a day.

Large Pills: 1 pill, 2 times a day. (Each large pills weighs 9 grams.)

Quan Lu Wan is produced as "Alrodeer Pills" by the Hangzhou Chinese Medicine Works, Hangzhou, China, in bottles of 100 small pills.

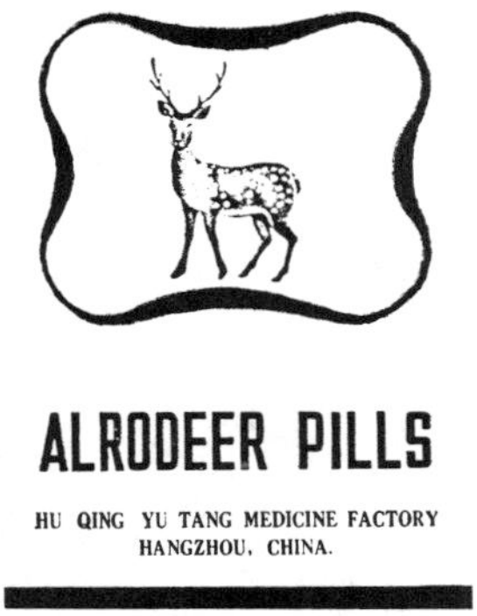

ALRODEER PILLS
HU QING YU TANG MEDICINE FACTORY
HANGZHOU, CHINA.

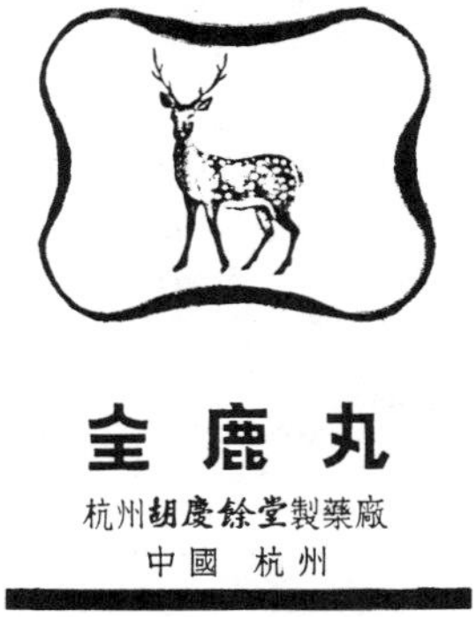

There are 36 ingredients; the most important ones are listed below in 6 groups according to function.

Pinyin Name	Pharmaceutical Name	Percent	TCM Function
Group 1			
Lu Rou	Deer meat	39.95	Strengthen Yang and Kidney Jing;
Lu Rong	Cornu Cervi Parvum		Nourish Qi and Blood
	(Velvet of Young Deer Horn)	0.5	
Lu Wei	Deer Penis and Testicle	0.25	
Lu Shen	Deer Kidney	0.37	
Lu Jiao Jiao	Cornu Cervi Colla		
	(Gelatin from Mature Deer Horn)	1.0	
Group 2			
	Ba Zhen Tang (Eight Precious Ingredients with Huang Qi instead of Bai Shao)		
Ren Shen	Radix Ginseng	2.0	Nourish Qi and Blood
Bai Zhu	Rhizoma Atractylodis Macrocephalae	2.0	
Fu Ling	Sclerotium Poriae Cocos	2.0	
Gan Cao	Radix Glycyrrhizae Uralensis	2.0	
Dang Gui	Radix Angelicae Sinensis	2.0	
Chuan Xiong	Radix Ligustici Wallichii	2.0	
Sheng Di	Radix Rehmanniae Glutinosae	2.0	
Shou Di	Radix Rehmanniae Glutinosae Conquitae	2.0	
Huang Qi	Radix Astragali	2.0	
Group 3			
Gou Qi Zi	Fructus Lycii Chinensis	2.0	Strengthen Liver and Kidney;
Du Zhong	Cortex Eucommiae Ulmoidis	2.0	Strengthen tendons and bones
Niu Xi	Radix Achyranthis Bidentatae	2.0	
Xu Duan	Radix Dipsaci	2.0	
Group 4			
Rou Cong Rong	Herba Cistanches	2.0	Strengthen Kidney Yang; Stop
Suo Yang	Herba Cynomorii Songarici	2.0	spermatorrhea
Ba Ji Tian	Radix Morindae Officinalis	2.0	
Group 5			
Tian Men Dong	Tuber Asparagi Cochinchinensis	2.0	Moisten Yin; Calm the Spirit
Mai Men Dong	Tuber Ophiopogonis Japonici	2.0	
Wu Wei Zi	Fructus Schisandrae Chinensis	2.0	
Group 6			
Chen Xiang	Lignum Aquilariae	1.0	Regulate Flow of Qi in the
Chen Pi	Pericarpium Citri Reticulatae	2.0	Middle Warmer

Notes: 1. The name of this formula, Quan Lu Wan, translates to "complete deer." This reflects many of the ingredients from the deer which are used, including deer meat, deer horn, deer penis and testicle, deer kidney, etc.

2. This use of this formula is similar to that of #13.24, Ren Shen Lu Rong Wan. Thus, if one is not available, the other is frequently used instead.

3. The Patent Medicine, Shen Gui Lu Rong Wan, is similar to Quan Lu Wan. In China, however, Shen Gui Lu Rong Wan has two formulas made in two different provinces, Henan Province and Jiangxi Province. The two formulas are similar, but the formula made in Henan has a greater effect to Strengthen Kidney Yang; the formula made in Jiangxi has a greater effect to Strengthen Vital Qi, Nourish Blood and Nourish Liver Yin.

13.35 玉 泉 丸

Yu	Chuan	Wan
jade stone	fountain	pills

Source: The formula is from the writings of Ye Tian-shi, Qing Dynasty, 1644-1911.

Function: 1. Nourish Kidney Yin; Clear Def. Yin Heat
2. Stop thirst due to Def. Kidney Yin; Promote salivation

Application: 1. Use to treat excess thirst due to Def. Yin and damaged body fluids.

2. Use to treat diabetes of mild or moderate severity.

Dose: 6 grams, 4 times a day. Each bottle contains 120 grams.

Yu Chuan Wan is produced by the Chengdu Medicine Works, Chengdu, China, in bottles of 120 grams.

Pinyin Name	Pharmaceutical Name	Percent	TCM Function
Wu Wei Zi	Fructus Schisandrae Chinensis	8.4	Nourish Kidney Yin; Promote Salivation; Stop thirst
Sheng Di Huang	Radix Rehmanniae Glutinosae	29.8	Nourish Yin; Clear Empty Heat; Increase Body Fluid
Tian Hua Fen	Radix Trichosanthis	23	Moisten Dryness in Lung; Promote Salivation; Stop thirst
Ge Gen	Radix Puerariae	28.8	Clear Stomach Heat; Promote Salivation; Stop thirst
Gan Cao	Radix Glycyrrhizae Uralensis	10	Clear Heat in the Middle Warmer; Harmonize the other herbs

Notes: 1. In the Chinese Journal of Patent Medicines, (Zhong Cheng Yao Yen Jiou), 1981, No. 6, a study which used this medicine with diabetic patients reported that it helped to reduce the glucose levels in the blood and urine.

2. The Yu Chuan Wan produced by the Chengdu Medicine Works received a prize in 1981 from the Chinese Government for use of the highest quality herbs.

13.36

至	宝	三	鞭	丸
Zhi	**Bao**	**San**	**Bian**	**Wan**
maximum	valuable	three	herb name	pills

Function: 1. Promote production of Congenital Jing; Nourish Blood
2. Strengthen Qi; Increase brain function

Application: 1. Use to strengthen a patient who has general weakness associated with Def. Kidney syndrome. Symptoms: Dizziness, tinnitus, palpitations, shortness of breath, poor memory, premature aging including grey hair at a young age and appearing older than actual age.

2. Use to treat impotence and spermatorrhea.

Dose: 1 honey pill, once a day. Each honey pill weighs 9 grams.

Zhi Bao San Bian Wan is produced as "Tze Pao Sanpien Pills" by the Yantai Pharmaceutical Works, Chefoo, China, in boxes of 10 honey pills.

The major ingredients are listed below in 4 groups, according to function. The percents are not available.

Pinyin Name	Pharmaceutical Name	TCM Function
Group 1		
Ren Shen	Radix Ginseng	Strengthen Qi; Strengthen Spleen
Huang Qi	Radix Astragali	
Group 2		
Lu Rong	Cornu Cervi Parvum	Strengthen Kidney Yang
Hai Ma	Hippocampus	
Rou Gui	Cortex Cinnamomi Cassiae	
Chen Xiang	Lignum Aquilariae	
Ba Ji Tian	Radix Morindae Officinalis	
Yin Yang Huo	Herba Epimedii	
Hai Gou Shen	Testes et Penis Otoriae	
Lu Bian	Deer Testicle and Penis	
Guang Gou Bian	Dog Testicle and Penis	
Group 3		
Shang Zhu Yu	Fructus Corni Officinalis	Strengthen Kidney; Stop spermatorrhea
Group 4		
He Shou Wu	Radix Polygoni Multiflori	Strengthen Kidney Yin; Nourish Blood; Reverse grey hair

Notes: 1. The Patent Medicine, Nan Bao, is similar to Zhi Bao San Bian Wan.

2. The Patent Medicine, Zhi Bao Qiang Li San Bian Wan, is similar to Zhi Bao San Bian Wan. The name translates to "Extra Strength Zhi Bao San Bian Wan."

3. The Patent Medicine, Zhi Bao San Bian Jing, is a liquid form of Zhi Bao San Bian Wan; the effect is similar.

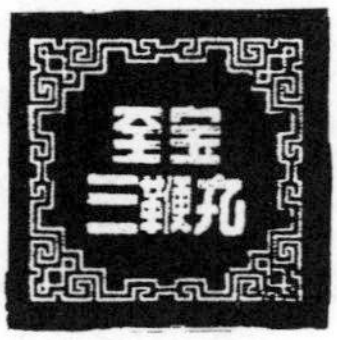

Chapter 14. Nourish Heart, Calm the Spirit

(Includes Patent Medicines used to promote relaxation; reduce anxiety and insomnia)

14.1 補 腦 丸

Bu	Nao	Wan
supplement	brain	pills

Function:
1. Supplement Blood
2. Supplement Heart and Kidney
3. Nourish the brain; Calm the Spirit

Application:

1. Use to treat symptoms due to Def. Heart Blood such as poor memory, uneasiness, palpitations and insomnia.

2. Use to treat symptoms due to Def. Liver Blood and Internal Wind such as headache and dizziness.

3. Some Western medicine disease applications include the following: Neurasthenia, neurosis, and other similar problems such as anxiety attacks, panic attacks and phobias.

Dose: 10 pills, 3 times a day.

Bu Nao Wan is produced as "Cerebral Tonic Pills" by the Xian Chinese Drug Pharmaceutical Works, Xian, China, in bottles of 300 pills.

Pinyin Name	Pharmaceutical Name	Percent	TCM Function
Dang Gui	Radix Angelicae Sinensis	10	Tonify Blood
Suan Zao Ren	Semen Zizyphi Spinosae	16	Nourish Heart and Liver; Calm the Spirit
Rou Cong Rong	Herba Cistanches	8	Tonify Kidney; Strengthen Kidney Yang
Bai Zi Ren	Semen Biotae Orientalis	6	Nourish Heart; Calm the Spirit
Tian Ma	Rhizoma Gastrodiae Elatae	4	Smooth Liver; Calm Internal Wind
Yuan Zhi	Radix Polygalae Tenuifoliae	4	Calm the Spirit
Hu Tao Ren	Semen Juglandis Regiae (Walnut Kernels)	8	Tonify Kidney
Tian Nan Xing	Rhizoma Arisaematis	4	Expel Wind Phlegm
Chang Pu	Rhizoma Acori Graminei	4	Open Orifices; Calm the Spirit
Gou Qi Zi	Fructus Lycii Chinensis	8	Soothe Liver; Calm Internal Wind
Hu Po	Succinum	4	Calm the Spirit
Long Chi	Dens Draconis	4	Tranquilize the Spirit
Wu Wei Zi	Fructus Schisandrae Chinensis	20	Strengthen Kidney and Heart Qi; Improve sleep and memory

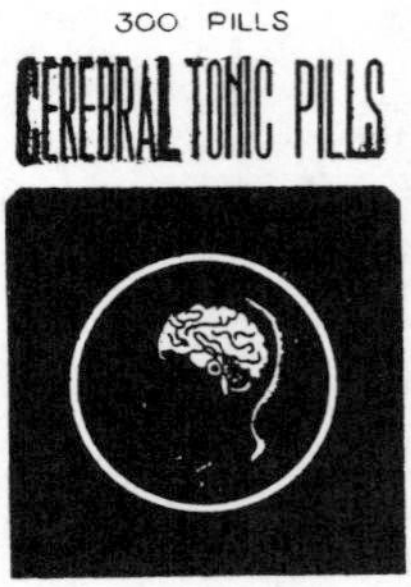

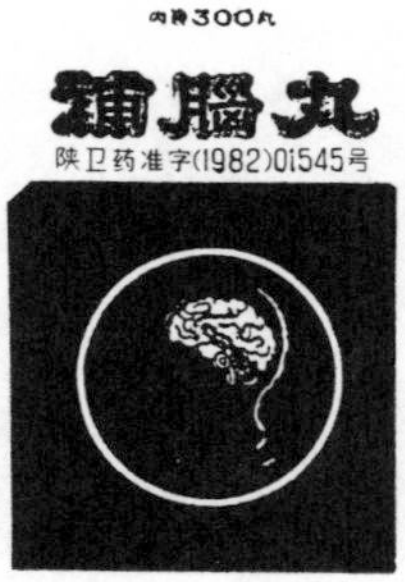

14.2 健 腦 丸

Jian	**Nao**	**Wan**
healthy	brain	pills

Function: 1. Nourish Heart; Tranquilize Spirit; Benefit wisdom

Application: 1. Use to treat Def. Heart, Def. Kidney, Def. Blood syndrome.
Symptoms: Poor memory, uneasiness, insomnia, palpitations, vertigo, tinnitus.

Use this in cases where there are Empty Heat signs from the Heart due to Def. Yin of the Kidney (uneasiness, palpitations, insomnia, night sweating, vertigo, tinnitus, poor memory.) In these cases, there is a Heart/Kidney imbalance where the Kidney fails to balance the Heart Fire causing the signs of Empty Heat.

2. Western medicine disease applications include the following: Meniere's syndrome (vertigo, tinnitus) with Empty Heat signs.

Dose: 10 pills, 3 times a day.

Jian Nao Wan is produced as "Healthy Brain Pills" by the Tsingtao Medicine Works, Tsingtao, China, in bottles of 300 pills.

Pinyin Name	Pharmaceutical Name	Percent	TCM Function
Suan Zao Ren	Semen Ziziphi Spinosae	18	Nourish Heart and Liver; Calm the Spirit
Shan Yao	Rhizoma Dioscoreae Oppositae	10	Strengthen Spleen; Strengthen Qi
Rou Cong Rong	Herba Cistanches	8	Tonify Kidney; Strengthen Kidney Yang
Wu Wei Zi	Fructus Schisandrae Chinensis	6	Strengthen Kidney and Heart Qi; Improve sleep and memory
Hu Po	Succinum	4	Calm the Spirit
Long Chi	Dens Draconis	4	Tranquilize the Spirit
Tian Ma	Rhizoma Gastrodiae Elatae	4	Smooth Liver; Calm Internal Wind
Ren Shen	Radix Ginseng	4	Tonify Qi
Dang Gui	Tadix Angelicae Sinensis	12	Tonify Blood
Gou Qi Zi	Fructus Lycii Chinensis	8	Soothe Liver; Calm Internal Wind
Yi Zhi Ren	Fructus Alpiniae Oxyphyllae	6	Warm the Kidney
Tian Zhu Huang	Concretio Silicea Bambusa	4	Clear Heat; Calm the Spirit
Jiu Jie Chang Pu	Rhizoma Anemondes Altaicae	4	Open Orifices; Calm the Spirit
Zhu Sha	Cinnabaris	4	Tranquilize the Spirit
Bai Zi Ren	Semen Biotae Orientalis	4	Nourish Heart; Calm the Spirit

Note: Case Report: An acupuncturist in Boston successfully used Jian Nao Wan with an obese teen-age girl who had an eating disorder. This helped the patient to change her attitude regarding her excessive eating.

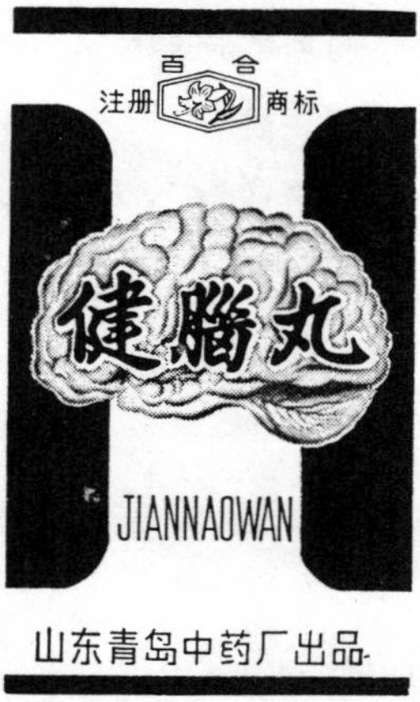
百合
注册 商标
健腦丸
JIANNAOWAN
山东青岛中药厂出品

14.3 天 麻 蜜 環 素

Tian	Ma	Mi	Huan	Su
-------Gastrodia-------		------name of a fungus-----		extract

Function: 1. Subside Liver Wind; Nourish Liver
2. Calm the Spirit; Tranquilize

Application: 1. Use to treat dizziness due to Liver Wind syndrome. Additional symptoms such as tinnitus and insomnia may also be present.

2. Use to treat numbness on the limbs.

3. Use to treat epileptic seizures

Dose: 3 to 5 tablets, 2 or 3 times a day, taken with warm water. The patient should take this for at least 15 days (one course). If there is no improvement after 2 courses, discontinue taking it. If it is effective, the patient should continue to take it.

Tian Ma Mi Huan Su is produced as "Tien Ma Mi Huan Su" by the People's Republic of China, in bottles of 36 capsules.

Pinyin Name	Pharmaceutical Name	Percent	TCM Function
Mi Huan powder		100	Soothe Liver; Calm Internal Wind

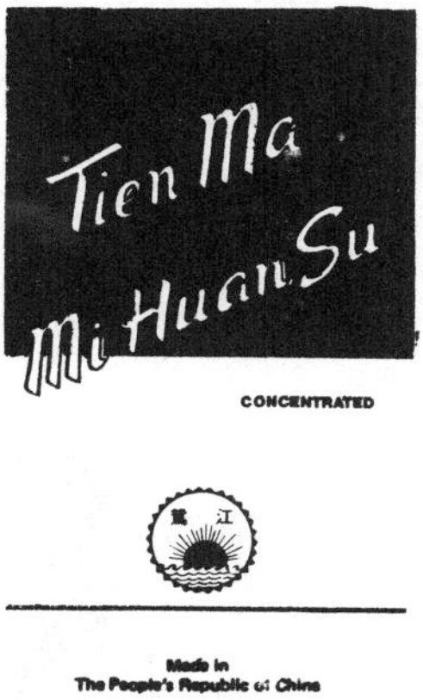

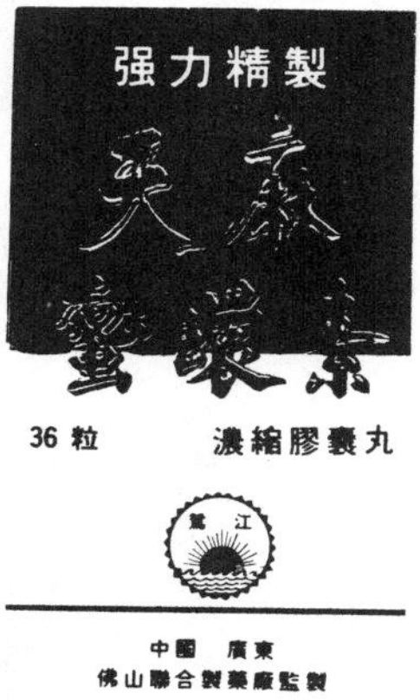

14.4 硃 砂 安 神 丸

Zhu	Sha	An	Shen	Wan
---------Cinnabar---------		calm	Spirit	pills

Source: Shou Shi Bao Yuan, (Book on Longevity and Protection of Health), Ming Dynasty, 1368-1644.

Function: 1. Calm the Heart Spirit
2. Clear Heat; Nourish Blood

Application: 1. Use to Clear Heart Fire which has damaged the Heart Blood and Heart Yin. Symptoms: Palpitations, uneasiness, nausea, feeling of heat in the chest, insomnia, nightmares. The Tongue is red; the Pulse is Thin and irregular.

2. Use to treat neurasthenia with the above-mentioned Heart Fire symptoms plus poor memory and mental depression.

3. Use to treat hysteria with the above-mentioned Heart Fire symptoms.

Caution: In China, this is a commonly used herbal formula, however, it is not used for a long period of time, nor is the dose increased. It may be used for two weeks, then stopped for one week; then, if necessary, resumed again for two weeks and stopped for one week. The ingredient Zhu Sha (Cinnabaris, 17.4%) is mercuric sulfide, a substance which should not be used over a long period of time, nor taken in large doses; it will be poisonous.

Dose: Adults: 6 pills, 3 times a day, with warm water after meals.

Zhu Sha An Shen Wan is produced as "Cinnabar Sedative Pills" by the Lanzhou Chinese Mediicne Works, Lanzhou, China, in bottles of 100 pills.

Pinyin Name	Pharmaceutical Name	Percent	TCM Function
Zhu Sha	Cinnabaris	17.4	Calm the spirit; Stop agitation
Huang Lian	Rhizoma Coptidis	8.8	Clear Heart Heat
Dang Gui	Radix Angelicae Sinensis	43.4	Strengthen Blood in Heart
Sheng Di	Radix Rehmanniae Glutinosae	26.1	Clear Heart Heat; Nourish Yin
Sheng Gan Cao	Radix Glycyrrhizae Uralensis (raw)	4.3	Clear Heart Heat; Strengthen Qi

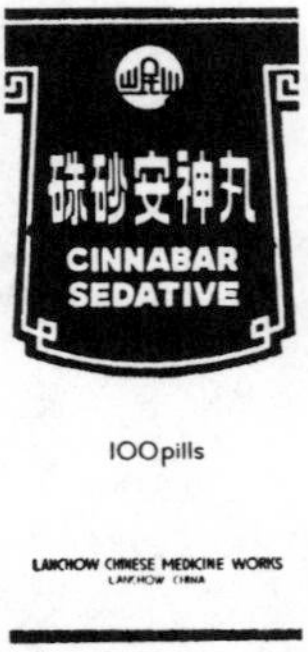

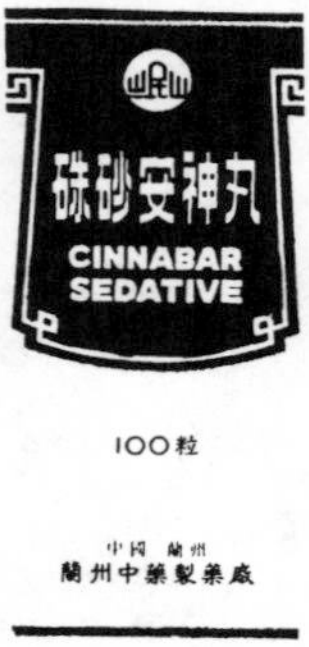

14.5 天 王 補 心 丹

天	王	補	心	丹
Tian	**Wang**	**Bu**	**Xin**	**Dan**
celestial	emperor	Nourish	Heart	pills

Source: Shi Yi De Xiao Fang, (Effective Formulas Tested by Physicians for Generations), Yuan Dynasty, 1279-1368.

Function: 1. Nourish Yin; Clear Heat
2. Tonify Heart; Calm the spirit

Application: 1. Use to treat Empty Fire due to Def. Kidney and Heart Yin. Symptoms: Palpitations, restlessness, uneasiness, insomnia, poor memory, short attention span, poor concentration, constipation, mouth and tongue ulcers. The Tongue is red with little or no Tongue coating; the Pulse is Thin and rapid.

2. Some Western medicine disease applications include the following: (Use this formula only in cases who have the above-mentioned Empty Fire symptoms due to Def. Kidney and Heart Yin.) Rheumatic valvular heart disease. (This formula will help to reduce the palpitations and other symptoms listed under #1, above.) Hyperthyroidism, neurasthenia, menopausal symptoms.

Dose: 8 pills, 3 times a day

Tian Wang Bu Xin Dan is produced as "Tien Wang Pu Hsin Tan" by the Lanzhou Fo Ci Pharmaceutical Factory, Lanzhou, China, in bottles of 200 pills.

Pinyin Name	Pharmaceutical Name	Percent	TCM Function
Sheng Di Huang	Radix Rehmanniae Glutinosae	29.63	Nourish Yin; Clear Heart Heat; Clear Kidney Heat
Dang Gui	Radix Angelicae Sinensis	7.41	Nourish Blood; Strengthen Heart
Wu Wei Zi	Fructus Schisandrae Chinensis	7.41	Nourish Heart; Strengthen Kidney
Suan Zao Ren	Semen Ziziphi Spinosae	7.41	Nourish Heart; Calm Spirit
Bai Zi Ren	Semen Biotae Orientalis	7.41	Nourish Heart; Calm Spirit; Promote bowel movement
Tian Men Dong	Tuber Asparagi Cochinchinensis	7.41	Nourish Yin; Clear Empty Heat
Mai Men Dong	Tuber Ophiopogonis Japonici	7.41	Nourish Yin; Clear Heart Heat
Xuan Shen	Radix Scrophulariae Ningpoensis	7.41	Nourish Yin; Clear Heat
Dan Shen	Radix Salviae Miltiorrhizae	3.7	Promote Blood circulation; Calm the Spirit; Stop agitation
Dang Shen	Radix Codonopsis Pilosulae	3.7	Strengthen Spleen; Tonify Qi
Fu Ling	Sclerotium Poriae Cocos	3.7	Strengthen Spleen; Calm the Heart and Spirit
Jie Geng	Radix Platycodi Grandiflori	3.7	Guides other herbs to Upper Warmer
Yuan Zhi	Radix Polygalae Tenuifoliae	3.7	Calm the Spirit; Pacify the Heart

Note: 1. Some formulas produced by different manufacturers may contain an additional two herbs, Zhu Sha and Shi Chang Pu.

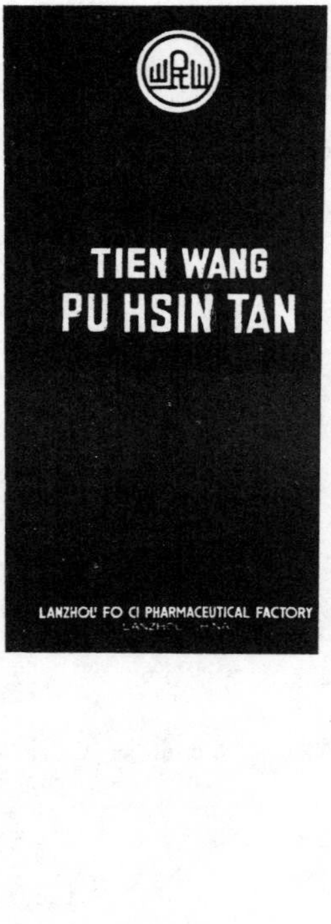
TIEN WANG
PU HSIN TAN
LANZHOU FO CI PHARMACEUTICAL FACTORY

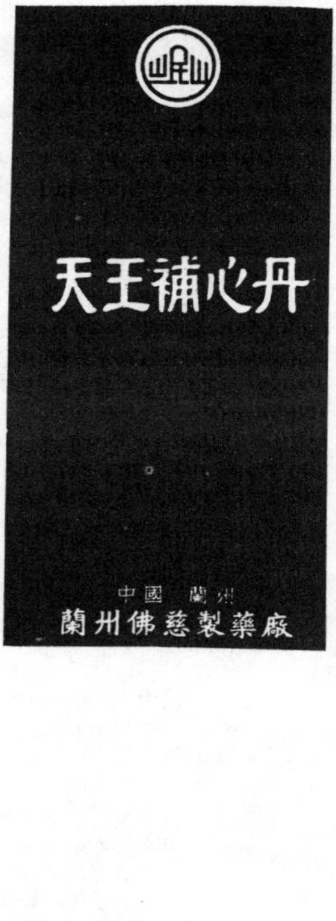
天王補心丹
中國 蘭州
蘭州佛慈製藥廠

14.6 柏 子 養 心 丸

柏	子	養	心	丸
Bai	**Zi**	**Yang**	**Xin**	**Wan**
-----------Biotae----------		Nourish	Heart	pills

Source: Zheng Zhi Zhun Sheng, (Standards for Diagnosis and Treatment), Ming Dynasty, 1368-1644.

Function: 1. Nourish Blood; Strengthen Heart
2. Tonify Qi; Calm spirit

Application: 1. Use to treat Def. Heart syndrome due to Def. Blood. Symptoms: Low energy, chills, cold limbs, palpitations, insomnia, headache, dizziness, poor memory, agitation, nightmares, a pale face.

2. Use to treat neurasthenia with the above-mentioned symptoms.

Dose: 8-10 pills, 2 times a day

Bai Zi Yang Xin Wan is produced as "Pai Tzu Yang Hsin Wan" by the Lanzhou Chinese Medicine Works, Lanzhou, China, in bottles of 200 pills.

Pinyin Name	Pharmaceutical Name	Percent	TCM Function
Dang Shen	Radix Codonopsis Pilosulae	3.14	Tonify Qi; Strengthen Spleen
Chuan Xiong	Radix Ligustici Wallichii	12.58	Promote Blood circulation; Move Stuck Qi; Stop headache
Rou Gui	Cortex Cinnamomi Cassiae	3.14	Strengthen Yang; Warm the Middle Warmer; Expel Cold; Stop pain
Fu Ling	Poria cocos	25.16	Strengthen Spleen; Promote urination; Tranquilize
Yuan Zhi	Radix Polygalae Tenuifoliae	3.14	Calm the Spirit; Pacify Heart
Wu Wei Zi	Fructus Schisandrae Chinensis	3.14	Strengthen Qi; Strengthen Kidney; Nourish Heart; Stop sweating
Gan Cao	Radix Glycyrrhizae Uralensis	1.26	Warm the Middle Warmer; Harmonize other herbs
Huang Qi	Radix Astragali	12.58	Strengthen Qi; Stop sweating
Dang Gui	Radix Angelicae Sinensis	12.58	Tonify Blood; Promote Blood circulation
Ban Xia Qu	Rhizoma Pinelliae Ternatae	12.58	Dry Dampness; Strengthen Spleen
Suan Zao Ren	Semen Ziziphi Spinosae	3.8	Nourish Heart; Strengthen Blood; Calm the Spirit
Bai Zi Ren	Semen Biotae Orientalis	3.14	Nourish Heart; Calm the Spirit
Zhu Sha	Cinnabaris	3.8	Clear Heart Heat; Tranquilize the Spirit

TRADE MARK

PAI TZU YANG HSIN WAN

200 pills

LANCHOW CHINESE MEDICINE WORKS
LANCHOW CHINA

岷山 商標

柏子養心丸

200粒

適 應

失眠，口舌乾燥。

中國 蘭州

蘭州佛慈製藥廠

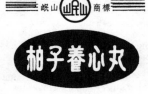

14.7 安 神 補 腦 丸

安	神	補	腦	丸
An	**Shen**	**Bu**	**Nao**	**Pian**
calm	Spirit	supplement	brain	tablets

Function:
1. Tranquilize the Spirit; Supplement the Heart
2. Nourish Kidney Yin and Liver Yin; Supplement Blood

Application: 1. Use to Strengthen Blood to treat Def. Blood which has produced Def. Liver Blood syndrome or Def. Heart Blood syndrome.

Use to treat Def. Liver Blood syndrome with the following symptoms: Headache, dizziness, vertigo, tinnitus. In TCM, when the Def. Liver Blood condition is present, the Def. Blood fails to Nourish the Liver and this thus gives rise to Liver Wind which rises upwards, thus producing symptoms which affect the head, including headache, dizziness and tinnitus.

Use to treat Def. Heart Blood syndrome with the following symptoms: Palpitations, insomnia, poor memory, uneasiness. In TCM, when the Def. Blood cannot adequately nourish the Heart (Blood is Yin), there is relative excess Yang, and this Heat disturbs the Heart causing palpitations, insomnia, poor memory, uneasiness, etc.

3. Some Western medicine disease applications include the following: (Cases who are treated with this formula should have the above-mentioned Def. Liver Blood or Def. Heart Blood symptomatology.) Neurasthenia, Meniere's syndrome, hyperthyroidism.

Dose: 4 tablets, 3 times a day.

An Shen Bu Nao Pian is produced as "Ansenpunaw Tablets" by the Chung Lien Drug Works, Hangzhou, China, in bottles of 100 coated tablets.

Pinyin Name	Pharmaceutical Name	Percent	TCM Function
Huang Jing	Rhizoma Polygonati	36.0	Strengthen Blood; Nourish Yin
Nu Zhen Zi	Fructus Ligustri Lucidi	36.0	Strengthen Liver and Kidney Yin; Extinguish Liver Wind
Dang Gui	Radix Angelicae Sinensis	27.4	Strengthen Blood; Promote Blood circulation
He Huan Pi	Cortex Albizziae Julibrissin	27.4	Calm the spirit; Smooth Liver
Han Lian Cao	Herba Ecliptae Prostratae	18.2	Nourish Liver and Kidney Yin; Extinguish Liver Wind
Suan Zao Ren	Semen Ziziphi Spinosae	18.2	Nourish Heart and Liver Yin; Calm the Spirit
Fu Ling	Sclerotium Poriae Cocos	11.5	Strengthen Spleen; Tranquilize the Spirit
He Shou Wu	Radix Polygoni Multiflori	11.5	Strengthen Liver and Kidney
Zhu Sha	Cinnabaris	6.9	Tranquilize; Calm the Heart Spirit

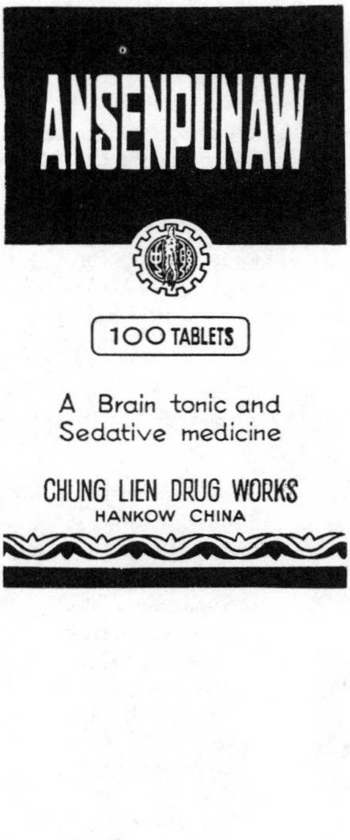
ANSENPUNAW
100 TABLETS
A Brain tonic and
Sedative medicine
CHUNG LIEN DRUG WORKS
HANKOW CHINA

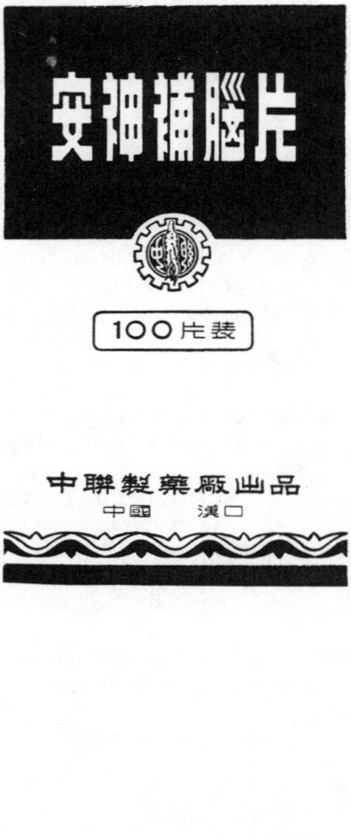
安神補腦片
100片裝
中聯製藥廠出品
中國 漢口

14.8 酸 棗 仁 湯 片

Suan	**Zao**	**Ren**	**Tang**	**Pian**
--------------------Ziziphi--------------------			decoction	tablets

Source: Jin Gui Yao Lue, (Synopsis of the Golden Chamber), Zhang Zhong Jing, 219 A.D.

Function: 1. Nourish Blood; Tranquilize the Spirit
2. Clear Heat; Stop uneasiness

Application: 1. Use to treat Empty Fire which has interferred with the Heart Spirit due to Def. Liver Blood. Symptoms: Uneasiness, insomnia, palpitations, nightmares, night sweating, dizziness, vertigo, dry mouth. The Pulse is Wiry, Thin, or Thin and rapid.

2. Some Western medicine disease applications include the following: (Cases who are treated with this formula should have the above-mentioned symptoms of Empty Fire and Def. Liver Blood.) Neurasthenia, climacteric or menopausal syndrome.

Dose: 2 or 3 pills, 3 times a day.

Suan Zao Ren Tang Pian is produced as "Tabellae Suanzaoren Tang" by the Sing-Kyn Drug House, Guangzhou, China, in bottles of 48 tablets.

Pinyin Name	Pharmaceutical Name	Percent	TCM Function
Suan Zao Ren	Semen Ziziphi Spinosae	50.0	Nourish Liver Blood; Tranquilize Heart; Calm the Spirit
Chuan Xiong	Radix Ligustici Wallichii	8.3	Promote Blood and Qi circulation; Soothe Liver
Fu Ling	Sclerotium Poriae Cocos	17.0	Tranquilize Heart
Zhi Mu	Radix Anemarrhenae Asphodeloidis	17.0	Nourish Yin; Clear Heat; Stop uneasiness
Gan Cao	Radix Glycyrrhizae Uralensis (raw)	8.3	Clear Heat; Harmonize other herbs

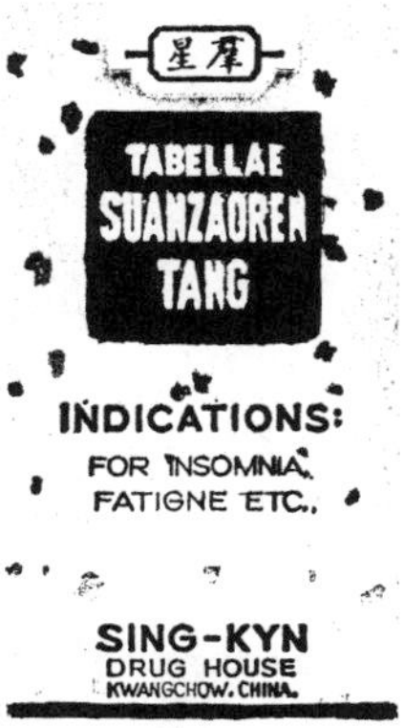

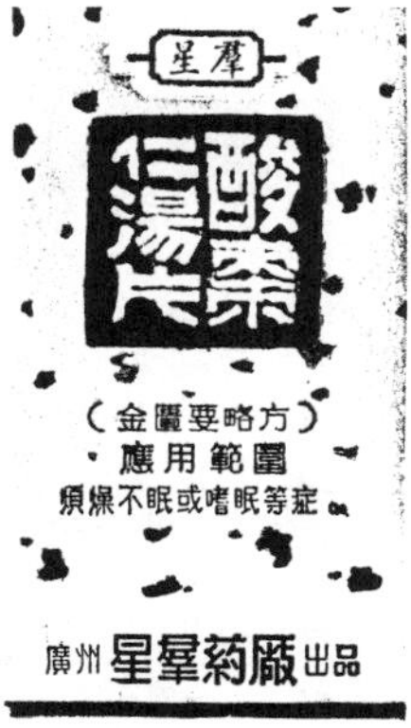

14.9 定 心 丸

Ding	Xin	Wan
stabilize	Heart	pills

Function: 1. Nourish Blood; Tranquilize the Spirit; Calm the Heart
2. Clear Heart Heat

Application: 1. Use to treat Heart syndrome due to Def. Heart Qi and Def. Heart Blood.
Symptoms: Palpitations, insomnia, poor memory, dizziness, vertigo, hot flashes, dry mouth, restlessness.

2. Some Western medicine disease applications include the following: (In order to use this formula, the case must also have the Def. Heart Syndrome symptoms mentioned above.) Sinus tachycardia;neurasthenia; pre-menstrual syndrome; climacteric psychosis or involutional psychosis.

Dose: 6 pills, 2 or 3 times a day

Ding Xin Wan is produced by the Min-Kang Drug Manufactory, I-Chang, China, in bottles of 100 pills.

Pinyin Name	Pharmaceutical Name	Percent	TCM Function
Dang Shen	Radix Codonopsis Pilosulae	4.6	Strengthen Qi; Nourish Spleen
Dang Gui	Radix Angelicae Sinensis	9.1	Tonify Blood; Promote Blood circulation
Fu Shen	Sclerotium Poriae Cocos Pararadicis	9.1	Calm the Spirit
Yuan Zhi	Radix Polygalae Tenuifoliae	9.1	Calm the Spirit;Tranquilize Heart
Suan Zao Ren	Semen Ziziphi Spinosae	9.1	Nourish Liver Blood; Tranquilize Heart; Calm the Spirit
Bai Zi Ren	Semen Biotae Orientalis	13.7	Nourish Heart; Calm the Spirit
Huang Qin	Radix Scutellariae Baicalensis	4.6	Clear Heat
Mai Men Dong	Tuber Ophiopogonis Japonici	9.1	Nourish Yin; Clear Heat Increase Body Fluid
Hu Po	Succinum	2.3	Calm the Spirit
	Medium to 100%		

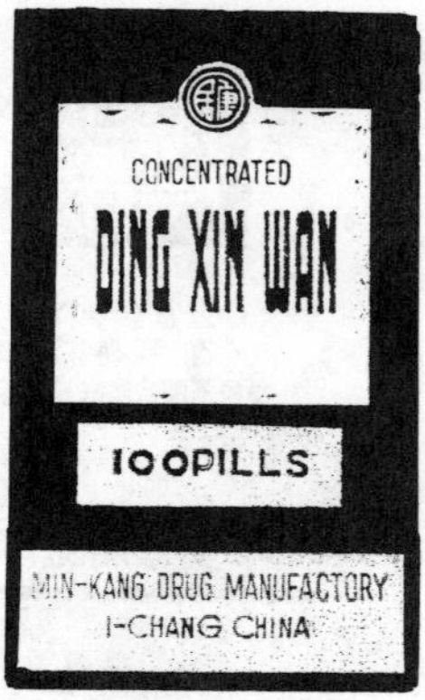

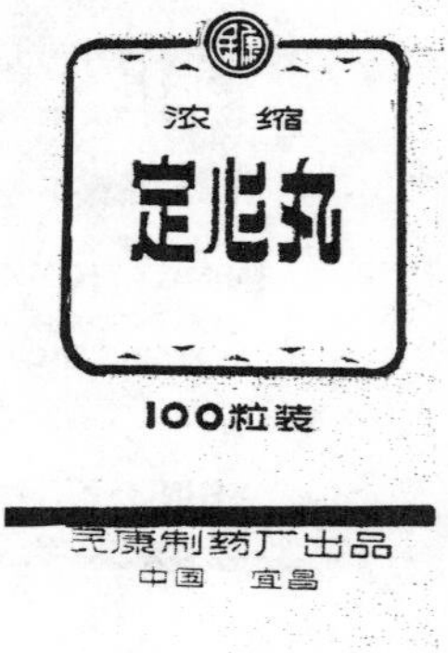

14.10 安 眠 片

An	Mian	Pian
peaceful	sleep	tablets

Function: 1. Calm the Spirit; Clear Heart Heat; Tranquilize; Strengthen Liver

Application: 1. Use to treat insomnia due to Deficient Heart Yin with Empty Heat which has disturbed the Spirit. Also use to treat symptoms such as agitation, anxiety, over-thinking, excess dreaming, and poor memory all due to Deficient Heart Yin.

2. Some Western medicine disease appplications include the following: (Note, the following disorders must be accompanied with the Deficient Heart Yin signs mentioned above.) Neurasthenia, panic attacks, depression.

Dose: 4 tablets, 3 times a day, taken with warm water.

An Mian Pian is produced as "Anmien Pien" by Hopei Province, China, in bottles of 60 coated tablets.

The contents are presented below in 4 separate groups, according to function. The percents are not available.

Pinyin Name	Pharmaceutical Name	TCM Function
Group 1		
Suan Zao Ren	Semen Ziziphi Spinosae	Nourish Blood; Smooth Liver Qi;
Yuan Zhi	Radix Polygalae Tenuifoliae	Calm the Spirit
Fu Ling	Sclerotium Poriae Cocos	
Group 2		
Zhi Zi	Fructus Gardeniae Jasminoidis	Clear Heart Heat; Calm the Spirit
Group 3		
Shen Qu	Massa Fermentata	Strengthen Spleen; Regulate digestion
Group 4		
Gan Cao	Radix Glycyrrhizae Uralensis	Harmonize other herbs; Strengthen Spleen

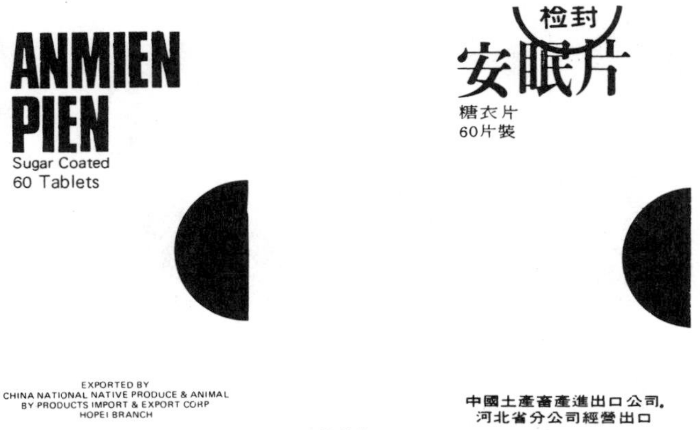

14.11 磁 朱 丸

磁	朱	丸
Ci	**Zhu**	**Wan**
Magnetite	Cinnabar	pills

Source: Qian Jin Yao Fang, (Important Formulas worth One Thousand Gold Pieces), Tang Dynasty, 618-907.

Function:
1. Calm the Spirit
2. Reduce Excess Yang due to Kidney/Heart Yin Disharmony
3. Improve vision

Application:

1. Use to treat Kidney/Heart Yin Disharmony. Symptoms: Palpitations, insomnia, dizziness, tinnitus, deafness, blurred vision, photophobia, restlessness, agitation.

2. Use to treat epileptic seizures. The effect may be better if it is combined with other medicines, such as those which can Stop Liver Wind (#6.1, Tian Ma Wan); or Calm the Spirit and Expel Phlegm (#14.1, Bu Nao Wan).

Dose: 5 or 6 pills, 2 times a day.

Ci Zhu Wan is produced by the Guangzhou Pharmaceutical Industry Co., Guangzhou, China, in bottles of 120 pills.

Pinyin Name	Pharmaceutical Name	Percent	TCM Function
Ci Shi	Magnetitum	28.8	Calm the Spirit; Strengthen Yin; Reduce Excess Yang; Improve vision
Zhu Sha	Cinnabaris	14.4	Clear Heart Heat; Calm the Spirit
Shen Qu	Massa Fermentata	56.8	Strengthen Spleen; Regulate Digestion; Prevent damage to Stomach Qi from two mineral ingredients; Used as a medium to hold the other ingredients

Part III. Bibliography

1. Liu De-Yi: Zhong Yao Cheng Yao Xue, (Traditional Chinese Patent Medicines Text). Tianjin: Tianjin Science and Technology Press, 1984.

2. Yie Xian-Chun: Chang Yong Zhong Cheng Yao, (Common Traditional Chinese Patent Medicines). Shanghai: The Shanghai People's Publishing House, 1976.

3. Zhong Yao Zhi Ji Shou Ci, (Handbook of Traditional Chinese Patent Medicines). Compiled by the Academy of Traditional Chinese Medicine, Institute of Chinese Materia Medica, Beijing. Beijing: People's Medical Publishing House, 1975.

4. Song Lian-Zhu, Tau Nai-Gui: Shi Yong Zhong Cheng Yao Shou Ce, (Practical Handbook of Chinese Patent Medicines). Jinan, Shendong Province: Shendong Science and Technology Press, 1985.

5. Jin Shi-Yuan: Zhong Cheng Yao De He Li Ying Yong, (The Proper Use of Traditional Chinese Patent Medicines). Beijing: The People's Medical Publishing House, 1984.

6. Chen Zhong-Rui, She Ji-Lin: Xiao Er Chang Yong Zhong Cheng Yao, (Common Traditional Chinese Patent Medicines for Children). Beijing: Intellectual Publishing House, 1983.

7. Beijing Shi Zhong Cao Yao Zhi Ji Xuan Bian, (The Selection of Traditional Chinese Patent Medicines in Beijing). Compiled by the Beijing Health Bureau. Beijing: The People's Medical Publishing House, 1973.

8. Beijing Shi Zhong Yao Tiao Ji Gui Cheng, (Rules for the Preparation of Traditional Chinese Herbal Formulas in Beijing). Compiled by the Beijing Health Bureau. Beijing: The Beijing Health Bureau Publishing Office, 1983.

9. Zhong Yao Xue, (Textbook of Herbal Medicine). Compiled by the Chengdu College of Traditional Chinese Medicine. Shanghai: Shanghai Science and Technology Press, 1978.

10. Zhong Yao Lin Chuang Yin Yong, (The Clinical Use of Traditional Chinese Medicine). Compiled by the Zhongshan Medical College. Guangdong: People's Publishing House,1975.

11. Fang Ji Xue, (Textbook of Traditional Chinese Medicine Formulas). Compiled by the Guangzhou Traditional Chinese Medicine College. Shanghai: Shanghai Science and Technology Press, 1979.

12. Zhong Cao Yao Jiao Xue Can Kao Zi Liao, (The Teacher's Guide for Traditional Chinese Medicine). Compiled by Beijing College of Traditional Chinese Medicine. Beijing: Beijing College of Traditional Chinese Medicine, 1982.

13. Zhong Yi Fu Ke Xue, (Traditional Chinese Medicine Text for Gynecology). Compiled by The Hubei College of Traditional Chinese Medicine. Shanghai: Shanghai Science and Technology Press, 1984.

14. Beijing Shi Zhong Yao Cheng Feng Xuan Ji, (The Beijing Selection of Traditional Chinese Patent Medicines). Compiled by the Beijing Public Health Bureau. Beijing: Beijing Science and Technology Press, 1959.

15. Zhong Yi Da Ci Dian, (Dictionary of Traditional Chinese Medicine). Compiled by the Beijing Academy of Traditional Chinese Medicine. Beijing: People's Medical Publishing House, 1982.

16. Nei Ke Xue, (Traditional Chinese Medicine Textbook of Internal Medicine). Compiled by the Shanghai College of Traditional Chinese Medicine. Shanghai: Shanghai Science and Technology Press, 1979.

17. Zhong Yi Er Ke Xue, (Traditional Chinese Medicine Textbook of Pediatrics). Compiled by the Shanghai College of Traditional Chinese Medicine. Shanghai: Shanghai Science and Technology Press, 1984.

18. Zhong Yi Shang Ke Xue, (Textbook of Traditional Chinese Medicine for Treating Trauma). Compiled by the Gunagzhou College of Traditional Chinese Medicine. Shanghai: Shanghai Science and Technology Press, 1981.

19. Wai Ke Xue, (Traditional Chinese Medicine Textbook of Surgery). Compiled by the Guangzhou College of Traditional Chinese Medicine. Shanghai: Shanghai Science and Technology Press, 1983.

20. A Concise Chinese-English Dictionary of Medicine. Compiled by the Beijing Medical College. Beijing: People's Medical Publishing House, 1982.

21. English-Chinese Glossary of Basic Medical Terms. Beijing: People's Medical Publishing House, 1975.

22. Zhong Yi Ming Ci Shu Yu Xuan Shi, (Explanation of Traditional Chinese Medicine Terminology). Compiled by the Beijing Academy of Traditional Chinese Medicine. Beijing: People's Medical Publishing House, 1978.

23. Zhu, Mei: Lao Zhong Yi Zhu Mei Jing Yen Fang, (Effective Traditional Chinese Medicine Formulas of Dr. Mei Zhu) (Senior Physician, Xuan Wu Traditional Chinese Medicine Hospital). Beijing: In Preparation.

24. Bensky, Dan and Gamble, Andrew: Chinese Herbal Medicine MATERIA MEDICA. Seattle: Eastland Press, 1986.

25. Kaptchuk, Ted: The Web That Has No Weaver, Understanding Chinese Medicine. New York: Congden and Weed, 1983.

26. Dharmananda, S: Prescriptions on Silk and Paper: The History and Development of Chinese Patent Medicines. Portland, Oregon, Institute for Traditional Medicine and Preventive Health Care, 1989.

27. Fratkin, J: Chinese Herbal Patent Formulas, A Practical Guide. Portland, Oregon, Institute for Traditional Medicine and Preventive Health Care, 1986.

28. The Merck Manual of Diagnosis and Therapy. Edited by Robert Berkow and John H. Talbott. Rahway, New Jersey: Merck Sharp & Dohme Research Laboratories, 1977.

29. Bensky, Dan and Barolet, Randall: CHINESE HERBAL MEDICINE Formulas & Strategies. Seattle: Eastland Press, 1990.

Part IV. List of Some Stores in the U.S. where the Chinese Patent Medicines may be purchased

Boston, Massachusetts

PPI Pharmacy (Speak English)
78 Essex Street
Chinatown, Boston, MA 02111
(617) 426-5565

Cheng Kwong Market
73-79 Essex Street
Chinatown, Boston
(617) 482-3231

Vinh Kan Ginseng Co.
675 Washington Street
Chinatown, Boston
(617) 338-9028

Kwong Ming Co.
8A Tyler Street
Chinatown, Boston
(617) 451-9168

Golden Import
46 Beach Street
Chinatown, Boston
(617) 350-7001

Lee Yuen Cheung Co.
27A Tyler Street
Chinatown, Boston
(617) 482-5322

Los Angeles, California

Essential Chinese Herbs
646 N. Spring Street
Chinatown, L.A., CA 90012
(213) 680-1374

Wing Fung Tai Ginseng, Inc.
833 N. Broadway
Chinatown, L.A., CA 90012
(213) 617-0699

New York, N.Y.

BAC-AI Pharmacy
216B Canal Street
Chinatown, N.Y., N.Y. 10013
(212) 513-1344

San Francisco, California

North South China Herb Co.
1556 Stockton Street
Chinatown, S.F., CA 94134
(415) 421-4907

Chicago, Illinois

Wah Hon Herb Co.
2402 South Wentworth
Old Chinatown, Chicago, IL 60613
(312) 842-0677

Wah Leung Herb Co.
4930 North Broadway
New Chinatown, Chicago, IL 60640
(312) 271-4922

Oakland, California

nuherbs co., specializing in imported herbs, herbal formulas, acupuncture supplies and reference books:

Note, nuherbs sells only to certified health professionals, pharmacies (or health food stores acting as pharmacies) and medical or acupuncture students. Proof of certification, or a health care practice is required.

Wholesale

nuherbs co.
3820 Penniman Avenue
Oakland, California 94619
(800) 233-4307 or (415) 534-HERBS
FAX (415) 534-4384 TELEX 338139 HQ OAK

Retail

Draline Tong
1003 Webster Street
Oakland, California 94607
(415) 465-6544

Washington, D.C., Northern VA

China Herbs, Eden Center (7 Corners)
6763 Wilson Blvd.
Falls Church, Virginia 22044
(703) 536-3339

Note: Several formulas listed in this book are also available in the **Zand** product line:
McZand Herbal, Inc., P.O. Box 5312
Santa Monica, CA 90409 (213) 392-0404

Note: Some of these herbal formulas are now produced in the U.S., in formulas developed by Ted Kaptchuk, O.M.D. They are available in liquid or tablet form, under the label, **Jade Pharmacy**. For more information, see below:

Crane Enterprises, 45 Samoset Ave., RFD 1,
Plymouth, MA 02360 1-800-227-4118

K'an Herb Company, 2425 Porter Street, Suite 18
Soquel, CA 95073 1-800-543-5233 (408) 462-9915
FAX: 408-479-9118

Part V. Some Patent Medicines which may be Helpful when Travelling

1. **Sudden onset sore throat, common cold, flu (associated with Wind-Heat)** Early stage, at the first signs.
   #1.4 Yin Chiao Jie Du Pian, PLUS #7.8 Niu Huang Jie Du Pian (especially for sore throat);
   OR #1.11 Zhong Gan Ling, OR #7.9 Liu Shen Wan (excellent for sore throat if #7.8 is not effective).
The Liu Shen Wan bottle is very small, only 3/4" high, containing 100 tiny pills, enough for 3 days. It may be combined with #1.4 Yin Chiao Jie Du Pian. Symptoms are often relieved within 24 to 48 hours, but the herbs should be taken for a full day after feeling well. If laryngitis is present, #7.13 Hou Yan Wan.

2. **Sudden onset chills, headache, stuffy nose, with or without fever (associated with Wind-Cold)**
   #1.1 Chuan Xiong Cha Tiao Wan

3. **Rhinitis and nasal sinusitis** #1.10 Bi Yan Pian, OR #1.12 Bi Min Gan Wan

4. **Loud cough (yellow sputum) following an Upper Respiratory Infection (associated with Lung Heat)**
   #3.3 Ma Xing Zhi Ke Pian, which may be combined with #3.5 Jie Geng, if necessary;
   OR #3.4 Qing Fei Yi Huo Pian, OR #3.1 Chuan Bei Jing Pian (with abundant expectoration)

5. **Motion sickness, nausea (especially in the summer, due to Summer Heat and Dampness)** #2.3 Ren Dan

6. **Sports Injury which may be associated with skiing accident, tennis, running, etc.**
   #4.7 Xiao Huo Luo Dan, AND #4.11 Bao Zhen Gao (herbal plaster)

7. **Itching (sudden onset, associated with Wind)** #6.2 Hua She Jie Yang Wan, OR Chuan Shan Jia Chu Shi Ching Du Wan (Armadillo Counter Poison Pill, see #6.2, Notes)

8. **Acute gastroenteritis, diarrhea (especially in the summer, associated with Dampness and Wind-Cold)**
   #2.1 Huo Xiang Zheng Qi Wan OR #2.5 Kang Ning Wan ("Pill Curing")

9. **Serious diarrhea including amebic dysentery**
   #7.4 Huang Lian Su Pian, OR #7.27 Chuan Xin Lian Kang Yan Pian

10. **Constipation** #9.3 Run Chang Wan

11. **Burns** #7.33 Jing Wan Hong (ointment)

12. **Urinary Tract Infection (Damp Heat in the Lower Warmer)**
    #10.1 Shi Ling Tong Pian (also used for kidney stones or gallstones),
    OR #7.27 Chuan Xin Lian Kang Yan Pian (also helpful as preventative when sitting for long periods)

13. **Chronic poor digestion (associated with Def. Spleen/Stomach Qi)** #11.4 Xiang Sha Liu Jun Wan

14. **Menstrual Disorders** Heavy Bleeding #12.10 Yun Nan Bai Yao; Irregular Menstruation #12.12 Wu Ji Bai Feng Wan; Breast distension #11.1 Shu Gan Wan (Stuck Liver Qi); PMS #11.9 Xiao Yao Wan (Stuck Liver Qi)

15. **Leucorrhea** Yellow, due to acute infection (associated with Damp Heat) #7.7 Yu Dai Wan;
    White, (associated with Def. Qi and Def. Blood) #12.11 Qian Jin Zhi Dai Wan

16. **Fatigue (associated with Def. Qi)** These may be used when extra energy is needed for long tours or long lectures. #13.1 Ling Zhi Feng Wan Jiang, OR Ren Shen Feng Wang Jiang (See Notes, #13.1)

17. **Insomnia (due to Def. Heart Qi, Def. Heart Blood)** #14.7 An Shen Bu Nao Wan, OR #14.9 Ding Xin Wan

Part VI. Alphabetical Index of the Patent Medicines

(Includes Alternate Chinese and English Spellings)

Part VII. Index of Medical Terms and Disorders Treated with the Patent Medicines

Each medical term or disease listed below is followed by the Patent Medicine Number in this book where the Chinese herbal formula is further discussed; i.e. 12.15 refers to Chapter 12, Patent Medicine Number 15.

Definitions for some Chinese Medical Terms are included in Part VII; for more information, see Kaptchuk T: The Web That Has No Weaver, Understanding Chinese Medicine. New York: Congden and Weed, 1983.

The information listed below is based on historical information and is not meant to replace medical advice.

A

B

C

D

E

F

G

H

J

K

L

M

N

O

P

R

S

T

U

V

Part VIII. Brief Definitions of some Traditional Chinese Medicine Terms

Most of these definitions are cited from Kaptchuk T: The Web That Has No Weaver, Understanding Chinese Medicine. New York: Congden and Weed, 1983.

Damp Heat - Collection of Dampness and Heat, often resulting in infection (bacterial or viral).

Def. - Deficient, see below.

Deficient Blood - A general pattern of dizziness; pale, lustreless face; pale lips; dry skin or hair; scant menses; pale Tongue material; thin Pulse.

Deficient Qi - General weakness; pale, bright face; shallow respiration; low or soft voice; spontaneous sweating; pale Tongue material; Empty, weak Pulse.

Deficient Yang - Similar to Deficient Qi but with signs of Interior Cold, including cold limbs; aversion to cold; puffy Tongue; slow Pulse.

Deficient Yin - Similar to Deficient Blood, but characterized by "appearance of Heat," including agitated manner; red cheeks; warm palms and soles; night sweats; red Tongue material and rapid, thin Pulse.

Empty Fire - In Excess/Heat conditions where the "Fire" often rises to the head, and there are signs such as splitting headaches; dizziness; red face and eyes; dry mouth; deafness or sudden ringing in the ears. In addition, irritability, frequent anger and insomnia may be present, as well as constipation; dark, scanty urine; red Tongue with rough, yellow moss; and a rapid and full, as well as Wiry Pulse.

This pattern is often seen in Western medicine as essential hypertension, migraine headaches, bleeding of the upper digestive tract, menopausal complaints; eye diseases such as acute conjunctivitis and glaucoma; or ear disturbances such as labyrinthitis, Meniere's disease, or otitis.

Jing - The Substance, or Essence, that underlies all organic life and is the source of organic change. It is thought of as fluidlike, and is supportive, nutritive and is the basis of reproduction and development.

Lower Warmer - Anatomical location referring to the abdominal area below the navel, especially encompassing the Kidney and Liver. (The location of the Liver is related to its Meridian pathway in the lower groin.) The condition of Damp Heat in the Lower Warmer may refer, for example, to an infectious process in the large intestine (dysentery) or in the bladder (urinary tract infection).

Middle Warmer - Anatomical area below the chest, but above the navel, including the Spleen and Stomach. In Traditional Chinese Medicine theory, the term Spleen/Stomach disharmony often refers to a variety of digestive disorders.

OPI - Outside Pernicious Influence - Outside factor precipitating a sudden onset of acute illness. In Western medicine terms this frequently refers to onset of an acute infectious process, such as that seen with the common cold or flu (OPI Wind-Cold or OPI Wind-Heat). See Part II, Chapter 1.

Orifices - The sense organs of the head, including eyes, ears, nose and mouth. In conditions where the orifices are "closed," there is unconsciousness. Fratkin, J, Chinese Herbal Patent Formulas, 1986, 330.

Qi - (pronounced "chee"as in cheese), does not translate well, into one English word. Chinese thought does not distinguish between matter and energy, but Qi is considered matter on the verge of becoming energy, or energy at the point of materializing (Kaptchuk, p. 35). In Traditional Chinese Medicine theory, it is often referred to as the "energy" present in the Meridians and the organs of the body.

Stagnation of Blood (or Congealed Blood) - The Blood has become obstructed and is not flowing smoothly. There is sharp, stabbing pain accompanied by tumors, cysts or swelling of the Organs (most commonly the Liver).

Stagnation of Qi (or Stuck Qi) - The normal movement of Qi is impaired, where it does not flow through the body in a smooth and orderly fashion. Stagnant Qi in the limbs and Meridians may be the origins of pain and aches in the body. Stagnation of Qi in the Lungs may result in coughing and dyspnea. Stagnation of Qi in the Liver may result in distension in the ribs and abdomen, or elsewhere, including breast distension.

Upper Warmer - Anatomical area including the head and chest.

Wei Stage of Febrile Disease - The first stage of Four Stages of Febrile Disease. The Wei Qi is the protective Qi of the body. This stage develops when an OPI is in the first depth of the body, with symptoms such as fever, a slight fear of cold, headache, coughing, slight thirst, with or without perspiration. It is often an early stage of OPI Wind-Heat syndrome, seen with the common cold or flu.

Wei Syndrome (Wei Zheng) - Weakness and eventual wasting of the musculature, especially of the lower extremities, and the resultant impairment of motor function. Bensky and Gamble, 1986, p. 694

Wind - In Traditional Chinese Medicine theory, this refers to anything that has sudden onset and movement.

This may refer to sudden onset from an Outside Factor, such as the common cold or flu (OPI Wind-Cold or Wind-Heat) as seen in an infectious or contagious disease. See Chapter 1.

Or, this may refer to sudden onset from the inside, such as Internal Wind (often referred to as Liver Wind), where there is dizziness, tinnitus, numbness of the limbs, tremors, convulsions and stroke (apoplexy). See Chapter 6.

Because Wind is associated with movement, it is often recognized by signs that move from place to place, such as itching or skin eruptions that change location, spasms, tremors of the limbs, twitching, dizziness or tetany. Chapter 6.

Wind-Cold - An OPI condition (acute, infectious disease) characterized by headache; soreness due to obstructed Meridians; relatively severe chills; low fever; white, moist Tongue moss; floating, tight Pulse. See Chapter 1, A.

Wind-Heat - An OPI condition (acute, infectious disease) similar to Wind-Cold, however the fever tends to be higher and the chills are less pronounced; the Pulse is floating and fast; the Tongue is dry and reddish, with a yellow moss. See Chapter 1, B.

Definitions of Some Organ Functions in Traditional Chinese Medicine which Differ Greatly from their Organ Functions in Western Medicine

Heart - The Heart regulates the flow of Blood and stores and rules the Shen (Spirit). When the Shen is disturbed, the individual may show symptoms such as insomnia, excessive dreaming or forgetfulness. More serious disorders include hysteria, irrational behavior, insanity and delirium. See Chapter 14.

The tongue is closely related to the Heart Qi and Blood. Pathological changes of the tongue such as inflammations or ulcerations can often be treated by acupuncture or herbal therapy directed at the Heart.

Pericardium - The Pericardium is the outer protective shield of the Heart. In Traditional Chinese Medicine theory, the Pericardium is not distinguished from the Heart, except that it is the first line of defense against an OPI attacking the Heart. See Chapter 5.

Spleen - The Spleen is the primary link in the process by which food is transformed into Qi and Blood; it is considered the organ of digestion. If the Spleen is in disharmony, there may be Deficient Qi or Deficient Blood. If digestion is affected, adbominal distension or pain, diarrhea, or anorexia may be present. See Chapter 11.

The Spleen also keeps the Blood flowing in its proper paths. The Spleen Qi holds the Blood in place. When the Spleen Qi is weak, such symptoms as vomiting blood, blood in the stool, blood under the skin, menorrhagia or uterine bleeding may be present. Many chronic bleeding disorders are treated through the Spleen in Traditional Chinese Medicine theory. See Chapter 12.

The Spleen transports Blood and Qi to the muscles and flesh. Consequently, the movement of the muscles, flesh and the four limbs, depends on the function of the Spleen. Muscle tone often indicates the relative strength or weakness of the Spleen.

The mouth and lips are closely related to the Spleen. If the Spleen is weak, the mouth will be insensitive to taste and the lips will be pale.

Liver - The Liver moves the Qi and Blood in all directions, sending them to every part of the body. When there is an interruption in the smooth movement of Qi, either Stagnant Qi or Congealed Blood can develop with symptoms such as pain, or distension in the flanks, swollen or painful breasts and genitals, or lower abdominal pain. See Chapter 11.

If the Liver adjusting function affects the Spleen or Stomach, digestive problems may be present such as abdominal pain, nausea, belching, intestinal rumbling or diarrhea.

The Liver function also includes control of bile secretion. If this is impaired, such symptoms as jaundice, bitter taste in the mouth, vomiting of yellow fluid, distension of the flanks, or loss of appetite may be present.

The Liver also harmonizes the emotions. Anger and emotional frustration are especially associated with the Liver.

The Liver stores the Blood and disharmony here may result in two types of symptoms:
1) rough and dry eyes where there is insufficient Blood to nourish the eyes and
2) unusually heavy menstrual flow where the Blood is not stored properly.

The Liver controls proper movement of all the tendons (and ligaments). Liver disharmony may result in symptoms such as spasms, numbness of the limbs, and difficulty in bending or stretching; the nails may be thin, brittle, and pale.

The Liver has a special relationship to the function of the eyes. Many disorders of the eyes and vision are considered to be related to the Liver function.

Kidneys - The Kidneys store the Jing (source of life and of individual development); and control birth, development, and maturation. Reproductive problems such as sterility or impotence and developmental disorders such as retarded growth or lack of sexual maturation are seen as dysfunctions of the Kidney Jing. See Chapter 13.

The Kidneys control the entire process of Water movement.

The Kidneys control the bones and produce the marrow. In a child, insufficient Kidney Jing may result in soft bones or incomplete closure of the bones of the skull. In an adult, insufficient Kidney Jing can produce weak legs and knees, brittle bones, or stiffness of the spine.

The Kidneys control the teeth. When the teeth develop poorly, or fall out, this may be related to insufficient Kidney Jing.

The Kidney Jing also controls the moistness and vitality of head hair. The loss of hair associated with aging is related to weakness of the Kidney Jing.

The Kidneys have a special relationship to the Lungs in controlling normal breathing. Kidney disharmonies may result in respiratory problems, especially chronic asthma.

The term Kidney Yin refers to the internal fluid or overall moisturizing function of the Kidneys.

The term Kidney Yang refers to the internal "fire" or overall warming function of the Kidneys.

Quotes from Reviews of

Outline Guide to Chinese Herbal Patent Medicines in Pill Form
- with Sample Pictures of the Boxes

"This comprehensive introduction to Chinese herbal medicine has the field to itself. Nothing else of this scope is available for the general public...Should be in the library of any health-conscious reader."

The Book Reader, September/October, 1990

"This extraordinary book introduces the reader to a world of medical treatment practically unknown in the Western world...This book does not dally with philosophical discussions which may be found in other herbalist manuals; it is a rigorous and thorough presentation of herbal compounds used successfully for many hundreds of years."

Arizona Networking News, Fall, 1990

"This is a uniquely practical, bridge-builder of a book that's meant to be carried along to the Chinese pharmacy."

EastWest Journal, January, 1991, p. 76

Some Common Patent Medicines which may be Helpful when Travelling......Page 344

List of Some Stores in the U.S. where Chinese Patent Medicines may be purchased......
Page 343

Complete Medical Index......Pages 349-368